Anesthesia for Cesarean Section

Giorgio Capogna

Editor

Anesthesia for Cesarean Section

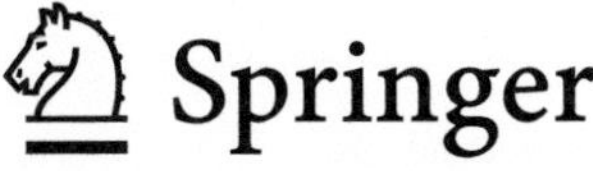 Springer

Editor
Giorgio Capogna
Department of Anesthesiolgy
Città di Roma Hospital
Rome, Italy

ISBN 978-3-319-82489-5   ISBN 978-3-319-42053-0   (eBook)
DOI 10.1007/978-3-319-42053-0

Printed on acid-free paper

This Springer imprint is published by Springer Nature
The registered company is Springer International Publishing AG
The registered company address is: Gewerbestrasse 11, 6330 Cham, Switzerland

Preface

In 1849 Charles Meigs affirmed that "no man has a right to subject a living, breathing, human creature to so great a hazard as that attending the caesarean section." Nowadays, more than 150 years later, cesarean section is probably the most common surgical procedure in the world and considered so safe and convenient that obstetricians have to deal with the controversial issue of the cesarean section on maternal request. Anesthesia, in parallel, has changed enormously from an "out of label" risky procedure to something that is well established with no, or very minimal, maternal and neonatal side effects.

This book describes the current standard practice of anesthesia for cesarean section through the clinical experience of well-known European experts in this field. The core message throughout is that even if cesarean section is a surgical procedure it is still a "delivery" and not only a "section," first and foremost a birth not just an operation. The anesthesiologist should provide not only a "pain free" surgery but also a "side effects free" anesthesia by choosing the right drugs and the appropriate techniques tailor made for the parturient. In this way the childbirth experience, even if in the operating theater, will be more human and extraordinary thanks to the holistic approach of the whole clinical team, of which the anesthesiologist is an indispensable member.

Rome, Italy   Giorgio Capogna

Contents

An Opening for the Life

1

Paolo Mazzarello

1.1 Twin Tragedies

The history of cesarean section is a long chain of tragedies for the mother and the baby [1, 2]. The origins of this surgical procedure—opening of the abdomen to extract the fetus—are lost in the mists of the past and fade into folklore, mythos, and legend of ancient societies [3–5]. According to Greek mythology, the god of medicine, Asclepius, was born directly from the cut of the abdomen of his mother, the nymph Coronis. A similar birth had the god of wine and religious ecstasy, Dionysus, extracted by Zeus from the womb of the mortal Semele, after her death. The legends on the unnatural birth through the abdomen cut pervade also the Eastern Hindu and Buddhist cultures. According to a tradition, Buddha saw the light through a cesarean section performed on his mother Maya. Also in literary Persian culture there are references to this type of operation. In the poem *Shahnameh* the beloved Persian poet Ferdowsi describes the mythical hero Rostam's birth through a cesarean section.

In fact, the first references to an abdominal birth from a deceased woman are probably in the Babylonian world, but we have no technical indication on how the operation could have been carried out [5]. However, it is evident that in ancient time this kind of delivery, when made, was always practised after the death of the mother. In the Roman world, the cesarean section was regulated by the *lex regia* attributed to the king Numa Pompilius although we do not know if and for how long it was applied. This law prohibited "the burial of the corpse of a pregnant woman before the child was extracted." Among the few Roman historical figures who, according to tradition, would have come to the world via cesarean section, on the testimony of Pliny the Elder, there was Publius Cornelius Scipio Africanus, the general who

P. Mazzarello
Department of Brain and Behavioral Sciences, and University Museum System,
University of Pavia, Strada Nuova, 65, I-27100 Pavia, Italy
e-mail: paolo.mazzarello@unipv.it

G. Capogna (ed.), *Anesthesia for Cesarean Section*,
DOI 10.1007/978-3-319-42053-0_1

defeated Hannibal at the battle of Zama. Contrary to what has long been believed, there are no real evidences that Julius Caesar was born by a cesarean delivery, a myth that is disproved by the fact that his mother survived for many years after his birth. Caesar's alleged extraordinary delivery was long considered the source of origin of the term "cesarean" and probably was based on a wrongful interpretation of the writings of Pliny the Elder [5]. In fact, both in the Roman world and in the medieval period, the term was never used. In medical, literary, and theological texts, the terms used were "extraction" or "cutting" to describe or indicate the intervention.

The Church elevated to the rank of the patron saint of women in labor Margaret of Antioch, who, according to tradition, lived in the third century A.D. At the age of 15, around 290, the young girl was sentenced to death because of her Christian faith. In the cell where she was held the devil appeared in the form of a dragon and then swallowed her alive. But she defeated the monster tearing his belly with a cross that she held in her hands, freeing herself through a sort of cesarean section *from inside*. For this reason, she became the patron saint of expectant women (especially in difficult labor). Her holy memory survived the generations, and her figure is still venerated by the Catholic and the Orthodox Churches.

Only in the late Middle Ages, cesarean section became an operative act on the female body described by medicine. The Catholic Church also expressed interest in this surgical intervention to be performed on pregnant women immediately after death. This created the possibility to save from damnation the souls of unborn children through baptism. The unnatural and extraordinary birth from the womb was thus the precondition of true birth, that is, the spiritual one. Odon de Sully, who was archbishop of Paris between 1196 and 1208, issued an order in this regard which expressly prescribed: "The women who die during childbirth are opened, if it is considered that the child is still alive, providing that it is carefully ascertained their death." [6]. The incision of the abdomen of a pregnant woman after the death was a Christian religious duty even according to St. Thomas author of the *Summa Theologiae* (III, q. 68, a. 11): "si tamen mater mortua fuerit, vivente prole in utero, debet aperire ut puer baptizetur" ("however, if the mother is dead while the offspring is still alive in her womb, you have to open it to ensure that the child is baptized"). The practice of extraction of a postmortem fetus was approved by several religious councils and defined with some details. The woman underwent the operation immediately after her death and the child who showed signs of life had to be quickly baptized, while he had to be buried in unconsecrated ground if stillborn. The ecclesiastical rules on the cesarean section were only expressed on the general indications plane and their practical application depended on local circumstances such as the availability of a surgeon who could operate. However, we have no documentary evidence of its widespread circulation although it is described in the works of several physicians and surgeons of the time. According to Guy de Chauliac, author in the fourteenth century of *Chirurgia Magna*, the operation was performed cutting the left side of the abdomen to facilitate access to the fetus and avoiding the liver. In the work, it is suggested to keep open the mouth of the mother (and her vagina) to facilitate air circulation and respiration of the fetus. The ecclesiastical regulations advising cesarean section on women who died during delivery were resumed in the climate of sacramental rigor that followed the Council of Trent. In 1582, the practice was made compulsory in his diocese by Carlo Borromeo, archbishop of Milan, and then extended to the entire Catholic world by Pope Paul V in 1614.

The publication in 1745 of the first edition of the work *Embriologia sacra* of the Sicilian priest Francesco Emanuele Cangiamila, gave a great impetus to the spread of knowledge of the *postmortem* cesarean section. The work of Cangiamila—translated in Latin, Spanish, French, Portuguese, and German—was addressed to the civil authorities and especially to the parish priests who were often at the bedside of the pregnant woman in danger of death so that the surgeons and midwives could perform a cesarean section as soon as the woman had died. According to Cangiamila, it was even a duty of the same priests to perform such an operation when no one else was able to perform it. In this way, cesarean section would have saved—both materially and spiritually—a newborn otherwise condemned to limbo (according to the Catholic Church, the afterlife condition of those who died without baptism).

References to cesarean section on a *living* woman began to appear in the medical texts in the sixteenth century. It was the French surgeon François Rousset in 1581 to introduce the "cesarean" expression in the work *Traitte nouveau de l'hysterotomotokie, ou enfantement caesarien*, who intended to promote the operation on a living woman in cases where childbirth was prevented by natural means. It was in this text that the term was placed in relation both to Julius Caesar and to the Latin verb *caedere* meaning "to cut." According to the surgical technique described by Rousset, the woman, sitting tight on the bed and supported by two strong assistants, was cut on the abdomen to the left along the paramedian line, to avoid the navel hardened by scar tissue. Then, the operator went on to the section of the underlying uterus supporting it with one hand, taking care, when cutting, to not hurt the baby. Finally, the organ was returned to its position without sewing it, while the abdominal wall was sutured. At the basis of this procedure there was the belief that the uterus, for its contraction capacity, was able to stop the bleeding and spontaneously heal: unfortunately this erroneous indication was the cause of many tragedies in the three centuries to come. Rousset actually wrote an entire treatise on an intervention that, apparently, he never performed in the first person, and that did not even exist as a reasonable possibility of physicians and surgeons of the time. His testimonies seem to lack credibility and do not appear to be based on objective reality of the facts. However, his book was rightly seen as a sort of founding act of the cesarean procedure in the living woman and made Rousset as "the inventor of the cesarean section." The book was translated into Latin in 1586 by Gaspard Bauhin who, in an appendix, told a story from the early sixteenth century, destined to become famous in the texts of the history of medicine. A wife of a pig gelder (i.e., a person who performed castration of animals) named Jakob Nufer, was in labor for several days, but the midwives and local surgeons who had turns at her bedside had not been able to make her give birth. The man was skilled in using knives. Just when the situation seemed desperate and hopeless, he asked his wife, now destroyed by the continuous suffering, for permission to operate on her. The woman, oppressed with grief, exhausted and discouraged, welcomed as a sort of liberation the dramatic proposal. Nufer laid her down on the kitchen table, then cut the engraved belly with a knife or a razor and pulled out a live child. The woman was saved and, as reported by Bauhin, continued to give birth in the following years. Another indirect testimony of a cesarean section is found in the famous work *La comare o ricoglitrice* (1596) written by the Italian physician Scipione Mercurio who claimed to have visited two women— during a trip to France—who presented abdominal scars as a consequence of the operation. A documented case of cesarean section was performed in Wittenberg on 21–22 April 1610, by the Saxon surgeon Jeremias Trautmann assisted by two midwives [5, 7]. Initially, the operation went well: the child was saved (and later lived at least nine years), and the woman seemed to recover. But then, some terrible delayed complications appeared that led to the death of the mother by infection or embolism, almost 25 days after birth. Autopsy, however, revealed that the uterus was repaired and healed. Subsequently, there were other documented cesarean operations on living women; however, this surgical intervention was considered an exceptional experience and remained in the deep memory of those who had done it. In fact two complications were almost always fatal: the early *postpartum* hemorrhage and the development of infections. Despite the tragedies that came with it, the intervention of cesarean section on a living woman slowly became widespread throughout Europe. But its primary purpose was to save the baby and to free the mother from acute suffering even though she did not have much chance to survive. Anyway cesarean delivery, although rarely, could also lead to a double success: the safety of mother and child. These cases with a favorable outcome appeared, however, to be accidental events, inexplicable, real strokes of luck that happened to some obstetrician or surgeon marked by a lucky star. According to statistics compiled for Italy between 1780 and 1875 by the historian of medicine and pharmacologist at the University of Pavia, Alfonso Corradi, the global maternal mortality rate, estimated in 158 cesarean interventions, was approximately 67%, but deaths in the hospital arrivals touched 88% of the operated pregnant women [8]. Terrible statistic that certainly overstated the successful cases because it was based on medical reports that tended to particularly emphasize the safe interventions, which gave fame and prestige to surgeons. Of course, the examples in which both protagonists of the birth, the baby and the mother, were saved together, were very few. It is also likely that in some registered successful cases, the statistics did not take account of the negative evolution after few days from the operation. The dangerousness of the intervention frightened the best surgeons. When they were found to face difficult situations, with pregnant women belonging to influential families, they preferred to avoid the risks of the cesarean cut. Called in the summer 1790 in the presence of the governor Johann Joseph von Wilzeck, minister plenipotentiary for the Austrian Lombardy, that had the prey wife to the pains of a difficult birth, the famous surgeon Giovanni Battista Palletta refused to intervene with a cesarean cut. At the end, the woman, imploring to be freed by the pains, succeeded in making herself operated, but owed succumb to the intervention, as it happened to her child [9]. Despite the positive cases, or partially positive in which only one of the two protagonists had survived, the birth with cesarean cut was the ghost that wandered in the mind of every obstetric, a sort of "synonymous of death for the woman." It was "an *extrema ratio* that aroused terror,", and to avoid it the obstetricians didn't hesitate to sacrifice the fetus, with embryotomy, as soon as it was possible. Because sometimes the embryotomy also was difficult or unattainable as a consequence of the difficulties of access along the narrow passages of a basin seriously deformed. It doesn't surprise therefore that, in an important university obstetric clinic as that of the San Matteo Hospital in Pavia, "not a mother had been saved in one century with the cesarean cut" [10].

Things began to change, just in Pavia, in May 1876.

1.2   The Revolutionary Intervention of Edoardo Porro

In April 1876 a 25-year-old woman, Giulia Cavallini, reached the obstetric clinic of San Matteo Hospital Pavia, 8 months pregnant. Born in Adria, a small Italian town in the province of Rovigo in the Veneto region, the woman had met a singer from Pavia who had made her pregnant and married her on the same day she was admitted to hospital. Physical examination immediately disclosed a dramatic situation: the woman was 1 m 48 cm tall and had a severely deformed pelvis that made natural delivery impossible. Edoardo Porro, professor of obstetrics at the University of Pavia, took charge of operating on the woman and tackled her clinical situation as a scientific and human challenge. Suffering from syphilis contracted in Milan during an obstetric operation on a woman with the illness, Porro was quite a character. He had fought with Garibaldi in Trentino (1866) and in Mentana (1867) near Rome before deciding to devote his life to practising obstetrics in the most deprived areas, but he still found time to pursue his research activity [1, 11]. In 1875, Porro had been appointed to the chair of obstetrics at Pavia University and was head of the maternity division when Giulia Cavallini appeared on the scene. Instead of giving up, as other obstetricians would have done in similar circumstances, undertaking a cesarean section with the main purpose to save the baby, Porro managed to reverse the woman's tragic destiny with surgical ingenuity, adopting a simple innovation that allowed him to save both mother and baby. In his early years as obstetrician, Edoardo Porro had been intrigued by a surgical paradox: the strange contrast between the high mortality rate of cesarean section and the generally positive results of laparotomy outside the period of pregnancy. Why opening the abdomen at the end of pregnancy was mortal, whereas cutting a non-pregnant woman meant saving her life? Porro was impressed by these contradictory experiences. It was logical to wonder where this difference stemmed. Strangely no obstetrician had clearly posed the question, or maybe no one had drawn the right conclusions. Instead the mind of Porro began to take shape of a response. Indeed, when placed correctly, the solution of the question seemed almost automatic. The uterus left in place was the source of origin of the chain of tragic consequences for the life of the woman. It became a wounded body inside the abdomen, the front door of the septic processes and source of unstoppable hemorrhagic manifestations. In addition, "the uterus section surfaces" could still come into contact with the infected air "by the way of the vaginal canal" as a result of the woman's movements. From this source it was unleashed peritonitis. If these were the facts, almost automatic was the practical conclusion. After the cesarean section, it was necessary to remove the "uterus-ovarian mass," thus eliminating a terrible septic focus and an uncontrollable source of bleeding. The secret was to remove the fetus, then to constrict the neck of the uterus with a *serre-noeud* of Cintrat in order to stop the circulation to the organ, then to perform a (subtotal) hysterectomy and a bilateral salpingectomy-oophorectomy. Finally, Porro sutured the stump of the neck at the abdominal wall, between the wound edges, to avoid infecting the pelvic cavity with septic fluids. In this way the two causes of post-cesarean death were eliminated or decreased: the source of hemorrhagic extravasation and, moreover, the likelihood of infections. So, a scientifically planned and well thought-out cesarean section, programmed to save both the mother and the child, was fully successful and gave to the world of medicine an obstetric procedure immediately adopted in hospitals all over the world. Nonetheless, Porro's operation made the woman sterile because her uterus has been removed during surgery. This fact raised some criticisms as the operation was deemed immoral by those who claimed it was ethically justified to jeopardize a woman's life given the poor chances of saving her, as long as her reproductive ability was preserved. So Porro turned to the bishop of Pavia, Lucido Maria Parocchi (later cardinal vicar of Rome), as a moral authority of the town, for his ethical opinion. The prelate skillfully solved the question claiming that as many theologians had tolerated the castration of young men destined to be choir singers in Roman chapels (e.g., the Sistine Chapel), for the obstetricians there were even more reasons to allow the sterilization procedure that Porro had adopted to save two human lives [20, 1].

The new era of obstetrics under the sign of a double healing for cesarean section had, however, a difficult initial development. Porro's success with the double safety of the mother and child was a guarantee that the operation could constitute a real solution. But the first obstetricians that applied the method, after its inventor, had unfavorable results because the patients came to the operating table in a desperate condition: they were cachectic or childbirth was retarded by too many hours of labor. However, the surgical technique rapidly spread all over Europe, the United States, Russia, and Mexico; particularly successful was the application in England where it was adopted by Russell Alexander Simpson, Clement Godson, and Lawson Tait [12–15]. The method continued to be widely used in the 25 years after its invention. In 1901 a pupil of Porro, the obstetrician Ettore Truzzi, compiled a detailed table with the number of maternal deaths, year after year, following the intervention devised by his master, gathering in total 1097 cases. In the first 15 years he recorded high rates of mortality, but since 1890 there was a sharp decline, with annual rates ranging from 9% to about 20% [16]. Often the unfortunate result was due to the poor condition of women undergoing cesarean section, according to Porro. The operation became safe if performed in a planned way early in labor. Despite these impressive results, the frequency with which they used the method decreased significantly after 1900. Another technical innovation made him progressively obsolete: the *conservative* cesarean section.

1.3   The Conservative Cesarean Section

From the origins of the cesarean section on a living woman, to suture a uterine breach was considered an arduous and harmful operation. The obstetrician thought that the uterine motions were able to produce a spontaneous hemostasis and so he left the free organ to develop its spasmodic movements. But sepsis or severe bleeding complications were the rule.

Attempts to suture the uterine incision after cesarean section, however, date back to the eighteenth century. The obstetrician Jean Lebas, who was teaching in Montpellier, was one of the first—if not the first—to suture the uterus in 1769; the woman survived and returned to her occupations. The example of Lebas however, was not followed except occasionally and with disappointing results. Uterine suture "was prescribed by the obstetrics and the operation was equivalent to almost a condemnation of the mother." [17]

The essential progress in modern obstetrics of the cesarean section is due to the German obstetrician Max Sänger, who in 1882 introduced the efficient sutures with silver threads of the muscular plane that induced only minimal tissue reaction and avoided affecting the mucosa. His merit was also to awaken the community of obstetricians about the possibility of performing the cesarean surgery without irreversibly mutilating the woman generating capacity. A turning point had, however, already occurred in 1881 when Ferdinand Adolph Kehrer, based on a precise anatomical and histological study, decided to perform a cross-section in the lower segment of the uterus, thinner and less vascularized, along the trend of muscle fibers. With this surgical choice the bleeding was minimized. The double contribution on suture procedures and the site of cutting by Sänger and Kehrer, and the diffusion of asepsis, generated a progress to which concurred many obstetricians with a drastic reduction in mortality from cesarean delivery during the twentieth century [1, 5, 18, 19].

From a destructive intervention that "extinguished the sources of life" [17], cesarean delivery had now turned into a conservative procedure that left substantially intact the possibility of future fertility. So, this operation came in the twentieth century, beginning a story of progress and reduction in mortality up to the current situation that could almost be described as the era of the cesarean section "on demand" [5].

References

1. Mazzarello P. E si salvò anche la madre. L'evento che rivoluzionò il parto cesareo. Torino: Bollati Boringhieri; 2015.
2. Young JH. Caesarean Section. The History and Development of the Operation from Earliest Times. London: Lewis; 1944.
3. Crainz F. Il taglio cesareo nel mito e nella leggenda. Roma: Tipografia Julia; 1986.
4. Dongen PWJ. Caesarean section—etymology and early history. South Afr J Obstet Gynaecol. 2009;15:62–6.
5. Lurie S. The history of cesarean section. New York: Nova Science Publishers; 2013.

6. Filippini NM. La nascita straordinaria. Tra madre e figliola rivoluzione del taglio cesareo (sec. XVIII-XIX). Milano: FrancoAngeli; 1995.

7. Kraatz H. Der Wittenberger Kaiserschnitt des Jeremias Trautmann im Jahre 1610—eine historische Reminiszenz. Deutsches Gesundheitswesen. 1958;13:169–72.

8. Corradi A. Dell'ostetricia in Italia dalla metà del secolo scorso fino al presente. Bologna: Gamberini e Parmeggiani; 1874.

9. Fiammazzo A. Nuovo contributo alla biografia di Lorenzo Mascheroni, parte seconda, Il Mascheroni a Pavia, a Milano, a Parigi. La corrispondenza del Mascheroni col conte Girolamo Fogaccia. Bergamo: Istituto Italiano d'Arti Grafiche; 1904.

10. Mangiagalli L. Commemorazione del M.E. Edoardo Porro. Rendiconti del Reale Istituto Lombardo di Scienze e Lettere. 1905;38(serie II):77–84.

11. Cani V. Porro Edoardo. Dizionario Biografico degli Italiani. Roma: Istituto Enciclopedia Treccani; 2016.

12. Godson C. Porro's operation. Br Med J. 1884;I:142–59.

13. Godson C. Porro's operation. Br Med J. 1891;II:793–5.

14. Simpson RA. Case of Caesarean hystero-oöphorectomy, or Porro's operation: with remarks. Br Med J. 1881;I:956–8.

15. Tait L. An address on the surgical aspect of impacted labour. Br Med J. 1890;I:657–61.

16. Truzzi E. L'operazione cesarea Porro. Roma: Officina Poligrafica Romana; 1901.

17. Mangiagalli L. L'Ostetricia nel Secolo XIX. Ann Ostet Ginecol. 1900;22:1029–48.

18. Forleo R, Forleo P. Fondamenti di storia della Ostetricia e Ginecologia. Roma: Verduci Editore; 2009.

19. Todman D. A history of caesarean section: from ancient world to the modern era. Aust N Z J Obstet Gynaecol. 2007;47:357–61.

20. Porro E. Dell'amputazione utero-ovarico come complemento di taglio cesareo. Annali Universali di Medicina e Chirurgia. 1876;237:289–349.

Epidemiology, Indications, and Surgical Techniques

2

Paolo Gastaldi

2.1 Epidemiology

The labour room is a multiprofessional environment; it is complex by definition. The woman and the fetus are the main players on the scene. The midwife, gynecologist, anaesthetist, neonatologist, nurse, and the assistant share critical decisions about two human beings' lives.

Until half a century ago, cesarean section was rare. It was a dangerous operation for at least three reasons: poor surgical technique, risk of sepsis, and no anesthesia. Many women died during or soon after a cesarean section. Evolution of medicine changed this practice.

The World Health Organization declared in 1985, in Fortaleza, Brazil, that *'there is no justification for any reason to have a cesarean section rate higher than 10–15%'* [1].

An appropriate cesarean section prevents maternal and perinatal complications. There is no benefit for women or infants who do not need the procedure. The complications have a negative effect on a woman's health.

In 2015, WHO published a systematic review of the studies in the scientific literature to analyse the association between cesarean section rates and maternal, perinatal, and infant outcomes. A panel of international experts agreed on this statement [2].

> Caesarean sections are effective in saving maternal and infant lives, but only when they are required for medically indicated reasons. At population level, caesarean section rates higher than 10% are not associated with reductions in maternal and newborn mortality rates.
>
> Caesarean sections can cause significant and sometimes permanent complications, disability or death particularly in settings that lack the facilities and/or capacity to properly conduct safe surgery and treat surgical complications.

P. Gastaldi
UOC Ostetricia e Ginecologia, Ospedale Santo Spirito Roma, Rome, Italy
e-mail: gastaldi.paolo@gmail.com

© Springer International Publishing Switzerland 2017
G. Capogna (ed.), *Anesthesia for Cesarean Section*,
DOI 10.1007/978-3-319-42053-0_2

Caesarean sections should ideally only be undertaken when medically necessary. Every effort should be made to provide caesarean sections to women in need, rather than striving to achieve a specific rate. The effects of caesarean section rates on other outcomes, such as maternal and perinatal morbidity, pediatric outcomes, and psychological or social well-being are still unclear. More research is needed to understand the health effects of caesarean section on immediate and future outcomes.

An historical study on graphic analysis of labour in 1954 included 100 women with spontaneous labour. Of these women, 64 had an operative vaginal birth with forceps and one had a cesarean section [3].

The rate of cesarean section increased steeply during last decades. Urbanization, childbirth in hospital, reduction of homebirths, consultant-led maternity and the exclusion of midwives from clinical decisions, and induction of labour are possible causes of the increase of this operation [4, 5].

The obstetric population has changed. Many women live their pregnancy later in life. Average body mass index of the mother and fetal weight have increased [6].

The proportion of births by cesarean section has been proposed as an indicator for measuring access, availability, or appropriateness of medical care, as well as for monitoring changes in maternal mortality. A study of births by cesarean section estimated in 2007 at national, regional, and global levels with data from 126 countries, 89% of world live births. The global rate of cesarean section was 15%. In more developed countries, it was 21.1%, in less developed countries 14.3%, and in least developed countries 2% [7].

Repeat cesarean deliveries in the United States account for one third of the cesarean sections.

The most common indications for primary cesarean delivery, in a recent population study, were labour dystocia, abnormal or indeterminate fetal heart rate tracing, fetal malpresentation, multiple gestation, and suspected fetal macrosomia [8].

WHO proposed in 2014 the Robson classification system as a global standard for assessing, monitoring and comparing cesarean section rates within healthcare facilities over time, and between facilities [9].

2.2 Indications

2.2.1 Introduction

During pregnancy every woman is eager to know whether natural childbirth is possible for her. The obstetrician, midwife or doctor, has the duty to plan childbirth with her.

There are situations in which natural childbirth is contraindicated but most of the time the decision is difficult. Often it is necessary to wait for labour to decide.

The childbirth is natural or operative (Fig. 2.1). Natural is vaginal. Operative is both vaginal or abdominal. Operative vaginal childbirth is performed with forceps or with vacuum. There are more devices but these are universal. Operative abdominal childbirth is cesarean.

Fig. 2.1 Childbirth option

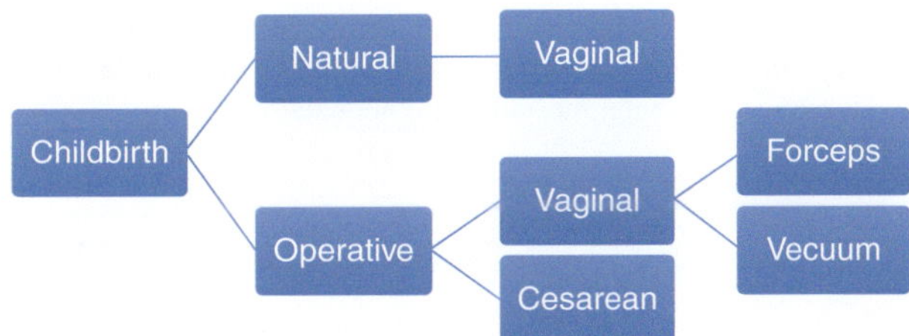

2.2.2 Classification

Classification of the indications for cesarean section is not simple. There are lots of categories. The most used is emergency or elective cesarean section. Using temporal criteria, cesarean section is prelabour or intrapartum.

A recent concept is planned or unplanned [9]. Planned cesarean section is at all times a prelabour decision. The indication is maternal, fetal, or both. A planned cesarean section sometimes becomes an emergency operation.

Unplanned is always urgent. It often regards obstetric care in labour. Fetal distress, maternal complications, and failure to progress in labour are indications that open a discussion among professionals in labour room. Cardiotocography and partogram are tools to be used wisely to agree on the indication of an emergency cesarean section.

Indications for a planned cesarean section have evolved over the last decades. Some indications are absolute, others are relative. Evidence-based medicine is a method to counsel women. Maternal request is a crisis between a woman's auto determination and midwifery which would suggest a natural childbirth.

2.2.3 Planned Cesarean Section

The indications for a planned cesarean section are seldom absolute and need to be discussed with the woman and her expectations (Fig. 2.2) [9].

2.2.3.1 Breech Presentation

Breech presentation is not purely coincidental [10]. It is frequent in preterm births. Some malformations prevent proper rotation of the fetus to the cephalic presentation. Uterine anomalies, such as bicornate uterus, may prevent cephalic presentation of the fetus. It is good practice to search for a cause. Breech presentation at term is an indication for one out of ten cesarean sections [11, 12]. External cephalic version, moxibustion, and posture are interventions that promote cephalic version [11, 13–16]. External cephalic version has recognized complications: transient bradycardia and other fetal heart rate abnormalities, placental abruption, vaginal bleeding, induction of labour.

Evidence-based medicine [9]

Women who have an uncomplicated singleton breech pregnancy at 36 weeks gestation should be offered external cephalic version. Exceptions include women in labour and women with a uterine scar or abnormality, fetal compromise, ruptured membranes, vaginal bleeding, or medical conditions.

Pregnant women with a singleton breech presentation at term, for whom external cephalic version is contraindicated or has been unsuccessful, should be offered CS because it reduces perinatal mortality and neonatal morbidity.

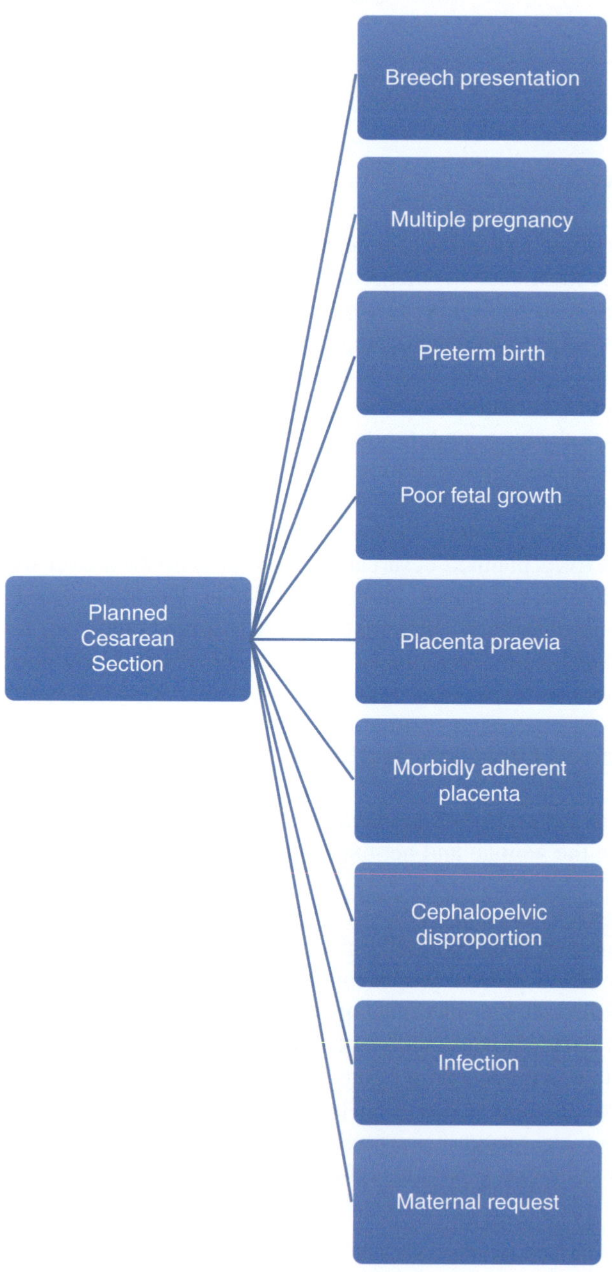

Fig. 2.2 Planned cesarean section

2.2.3.2 Multiple Pregnancy

In the last decades, artificial reproductive technology has increased the incidence of multiple pregnancy [17, 18]. Multiple pregnancy is associated with preterm birth and low birth weight [19–23]. The complexity of placental circulation in monochorionic twin pregnancy is a risk for a discordant growth. Second-born twin has a specific risk of complications during childbirth.

The management of the complications of multiple pregnancy, such as pre-eclampsia, influences the mode of delivery. Cephalic presentation of the first twin is a possible indication for a trial of labour [24]. The evidence is not conclusive.

> Evidence-based medicine [9]
>
> In otherwise uncomplicated twin pregnancies at term where the presentation of the first twin is cephalic, perinatal morbidity and mortality is increased for the second twin. However, the effect of planned CS in improving outcome for the second twin remains uncertain and therefore CS should not routinely be offered outside a research context.
>
> In twin pregnancies where the first twin is not cephalic, the effect of CS in improving outcome is uncertain, but current practice is to offer a planned CS.

2.2.3.3 Preterm Birth

The premature prelabour rupture of membranes determines preterm birth. The decision on the mode of delivery is not straightforward [25–27]. Pre-eclampsia, HELLP syndrome, and other maternal complications are an indication to expedite birth. Fetal compromise may induce a decision for preterm birth. There is no evidence that planned cesarean section changes the outcome of birth [28].

> Evidence-based medicine
>
> Preterm birth is associated with higher neonatal morbidity and mortality. However, the effect of planned CS in improving these outcomes remains uncertain and therefore CS should not routinely be offered outside a research context.

2.2.3.4 Poor Fetal Growth

Poor fetal growth is not always pathologic. It may be constitutional and there is no specific risk to anticipate childbirth [29–32]. Fetal growth restriction is pathologic. There is discordant growth with a significant difference between cephalic and abdominal circumference. The fetus is small for gestational age.

> Evidence-based medicine [9]
>
> The risk of neonatal morbidity and mortality is higher with 'small-for-gestational-age' babies. However, the effect of planned CS in improving these outcomes remains uncertain and therefore CS should not routinely be offered outside a research context.

2.2.3.5 Placenta Previa

The diagnosis of low-lying placenta changes with gestational age. It is necessary to repeat serial ultrasound scans to study the position of the placenta with respect to internal cervical os [19, 33]. Pulsed and Colour Doppler ultrasound give a detailed view of placental circulation. The major placenta previa, covering internal cervical os, is an absolute indication for cesarean section after the 36th week of pregnancy.

Evidence-based medicine [9]

Women with a placenta that partly or completely covers the internal cervical os (minor or major placenta previa) should be offered CS.

2.2.3.6 Morbidly Adherent Placenta

The risk of morbidly adherent placenta is increased after a previous cesarean section. Women with three or more previous cesarean sections have a risk of placenta previa of 1.8–3.7% and high risk of morbidly adherent placenta [34]. The most frequent complications are major obstetric hemorrhage, transfusion of large quantities of blood products, hysterectomy and admission to intensive care unit [35, 36]. Ultrasound, Colour flow mapping and MRI have increased early prenatal diagnosis [37].

Evidence-based medicine [9]

If low-lying placenta is confirmed at 32–34 weeks in women who have had a previous CS, offer colour-flow Doppler ultrasound as the first diagnostic test for morbidly adherent placenta.

If a colour-flow Doppler ultrasound scan result suggests morbidly adherent placenta, discuss with the woman the improved accuracy of magnetic resonance imaging (MRI) in addition to ultrasound to help diagnose morbidly adherent placenta and clarify the degree of invasion. Explain what to expect during an MRI procedure, inform the woman that current experience suggests that MRI is safe, but then there is a lack of evidence about any long-term risks to the baby; offer MRI if acceptable to the woman.

Discuss the interventions available for delivery with women suspected to have morbidly adherent placenta including cross-matching of blood and planned CS with a consultant obstetrician present.

When performing a CS for women suspected of having a morbidly adherent placenta, ensure that a consultant obstetrician and a consultant anaesthetist are present, an experienced paediatrician is present, a senior haematologist is available for advice, a critical care bed is available, and sufficient cross-matched blood and blood products are readily available.

2.2.4 Predicting Cesarean Section for Cephalopelvic Disproportion

The role of pelvimetry, shoe size, maternal height, and clinical and ultrasound estimation of fetal size to predict cephalopelvic disproportion is controversial [38, 39, 42].

Evidence-based medicine [9]

Pelvimetry is not useful in predicting 'failure to progress' in labour and should not be used in decision-making about mode of birth.

Shoe size, maternal height, and estimations of fetal size (ultrasound or clinical examination) do not accurately predict cephalopelvic disproportion and should not be used to predict 'failure to progress' during labour.

2.2.4.1 Mother to Child Transmission of Maternal Infections

The prevention of vertical transmission of maternal infections to the fetus influences the mode of delivery. The passage through the birth canal and direct contact with maternal vaginal and perineal secretions are a recognized cause of transmission of a maternal infection to the fetus. Cesarean section has been considered a preventive measure for some infections but evidence has a continuous evolution. There is new evidence for HIV [40–44], hepatitis B [45, 46], hepatitis C [47], and herpes virus infection [48–50].

Evidence-based medicine [9]

As early as possible give women with HIV information about the risks and benefits for them and their child of the HIV treatment options and mode of birth so that they can make an informed decision.

Do not offer a CS on the grounds of HIV status to prevent mother-to-child transmission of HIV to: women on highly active anti-retroviral therapy (HAART) with a viral load of less than 400 copies per ml or women on any anti-retroviral therapy with a viral load of less than 50 copies per ml. Inform women that in these circumstances the risk of HIV transmission is the same for a CS and a vaginal birth.

Consider either a vaginal birth or a CS for women on anti-retroviral therapy (ART) with a viral load of 50–400 copies per ml because there is insufficient evidence that a CS prevents mother-to-child transmission of HIV.

Offer a CS to women with HIV who are not receiving any anti-retroviral therapy or are receiving any anti-retroviral therapy and have a viral load of 400 copies per ml or more. Mother-to-child transmission of hepatitis B can be reduced if the baby receives immuno-globulin and vaccination. In these situations, pregnant women with hepatitis B should not be offered a planned CS because there is insufficient evidence that this reduces mother-to-child transmission of hepatitis B virus.

Women who are infected with hepatitis C should not be offered a planned CS because this does not reduce mother-to-child transmission of the virus.

Women with primary genital herpes simplex virus (HSV) infection occurring in the third trimester of pregnancy should be offered planned CS because it decreases the risk of neonatal HSV infection.

2.2.4.2 Maternal Request for Cesarean Section

To ask for a cesarean section without an obstetric indication is not a natural option for a woman close to term [19, 51]. Many women experience a preference for cesarean section. If they had a previous cesarean section or a previous negative outcome, or a complication in the current pregnancy or fear of childbirth, they think cesarean section is the safest way to give birth [52–54]. Respect to the woman's feelings is a duty for all those who attend her. The indication for a cesarean section on maternal request becomes effective after multidisciplinary counselling. Gynecologist, midwife, and anesthetist discuss the risks and benefits of cesarean section with her, comparing vaginal birth [55]. They offer referral to a specialist in mental health, who supports and certifies the maternal request and gives the alternative choice for a natural childbirth with active support.

Evidence-based medicine [9]

When a woman requests a CS, explore, discuss, and record the specific reasons for the request.

If a woman requests a CS when there is no other indication, discuss the overall risks and benefits of CS compared with vaginal birth and record that this discussion has taken place. Include a discussion with other members of the obstetric team (including the obstetrician, midwife, and anesthetist) if necessary to explore the reasons for the request, and to ensure the woman has accurate information.

When a woman requests a CS because she has anxiety about childbirth, offer referral to a healthcare professional with expertise in providing perinatal mental health support to help her address her anxiety in a supportive manner.

For women requesting a CS, if after discussion and offer of support (including perinatal mental health support for women with anxiety about childbirth), a vaginal birth is still not an acceptable option, offer a planned CS.

2.2.5   Unplanned Cesarean Section

Healthcare professionals in the labour room frequently assist a woman, who has no indication for a planned cesarean section.

Labour room is a teamwork. Decisions are shared among the members of the team. The midwife has the most important role. She is empathic with the woman and is her connection with the rest of the team. She is the team leader during natural childbirth.

The number of cesarean sections during labour is a quality index of the labour room performance. A third-level hospital has a greater number of unplanned cesarean sections than a less-equipped hospital.

The indications for unplanned cesarean section are often related to failure to progress in labour and fetal distress. There are maternal conditions, such as severe pre-eclampsia, in which a cesarean section comes after a trial of labour. Some factors reduce the likelihood of cesarean section.

2.2.5.1 Factors that Reduce the Likelihood of Cesarean Section

One-to-one support in labour room, induction of labour after 41 weeks, use of partogram during labour, consultant obstetrician who decides on cesarean section, and fetal blood sampling for abnormal heart rate pattern reduce the likelihood of cesarean section [56–64, 68].

Evidence-based medicine [9]

Women should be informed that continuous support during labour with or without prior training reduces the likelihood of CS.

Women with an uncomplicated pregnancy should be offered induction of labour beyond 41 weeks because this reduces the risk of perinatal mortality and the likelihood of CS.

A partogram with a four-hour action line should be used to monitor progress of labour of women in spontaneous labour with an uncomplicated singleton pregnancy at term because it reduces the likelihood of CS.

Consultant obstetricians should be involved in the decision-making for CS because this reduces the likelihood of CS.

Electronic fetal monitoring is associated with an increased likelihood of CS. When CS is contemplated because of an abnormal fetal heart rate pattern, in cases of suspected fetal acidosis, fetal blood sampling should be offered, if it is technically possible and there are no contraindications.

2.2.5.2 Failure to Progress in Labour

The partogram allows a graphic analysis of labour [61, 65, 66]. Failure to progress in labour is an indication for an unplanned cesarean section. The disorders of dilatation are prolonged latent phase, protracted active phase and arrest of cervical dilatation. The disorders of descent are failure to descent, protracted descent, and arrest of cervical dilatation (Table 2.1) (Fig. 2.3).

The three key words are failure, delay, and arrest [67]. Labour abnormalities derive from complex interaction between maternal body and fetal characteristics.

Table 2.1 Failure to progress in labour

Disorder	Dilatation	Descent
Failure	Prolonged latent phase	Failure of descent
Protraction	Protracted active phase	Protracted descent
Arrest	Arrest of dilatation	Arrest of descent

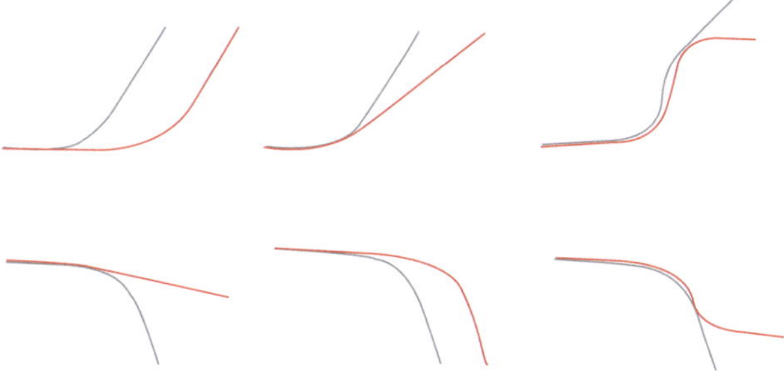

Fig. 2.3 The disorders of dilatation and descent

The decision for a cesarean section is clinical. A four-hour action line on the partogram is the standard to diagnose labour protraction [66, 67]. The most recent evidence is that dilatation progress takes up to six hours between 4 and 5 cm and up to three hours between 5 and 6 cm [5, 8] . After 6 cm labour accelerates and multiparous women are faster than nulliparous parturients. In many cases, active phase has no consistent pattern, but still a vaginal delivery is achieved with active phase not starting before 6 cm of dilatation. Labour protraction should not be based on an average starting point of active phase of labour or average duration of labour. In the presence of reassuring maternal and fetal conditions, a woman should be allowed to continue her labour.

It would be advisable to do a study that compares a partogram with and without an action line and its effect on maternal and neonatal well-being.

Evidence-based medicine [8]

Slow but progressive labor in the first stage of labor should not be indication for cesarean delivery.

Cervical dilatation of 6 cm should be considered threshold for active phase of most women in labor. Thus, before 6 cm of dilation is achieved, standards of active-phase progress should not be applied.

Cesarean delivery for active-phase arrest in first stage of labor should be reserved for women with >6 cm of dilatation with ruptured membranes who fail to progress despite four hours of adequate uterine activity, or at least six hours of oxytocin administration with inadequate uterine activity and no cervical change.

2.2.5.3 Fetal Distress

Fetal distress is not a specific notion. In clinical practice it means a not-reassuring fetal heart rate pattern recorded with cardiotocography in which a state of hypoxia and metabolic acidosis would be present [68].

There are transitory factors such as cord compression, maternal hypotension, maternal supine position, and uterine hyperstimulation. There are also permanent factors such as cord prolapse, complete placental abruption, and uterine rupture.

Cardiotocography only records two parameters: the fetal heart rate and contractions.

The four features of fetal heart rate that are scrutinized in a cardiotocograph are baseline heart activity, baseline variability, presence or absence of decelerations and presence of accelerations.

Cardiotocography is a screening test for perinatal asphyxia, not a diagnostic test or treatment [69–73]. There is a clear discrepancy between abnormalities in cardiotocographs and severe perinatal asphyxia, causing death or severe neurological impairment.

Cardiotocography has a good negative likelihood ratio; when normal the chance of hypoxia is low. It is moderately useful in predicting poor neonatal outcomes.

Some features of cardiotocographs may predict neonatal outcome or the surrogate measure of low umbilical cord blood pH: prolonged or severe bradycardia, decreased variability, decreased variability with no accelerations, decreased variability associated with variable or late decelerations or no accelerations, recurrent late decelerations with decreased variability, late decelerations, and variable decelerations [74–78].

The decision to change a woman's care in labour is delicate. The midwife and the doctor integrate the information of cardiotocographs with fetal blood sampling and fetal response to scalp stimulation. The care is empathic with the woman, her partner, and her family.

Evidence-based medicine [69]

Electronic fetal monitoring is associated with an increased likelihood of CS. When CS is contemplated because of an abnormal fetal heart rate pattern, in cases of suspected fetal acidosis, fetal blood sampling should be offered if it is technically possible and there are no contraindications.

If fetal scalp stimulation leads to an acceleration in fetal heart rate, regard this as a reassuring feature. Take this into account when reviewing the whole clinical picture.

Use the fetal heart rate response after fetal scalp stimulation during a vaginal examination to elicit information about fetal well-being if fetal blood sampling is unsuccessful or contraindicated.

2.2.5.4 Classification of Urgency

The classification of urgent cesarean section prevents any misunderstanding between healthcare professionals (Table 2.2). There are four grades of urgent cesarean section [9]. Some clinical conditions which determine **grade 1** cesarean sections are acute fetal bradycardia, cord prolapse, uterine rupture, or fetal blood sampling pH less than 7.2; **grade 2** cesarean section are antepartum hemorrhage or failure to progress in labor with maternal or fetal compromise; **grade 3** are failure to progress in labor with no maternal or fetal compromise or a woman booked for a planned cesarean section who is admitted with a prelabour rupture of membranes; **grade 4** are all cesarean sections carried out electively at a planned time to suit the mother and the clinicians.

The urgent cesarean section was measured with a three-colour code: red, orange, and green [79, 80]. The ideal decision-to-delivery time was 15 min for a red code, 30 min for an orange code, and 60 min for a green code. After six months of observation, mean decision-to-delivery interval was 31.7 min. Previously, it was 39.6 min.

Table 2.2 Urgency of cesarean section

Grade	Condition
1	Immediate threat to the life of the woman or fetus
2	Maternal or fetal compromise which was not immediately life-threatening
3	No maternal or fetal compromise but needs early delivery
4	Delivery timed to suit woman or staff

The NICE stated in 2011 that grade 1 and 2 cesarean sections must be performed as quickly as possible, grade 3, in most situations, within 75 min [9].

The decision to deliver in an interval of less than 15 min is often harmful for the woman and her fetus for an iatrogenic injury. This a treatment paradox.

2.3 Technique

2.3.1 Prerequisites

There are some evidence-based medicine prerequisites for cesarean section: agreement of the woman on the indication, informed consent; WHO surgical safety checklist; if appropriate, blood available for surgery; antacids and antiemetics available; achievement of anesthesia; prevention of aortocaval compression; neonatal resuscitation available; bladder empty with an indwelling catheter; operator appropriately experienced and skilled; prophylactic antibiotic and thrombo-prophylaxis [81].

2.3.2 WHO Surgical Safety Checklist

The three steps of WHO surgical safety checklist are: Sign In, Time out, Sign out [82] . It was the result of a prospective study in eight hospitals representing a variety of economic circumstances and diverse populations of patients participating in World Health Organization's Safe Surgery Saves Lives Program.

2.3.2.1 Sign In (for Cesarean Section)

Before induction of anesthesia, members of the team orally confirm that the patient has verified her identity, the surgical procedure and consent; the pulse oximeter is on the patient and functioning; all members of the team are aware of whether the patient has a known allergy; the patient's airway and risk of aspiration have been evaluated and appropriate equipment and assistance is available; if there is a risk of blood loss of at least 500 ml appropriate access and fluids are available.

2.3.2.2 Time Out (for Cesarean Section)

Before skin incision the entire team orally confirms that all team members have been introduced by name and role; confirms the patient's identity and procedure; reviews the anticipated critical events; surgeon reviews critical and unexpected steps, operative duration and anticipated blood loss; anesthesia staff review concerns specific to the patient; nursing staff review confirmation of sterility, equipment availability and other concerns; confirms that prophylactic antibiotics have been administered 60 min before incision is made or the antibiotics are not indicated; confirms that all imaging results for the correct patients are displayed in the operating room.

2.3.2.3 Sign Out (for Cesarean Section)

Before the patient leaves the operating room: nurse reviews items aloud with the team; name of the procedure as recorded; that the needle, sponge, and instrument counts are complete; whether there are any issues with equipment to be addressed; the surgeon, nurse, and anesthesia professionals review aloud the key concerns for the recovery and care of the patient.

2.3.3 Skin Incision

Surgical incisions for cesarean section are vertical and transverse [83–85]. The length must be adequate to perform a safe procedure. The incision should be approximately 15 cm long, as an 'Allis' clamp, laid on the skin.

2.3.3.1 Vertical Incision

This is a midline incision on the umbilical-pubic axis [84]. A vertical incision is a direct access to abdomen and pelvis. It is indicated for urgent cesarean section. A typical indication is a massive hemorrhage. The surgeon could practice a vertical incision for a perimortem cesarean section or when a patient is high risk for a coagulopathy or if she refuses a much-needed blood transfusion.

2.3.3.2 Pfannestiel's Incision

This is a lower transverse abdominal incision. It is slightly curved above the symphysis pubis. It involves dissection of subcutaneous layer and of anterior rectus sheath. This incision does not follow Langer's line, the natural orientation of collagen fibres in the dermis, parallel to the orientation of the underlying muscle fibres. It was introduced by Pfannestiel in 1896 and published in 1900 [86] . The extension of the incision into external and oblique muscles could damage ilioinguinal and iliohypogastric nerves. It may slow down an emergency cesarean section. It reduces the incidence of wound dehiscence. Wound hernias are uncommon. Instead postoperative haematomas and wound infections are possible [87–90].

2.3.3.3 Joel Cohen's Incision

It is a transverse incision, 3 cm below the line between the iliac anterior superior spines. It is higher than Pfannestiel's incision. It was introduced in 1954 for abdominal hysterectomy [87, 91, 92]. The opening of the subcutaneous tissue is not sharp. The surgeon incises the anterior rectus sheath in the midline for about 3 cm but does not separate rectus muscle from the sheath. The opening of the peritoneum is blunt and traction is in a transverse direction.

2.3.3.4 Maylard Incision

It is a high transverse incision with section of rectal muscles with cautery or surgical scalpel and ligature of inferior epigastric vessels [93, 94]. It is advisable to not separate rectus muscles from anterior rectus sheath. This incision is used for radical pelvic surgery.

> Evidence-based Medicine [9]
>
> CS should be performed using a transverse abdominal incision because this is associated with less postoperative pain and an improved cosmetic effect compared with a midline incision.
>
> The transverse incision of choice should be the Joel Cohen incision (a straight skin incision, 3 cm above the symphysis pubis; subsequent tissue layers are opened bluntly and, if necessary, extended with scissors and not a knife), because it is associated with shorter operating times and reduced postoperative febrile morbidity.
>
> The use of separate surgical knives to incise the skin and the deeper tissues at CS is not recommended because it does not decrease wound infection.

2.3.4 Uterine Incision

2.3.4.1 Low Transverse Incision

It is a transverse incision through the lower uterine segment. It was introduced in 1926 [95]. The loose fold of the peritoneum is incised, and the bladder is pushed down with care. The doyen's retractor exposes the uterine lower segment. Sometimes the uterus is rotated on the right side and its position is corrected before delivery of the fetus. The surgeon incises 2–3 cm in the middle to expose fetal membranes. Then he enlarges the depth and the width of opening with the blunt end of the scalpel or with fingers [96, 97]. The lateral extension of the incision may reach uterine vessels with a massive hemorrhage. The surgical extension on the upper segment usually is J-shaped or reverse T-shaped. In these cases, the scar is weaker than the incision limited to lower segment.

2.3.4.2 Low Vertical Incision

It is a vertical incision on the lower uterine segment [84]. It was introduced in 1922 [98]. It spares uterine vessels but is a real threat for the bladder. This incision needs a careful dissection of the bladder. It is an alternative when transverse incision is contraindicated by a medical reason, such as a fibroid.

2.3.4.3 Classical Incision

Classical incision is a vertical incision which involves upper uterine segment. The thickness of the myometrium poses a great risk for blood loss, infection and poor healing. Some conditions are a possible indication for a classical incision: preterm delivery before the formation of lower uterine segment [99]; premature rupture of membranes and transverse lie; transverse lie with back inferior; large cervical fibroid; severe adhesions in lower uterine segment; postmortem cesarean section; placenta previa with large vessels in lower segment.

Evidence-based medicine [9]

When there is a well-formed lower uterine segment, blunt rather than sharp extension of the uterine incision should be used because it reduces blood loss, incidence of postpartum hemorrhage, and the need for transfusion at CS.

2.3.5 Delivery of the Fetus

2.3.5.1 Cephalic Presentation

After uterine incision the operator tears fetal membranes with care. He introduces his hand into lower uterine cavity and elevates fetal head until it becomes visible through the incision. The active flexion of fetal head reduces its diameter. In transverse and posterior position, the operator must rotate fetal head as much as possible, in anterior position. The assistant applies fundal pressure. The collaboration between surgeon and assistant allows a minimal traction to deliver fetal head. The head comes out with an extension movement. Delivery of shoulders needs special care. A brachial plexus damage or palsy is possible as in normal childbirth. This a consequence of a reckless maneuver.

When fetal head is high in the uterus there is risk for excessive blood loss. A forceps or vacuum delivery is the solution. In literature there are specific vacuum cups for cesarean section.

Cesarean at full dilatation with a deeply engaged fetal head is a challenge. A third assistant raises fetal head from vagina to meet operator's hand. A pillow is an alternative device.

2.3.5.2 Face or Brow Cephalic Presentation

The head is deflexed. The operator places intrauterine hand behind occiput, flexes the head, rotates it to anterior or transverse position, and delivers it as usual (Table 2.3).

2.3.5.3 Frank Breech

The operator cups his hand around the bottom and delivers the breech by lateral flexion. When trunk is visible, leg is flexed rotating the femur laterally on fetal abdomen with index finger parallel to the femur. Then the conduct should be the same as in total breech extraction.

Table 2.3 Breech presentation

Breech	Legs and hip
Frank	Legs flexed at the hip extended at the knee
Complete	Legs flexed at the hip flexed at the knee
Footing	Legs extended at the hip extended at the knee
Kneeling	Legs extended at the hip flexed at the knee

2.3.5.4 Footling and Complete Breech

The operator holds one foot or both feet and so legs come first. He keeps the sacrum as anterior, as possible, to facilitate delivery.

2.3.5.5 Transverse Lie

The operator plans surgical approach according to the position of the fetus, location of the feet and of the placenta. The appraisal is both clinical and sonographic. A prolapse of shoulder is possible with a fetal hand coming first through uterine incision. Fetal extraction is not possible. The operator facilitates the hand inside the uterus.

2.3.5.6 Back Down Transverse Lie

The feet are in uterine fundus. It is important to follow the body of the fetus, finding the bottom and the legs. The delivery of posterior leg first keeps the back of the fetus in anterior position. Afterwards the operator may start a breech extraction as in footling breech presentation.

2.3.5.7 Back-up Transverse Lie

The operator follows the fetal body until the bottom and the legs. He grasps both feet and extracts them. Afterwards the operator may start a breech extraction as in footling breech presentation.

2.3.6 Delivery of the Placenta

The operator delivers the placenta with the help of uterine massage, 5 IU of oxytocin, intravenous or intramuscular, and gentle traction on the umbilical cord. This is Active Management of Third Stage of Labour [100–103]. Manual removal of the placenta is an alternative in the presence of heavy bleeding [104]. It has higher rate of postpartum endometritis and heavy bleeding than spontaneous delivery [105, 106].

> Evidence-based medicine [9]
>
> Oxytocin 5 IU by slow intravenous injection should be used at CS to encourage contraction of the uterus and to decrease blood loss.
>
> At CS, the placenta should be removed using controlled cord traction and not manual removal as this reduces the risk of endometritis.

2.3.7 Exteriorization of the Uterus

Exteriorization of the uterus during cesarean section may cause nausea and vomiting. Some women have strong postoperative pain. Venous air embolism is a rare complication. Exteriorization of the uterus does not reduce incidence of hemorrhage and infection [96, 107–109].

Evidence-based medicine [9]

Intraperitoneal repair of the uterus at CS should be undertaken. Exteriorization of the uterus is not recommended because it is associated with more pain and does not improve operative outcomes such as hemorrhage and infection.

2.3.8 Suturing of the Uterus

Kerr in 1926 recommended uterine closure in two layers [96] . Theoretically single-layer closure should cause less tissue damage and should take less operative time. Suture is either locking or non-locking. There are concerns about the integrity of the scar after a single layer suture of the uterus. Evidence is not conclusive [97, 110–115]. The closure of a classical incision is in three layers because of its thickness and vascularity [116].

Evidence-based medicine [9]

The effectiveness and safety of a single-layer closure of the uterine incision is uncertain. Except within a research context, the uterine incision should be sutured with two layers.

2.3.9 Peritoneal Closure

Non-closure of the visceral and parietal layer of the peritoneum is associated with less postoperative morbidity [117–120]. It reduces operative time and wound pain.

Evidence-based medicine [9]

Neither the visceral nor the parietal peritoneum should be sutured at CS because this reduces operating time and the need for postoperative analgesia, and improves maternal satisfaction.

2.3.10 Closure of the Skin

The suture of skin edges of the incision is either intracutaneous or subcuticular [84, 121, 122]. Subcuticular suture has a good cosmetic result. Cyanoacrylate, skin glue, is an alternative [123].

Evidence-based medicine [9]

Routine closure of the subcutaneous tissue space should not be used, unless the woman has more than 2 cm subcutaneous fat, because it does not reduce the incidence of wound infection.

Superficial wound drains should not be used at CS because they do not decrease the incidence of wound infection or wound haematoma.

Obstetricians should be aware that the effects of different suture materials or methods of skin closure at CS are not certain.

2.3.11 Misgav Ladach Technique

Misgav Ladach is a Jerusalem hospital. The technique for cesarean section is a combination of procedures. The result of non-randomized trials and randomized have demonstrated quicker postoperative recovery; reduction of febrile reactions, need for antibiotics, peritoneal adhesions, bleeding, and of postoperative pain, and shorter period before normal bowel function [84, 87, 92, 127].

There are important procedural aspects as follow:

1. Stretching of the skin to respect Langer's lines
2. Joel Cohen incision 17 cm long without involvement of the subcutaneous tissue
3. Short transverse incision about 2–3 cm through the fat down to the rectus sheath
4. Small transverse incision in the sheath
5. Transverse bilateral incision of the sheath with scissors, one blade under and one blade above, underneath the fat and subcutaneous tissue
6. Gentle cranio-caudal separation of the rectus sheath and rectus muscles
7. Stretching in a transverse way to open parietal peritoneum, using index fingers in a cranio-caudal direction to make a small hole
8. Identification of the lower uterine segment and of the bladder
9. Transverse incision of visceral peritoneum 10–12 cm in total and 1 cm above the bladder
10. Fritsch or doyen retractor
11. Small transverse incision in lower uterine segment
12. Transverse stretching of the hole with right thumb and left index finger
13. Two fingers below to release the head
14. Fundal pressure to bring the baby down
15. The fingers guide the head out of the uterine opening
16. Delivery of the baby
17. Manual removal of the placenta
18. Exteriorization of the upper uterus out of abdominal wound
19. Massage of the uterus
20. Cleaning of the inside of the uterus with a towel to remove remnants of membranes and to stimulate contraction and retraction of the uterus
21. Repair of uterine wall with one layer of continuous locked stitch
22. In special circumstances second layer with cross stitches
23. Visceral and parietal peritoneum unstitched
24. Artery forceps to grasp the fascia
25. Continuous running unlocking suture
26. Closure of the skin with two or three maximum mattress suture.

References

1. Appropriate technology for birth. Lancet. 1985;2(8452):436–7.
2. Betran AP, Torloni MR, Zhang JJ, Gülmezoglu AM. WHO Working Group on Caesarean Section WHO statement on caesarean section rates. BJOG. 2015;123(5):667–70. doi:10.1111/1471-0528.13526.
3. Friedman EA. The graphic analysis of labour. Am J Obstet Gynecol. 1954;68:1568.
4. Naji O, Abdallah Y, et al. Cesarean Birth: Surgical Techniques Glob Libr Women's Med. 2010. doi:10.3843/GLOWM.10133.

5. Zhang J, Landy HJ, Branch DW, Burkman R, Haberman S, Gregory KD, Hatjis CG, Ramirez MM, Bailit JL, Gonzalez-Quintero VH, Hibbard JU, Hoffman MK, Kominiarek M, Learman LA, Van Veldhuisen P, Troendle J, Reddy UM, Consortium on Safe Labor. Contemporary patterns of spontaneous labor with normal neonatal outcomes. Obstet Gynecol. 2010 Dec;116(6):1281–7.

6. Vahratian A, Troendle JF, Siega-Riz AM, Zhang J. Methodological challenges in studying labour progression in contemporary practice. Paediatr Perinat Epidemiol. 2006;20(1):72–8.

7. Betrán AP, Merialdi M, Lauer JA, et al. Rates of cesarean section: analysis of global, regional and national estimates. Paediatr Perinat Epidemiol. 2007 Mar;21(2):98–113.

8. ACOG/SMFM Obstetric Care Consensus. Safe prevention of the primary cesarean delivery. Obstet Gynecol. 2014;123:693–711.

9. National Collaborating Centre for Women's and Children's Health (UK). London: National Institute for Health and Care Excellence (UK). 2011 November Cesarean section

10. Royal College of Obstetricians and Gynaecologists. The management of breech presentation. Guideline no. 20. London: RCOG Press; 2001.

11. Hofmeyr GJ. External cephalic version facilitation for breech presentation at term. Cochrane Database Syst Rev. 2001;2:CD000184.

12. Hannah ME, Hannah WJ, Hewson SA, Hodnett ED, Saigal S, Willan AR. Planned caesarean section versus planned vaginal birth for breech presentation at term: a randomised multicentre trial. Lancet. 2000;356:1375–83.

13. Van Veelan AJ, Van Cappellen AW, Flu PK, Straub MJPF, Wallenburg HC. Effect of external cephalic version in late pregnancy on presentation at delivery: a randomized controlled trial. Br J Obstet Gynaecol. 1989;96:916–21.

14. Hofmeyr GJ. External cephalic version for breech presentation before term. Cochrane Database Syst Rev. 2001;2.

15. Hofmeyr GJ. Interventions to help external cephalic version for breech presentation at term. Cochrane Database Syst Rev. 2002;4.

16. Van Dorsten JP, Schifrin BS, Wallace RL. Randomized control trial of external cephalic version with tocolysis in late pregnancy. Am J Obstet Gynecol. 1981;141:417–24.

17. Office for National Statistics. Birth statistics: review of the registrar general on births and patterns of family building in England and Wales, 2002. London: Office for National Statistics; 2004.

18. National Collaborating Centre for Women's and Children's Health. Fertility: assessment and management for people with fertility problems. Clinical guideline. London: RCOG Press; 2004.

19. Thomas J, Paranjothy S. Royal college of obstetricians and Gynaecologists clinical effectiveness support unit. The National Sentinel Caesarean Section Audit Report. London: RCOG Press; 2001.

20. Petterson B, Nelson KB, Watson L, Stanley F. Twins, triplets, and cerebral palsy in births in Western Australia in the 1980s. BMJ. 1993;307:1239–43.

21. Rydhstrom H, Ingemarsson I. A case–control study of the effects of birth by caesarean section on intrapartum and neonatal mortality among twins weighing 1500–2499 g. Br J Obstet Gynaecol. 1991;98:249–53.

22. Rydhstrom H. Prognosis for twins with birth weight less than 1500 gm: the impact of cesarean section in relation to fetal presentation. Am J Obstet Gynecol. 1990;163:528–33.

23. Rydhstrom H. Prognosis for twins discordant in birth weight of 1.0 kg or more: the impact of cesarean section. J Perinat Med. 1990;18:31–7.

24. Crowther CA. Caesarean delivery for the second twin. Cochrane Database Syst Rev. 2000;2:CD000047.

25. Lumley J, Lester A, Renou P, Wood C. A failed RCT to determine the best method of delivery for very low birth weight infants. Control Clin Trials. 1985;6:120–7.

26. Confidential enquiry into stillbirths and deaths in infancy. An enquiry into the quality of care and its effect on the survival of babies born at 27–28 weeks. Project 27/28. London: TSO; 2003.

27. Murphy DJ, Sellers S, MacKenzie IZ, Yudkin PL, Johnson A. Case–control study of antenatal and intrapartum risk factors for cerbral palsy in very preterm singleton babies. Lancet. 1995;346:1449–54.

28. Topp M, Langhoff-Roos J, Uldall P. Preterm birth and cerebral palsy. Predictive value of pregnancy complications, mode of delivery, and Apgar scores. Acta Obstet Gynecol Scand. 1997;76:843–8.

29. Royal College of Obstetricians and Gynaecologists. The investigation and management of the small-for-gestational-age fetus. Guideline No. 31. London: RCOG Press; 2011.

30. GRIT Study Group. A randomised trial of timed delivery for the compromised preterm fetus: short term outcomes and Bayesian interpretation. BJOG. 2003;110:27–32.

31. Kinzler WL, Ananth CV, Smulian JC, Vintzileos AM. The effects of labor on infant mortality among small-for-gestational-age infants in the USA. J Matern Fetal Neonatal Med. 2002;12:201–6.

32. Levy BT, Dawson JD, Toth PP, Bowdler N. Predictors of neonatal resuscitation, low Apgar scores, and umbilical artery pH among growth-restricted neonates. Obstet Gynecol. 1998;91:909–16.

33. Lewsi G, Drife J, editors. Why mothers die 1997–1999. The fifth report of the confidential enquiries into maternal deaths in the United Kingdom. London: RCOG Press; 2001.

34. Guise JM, Eden K, Emeis C, Jonas DE, Morgan LC, Reuland D, Gilchrist M, Finkelstein J, Wiswanathan M, Lohr KN, Lyda-McDonald B. Vaginal birth after cesarean: new insights. Evid Rep Technol Assess. 2010;191:1–397.

35. Cantwell R, et al. Saving mothers' lives: reviewing maternal deaths to make motherhood safer 2006-2008. The eighth report of the confidential enquiries into maternal deaths in the United Kingdom. BJOG. 2011;118:1–203.

36. Warshak CR, Ramos GA, Eskander R, Benirschke K, Saenz CC, Kelly TF, Moore TR, Resnik R. Effect of predelivery diagnosis in 99 consecutive cases of placenta accreta. Obstet Gynecol. 2010;1:65–9.

37. Twickler DM, Lucas MJ, Balis AB, Santos-Ramos R, Martin L, Malone S, Rogers B. Color flow mapping for myometrial invasion in women with a prior cesarean delivery. J Matern Fetal Med. 2000;6:330–5.

38. Pattinson RE. Pelvimetry for fetal cephalic presentations at term. Cochrane Database Syst Rev 2001;3.

39. Gorman RE, Noble A, Andrews CM. The relationship between shoe size and mode of delivery. Midwifery Today Childbirth Educ. 1997;41:70–1.

40. National Collaborating Centre for Women's and Children's Health. Antenatal care: routine care for the healthy pregnant woman. London: National Institute for Health and Clinical Excellence (NICE); 2008.

41. Boer K, England K, Godfried MH, Thorne C. Mode of delivery in HIV-infected pregnant women and prevention of mother-to-child transmission: changing practices in Western Europe. HIV Med. 2010;11(6):368–78.

42. Warszawski J, Tubiana R, Le Chenadec J, Blanche S, Teglas JP, Dollfus C, Faye A, Burgard M, Rouzioux C, Mandelbrot L, ANRS French Perinatal Cohort. Mother-to-child HIV transmission despite antiretroviral therapy in the ANRS French perinatal cohort. AIDS. 2008;2:289–99.

43. Islam S, Oon V, Thomas P. Outcome of pregnancy in HIV-positive women planned for vaginal delivery under effective antiretroviral therapy. J Obstet Gynaecol. 2010;1:38–40.

44. Townsend CL, Cortina-Borja M, Peckham CS, de Ruiter A, Lyall H, Tookey PA. Low rates of mother-to-child transmission of HIV following effective pregnancy interventions in the United Kingdom and Ireland, 2000-2006. AIDS. 2008;8:973–81.

45. Wong VC, Ip HM, Reesink HW, Lelie PN, Reerink-Brongers EE, Yeung CY, et al. Prevention of the HBsAg carrier state in newborn infants of mothers who are chronic carriers of HBsAg and HBeAg by administration of hepatitis-B vaccine and hepatitis-B immunoglobulin. Double-blind randomised placebo-controlled study. Lancet. 1984;1:921–6.

46. Xu Z-Y, Liu C-B, Francis DP. Prevention of perinatal acquisition of hepatitis B virus carriage using vaccine: preliminary report of a randomized, double-blind placebo-controlled and comparative trial. Pediatrics. 1985;76:713–8.
47. European Paediatric Hepatitis C Virus Network. Effects of mode of delivery and infant feeding on the risk of mother-to-child transmission of hepatitis C virus. BJOG. 2001;108:371–7.
48. Randolph AG, Washington AE, Prober CG. Cesarean delivery for women presenting with genital herpes lesions. Efficacy, risks, and costs. JAMA. 1993;270:77–82.
49. Randolph AG, Hartshorn RM, Washington AE. Acyclovir prophylaxis in late pregnancy to prevent neonatal herpes: a cost-effectiveness analysis. Obstet Gynecol. 1996;88:603–10.
50. Scott LL, Alexander J. Cost-effectiveness of acyclovir suppression to prevent recurrent genital herpes in term pregnancy. Am J Perinatol. 1998;15:57–62.
51. Gamble JA, Creedy DK. Women's request for a cesarean section: a critique of the literature. Birth. 2000;27:256–63.
52. Benhamou D, Tecsy M, Parry N, Mercier FJ, Burg C. Audit of an early feeding program after cesarean delivery: patient wellbeing is increased. Can J Anaesth. 2002;49:814–9.
53. Jolly J, Walker J, Bhabra K. Subsequent obstetric performance related to primary mode of delivery. Br J Obstet Gynaecol. 1999;106:227–32.
54. Melender HL. Experiences of fears associated with pregnancy and childbirth: a study of 329 pregnant women. Birth. 2002;29:101–11.
55. Bewley S, Cockburn II J. The unfacts of 'request' caesarean section. BJOG. 2002;109:597–605.
56. Hodnett ED, Gates S, Hofmeyr GJ, Sakala C. Continuous support for women during childbirth. Cochrane Database Syst Rev. 2003;3.
57. Crowley P. Interventions for preventing or improving the outcome of delivery at or beyond term. Cochrane Database Syst Rev. 2003;(1).
58. Albers LL. The duration of labor in healthy women. J Perinatol. 1999;19:114–9.
59. Philpott RH, Castle WM. Cervicographs in the management of labour in primigravidae. J Obstet Gynaecol Br Commonw. 1972;79:592–8.
60. Philpott RH, Castle WM. Cervicographs in the management of labour in primigravidae. II. The action line and treatment of abnormal labour. J Obstet Gynaecol Br Commonw. 1972;79:599–602.
61. World Health Organization partograph in management of labour. World Health Organization maternal health and safe motherhood Programme. Lancet. 1994;343:1399–404.
62. Lavender T, Alfirevic Z, Walkinshaw S. Partogram action line study: a randomised trial. Br J Obstet Gynaecol. 1998;105:976–80.
63. Thacker SB, Stroup DF. Continuous electronic heart rate monitoring for fetal assessment during labor. Cochrane Database Syst Rev. 2000;1.
64. Vintzileos AM, Antsaklis A, Varvarigos I, Papas C, Sofatzis I, Montgomery JT. A randomized trial of intrapartum electronic fetal heart rate monitoring versus intermittent auscultation. Obstet Gynecol. 1993;81:899–907.
65. Lavender T, Alfirevic Z, Walkinshaw S. Partogram action line study: a randomised trial. BJOG. 1998;105(9):976–80.
66. Pattinson RC, Howarth GR, Mdluli W, et al. Aggressive or expectant management of labour: a randomised clinical trial. BJOG. 2003;110(5):457–61.
67. Schifrin BS, Cohen WR. Labor's dysfunctional lexicon. Obstet Gynecol. 1989;74(1):121–4.
68. National Collaborating Centre for Women's and Children's Health (UK). London: National Institute for Health and Care Excellence (UK); 2014 december Intrapartum Care Care of healthy women and their babies during childbirth Clinical Guideline 190 Methods, evidence and recommendations.
69. Larma JD, Silva AM, Holcroft CJ, Thompson RE, Donohue PK, Graham EM. Intrapartum electronic fetal heart rate monitoring and the identification of metabolic acidosis and hypoxic-ischemic encephalopathy. Am J Obstet Gynecol. 2007;197:301–8.
70. Sameshima H, Ikenoue T. Predictive value of late decelerations for fetal acidemia in unselective low-risk pregnancies. Am J Perinatol. 2005;22:19–23.

71. Hadar A, Sheiner E, Hallak M, Katz M, Mazor M, Shoham-Vardi I. Abnormal fetal heart rate tracing patterns during the first stage of labor: effect on perinatal outcome. Am J Obstet Gynecol. 2001;185:863–8.
72. Low JA, Victory R, Derrick EJ. Predictive value of electronic fetal monitoring for intrapartum fetal asphyxia with metabolic acidosis. Obstet Gynecol. 1999;93:285–91.
73. Nelson KB, Dambrosia JM, Ting TY, Grether JK. Uncertain value of electronic fetal monitoring in predicting cerebral palsy. N Engl J Med. 1996;334:613–8.
74. Cahill AG, Caughey AB, Roehl KA, Odibo AO, Macones GA. Terminal fetal heart decelerations and neonatal outcomes. Obstet Gynecol. 2013;122:1070–6.
75. Maso G, Businelli C, Piccoli M, Montico M, De SF, Sartore A, Alberico S. The clinical interpretation and significance of electronic fetal heart rate patterns 2 h before delivery: an institutional observational study. Arch Gynecol Obstet. 2012;286:1153–9.
76. Salim R, Garmi G, Nachum Z, Shalev E. The impact of non-significant variable decelerations appearing in the latent phase on delivery mode: a prospective cohort study. Reprod Biol Endocrinol. 2010;8:81.
77. Sheiner E, Hadar A, Hallak M, Katz M, Mazor M, Shoham-Vardi I. Clinical significance of fetal heart rate tracings during the second stage of labor. Obstet Gynecol. 2001;97:747–52.
78. Honjo S, Yamaguchi M. Umbilical artery blood acid-base analysis and fetal heart rate baseline in the second stage of labor. J Obstet Gynaecol Res. 2001;27:249–54.
79. Dupuis O, Sayegh I, Decullier E, Dupont C, Clément HJ, Berland M, Rudigoz RC. Red, orange and green caesarean sections: a new communication tool for on-call obstetricians. Eur J Obstet Gynecol Reprod Biol. 2008;140(2):206–11.
80. Tuffnell DJ, Wilkinson K, Beresford N. Interval between decision and delivery by caesarean section-are current standards achievable? Observational case series. BMJ. 2001;322(7298):1330–3.
81. Paterson Brown S, Howell C. Managing obstetric emergencies and trauma. 3rd ed. Cambridge: Cambridge University Press; 2014.
82. Haynes AB, Weiser TG, Berry WR, Lipsitz SR, Breizat AH, Dellinger EP, Herbosa T, Joseph S, Kibatala PL, Lapitan MC, Merry AF, Moorthy K, Reznick RK, Taylor B, Gawande AA. Safe Surgery Saves Lives Study Group.A surgical safety checklist to reduce morbidity and mortality in a global population. N Engl J Med. 2009;360(5):491–9.
83. Hema KR, Johanson R. Techniques for performing caesarean section. Best Pract Res Clin Obstet Gynaecol. 2001;15(1):17–47.
84. Burger JWA, van 't RM, Jeekel J. Abdominal incisions: techniques and postoperative complications. Scand J Surg. 2002;91:315–21.
85. Haeri AD. Comparisons of transverse and vertical skin incision for cesarean section. S Afr Med J. 1976;50:33–4.
86. Stark M, Finkel A. Comparison between the Joel Cohen and Pfannenstiel incisions in cesarean section. Eur J Obstet Gynecol Reprod Biol. 1994;53:121–2.
87. Sippo WC, Burghardt A, Gomez AC. Nerve entrapment after Pfannenstiel incision. Am J Obstet Gynecol. 1987;157:420–1.
88. Mowat J, Bonnar J. Abdominal wound dehiscence after cesarean delivery. Br Med J. 1971;2:256–7.
89. Biswas MM. Why not Pfannenstiel's incision? Obstet Gynecol. 1973;41:303–27.
90. Ellis H, PDJAD C-S. Abdominal incisions ± vertical or transverse? Postgrad Med J. 1984;60:407–10.
91. Wallin G, Fall O. Modi®ed Joel-Cohen technique for caesarean delivery. Br J Obstet Gynaecol. 1999;106:221–6.
92. Rock J, Jones III HW. TeLinde's operative gynecology. Philadelphia: Lippincott, Williams and Wilkins; 2003.
93. Helmkamp BF, Krebs HB. The Maylard incision in gynecologic surgery. Am J Obstet Gynecol. 1990;163:1554–7.
94. Ayers JW, Morley GW. Surgical incision for caesarean section. Obstet Gynecol. 1987;70:706–71.

95. Kerr JMM. The technique of cesarean section, with special reference to the lower uterine segment incision. Am J Obstet Gynecol. 1926;12:729–34.

96. Tully L, Gates S, Brocklehurst P, McKenzie-McHarg K, Ayers S. Surgical techniques used during caesarean section operations: results of a national survey of practice in the UK. Eur J Obstet Gynecol Reprod Biol. 2002;102:120–6.

97. Rodriguez AI, Porter KB, O'Brien WF. Blunt versus sharp expansion of the uterine incision in low-segment transverse cesarean section. Am J Obstet Gynecol. 1994;171:1022–5.

98. De Lee JB, Cornell EL. Low cervical caesarean sections (laparotrachelotomy). Results in one hundred and forty-®ve cases. JAMA. 1922;79:109–50.

99. Bethune M, Permezel M. The relationship between gestational age and the incidence of classical caesarean section. Aust N Z J Obstet Gynaecol. 1997;37:153–5.

100. Prendiville WJP, Elbourne D, McDonald SJ. Active versus expected management in the third stage of labour. Cochrane Database Syst Rev. 2000;3:CD000007.

101. Cotter AM, Ness A, Tolosa JE. Prophylactic oxytocin for the third stage of labour. Cochrane Database Syst Rev. 2001;4:CD001808.

102. McDonald SJ, Abbott JM, Higgins SP. Prophylactic ergometrine- oxytocin versus oxytocin for the third stage of labour. Cochrane Database Syst Rev. 2004;1:CD000201.

103. Gulmezoglu AM, Forna F, Villar J, Hofmeyr GJ. Prostaglandins for prevention of postpartum haemorrhage. Cochrane Database Syst Rev. 2007;3:CD000494.

104. Wilkinson C, Enkin MW. Manual removal of placenta at caesarean section. Cochrane Database Syst Rev. 2003;1:416.

105. Magann EF, Washburne JF, Harris RL, Bass JD, Duff WP, Morrison JC. Infectious morbidity, operative blood loss, and length of the operative procedure after cesarean delivery by method of placental removal and site of uterine repair. J Am Coll Surg. 1995;181:517–20.

106. McCurdy Jr CM, Magann EF, McCurdy CJ, Saltzman AK. The effect of placental management at cesarean delivery on operative blood loss. Am J Obstet Gynecol. 1992;167:1363–7.

107. Wilkinson C, Enkin MW. Uterine exteriorization versus intraperitoneal repair at caesarean section. Cochrane Database Syst Rev. 2000;2:CD000085.

108. Wahab MA, Karantzis P, Eccersley PS, et al. A randomised controlled study of uterine exteriorisation and repair at caesarean section. Br J Obstet Gynaecol. 1999;106:913–6.

109. Edi-Osagie EC, Hopkins RE, Ogbo V, Lockhat-Clegg F, Ayeko M, Akpala WO, et al. Uterine exteriorisation at caesarean section: influence on maternal morbidity. Br J Obstet Gynaecol. 1998;105:1070–8.

110. Pritchard JA, Macdonald PC. Cesarean section and cesarean hysterectomy. In: Pritchard JA, Macdonald PC, editors. Williams' obstetrics, 5th edn. New York: Appleton Century Crofts; 1976. pp. 903–923.

111. Enkin MW, Wilkinson, C. Single versus two layer suturing for closing the uterine incision at caesarean section. Cochrane Database Syst Rev. 2001;3.

112. Hauth JC, Owen J, Davis RO. Transverse uterine incision closure: one versus two layers. Am J Obstet Gynecol. 1992;167:1108–11.

113. Lal K, Tsomo P. Comparative study of single layer and conventional closure of uterine incision in cesarean section. Int J Obstet Gynaecol Obstet. 1988;27:349–52.

114. Bujold E, Bujold C, Hamilton EF, Harel F, Gauthier RJ. The impact of a single-layer or double- layer closure on the uterine rupture. Am J Obstet Gynecol. 2002;186:1326–30.

115. Chapman SJ, Owen J. One- versus two-layer closure of a low transverse cesarean: the next pregnancy. Obstet Gynecol. 1997;89:16–8.

116. Balat O, Atmaca R, Gokdeniz R. Three-layer closure technique at cesarean section: a prospective, randomized clinical trial. IMJ. 2000;7:299–301.

117. Wilkinson CS Enkin MW. Peritoneal non-closure at casarean section. Cochrane Database Syst Rev 2001;3.

118. Johanson RB. RCOG green top guideline no 23: peritoneal closure, 1998.

119. Galaal KA, Krolikowski A. A randomized controlled study of peritoneal closure at cesarean section. Saudi Med J. 2000;21:759–61.

120. Rafique Z, Shibli KU, Russell IF, Lindow SW. A randomised controlled trial of the closure or non-closure of peritoneum at caesarean section: effect on postoperative pain. BJOG. 2002;109:694–8.
121. Lindholt JS, Moller-Christensen T, Steel RE. The cosmetic outcome of the scar formation after cesarean section: percutaneous or intracutaneous suture? Acta Obstet Gynecol Scand. 1994;73:832–5.
122. Frishman GN, Schwartz T, Hogan JW. Closure of Pfannenstiel skin incisions. Staples vs subcuticular suture. J Reprod Med. 1997;42:627–30.
123. Gorozpe-Calvillo JI, Gonzalez-Villamil J, Santoyo-Haro S, Castaneda-Vivar JJ. Closure of the skin with cyanoacrylate in cesarean section. Ginecologia y Obstetricia de Mexico. 1999;67:491–6.
124. Stark M, Chavkin V, Kupfersztain C, et al. Evaluation of combinations of procedures in cesarean section. Int J Obstet Gynecol. 1995;48:273–6.
125. Robson MS. Classification of caesarean sections. Fetal Matern Med Rev. 2001;12(1):23–39.
126. Hanzal E, Kainz C, Hoffmann G, Deutinger J. An analysis of the prediction of cephalopelvic disproportion. Arch Gynecol Obstet. 1993;253:161–6.
127. Royal College of Obstetricians and Gynaecologists Clinical Effectiveness Support Unit. The use of electronic fetal monitoring: the use and interpretation of cardiotocography in intrapartum fetal monitoring. Evidence-based clinical guideline no. 8. London: RCOG Press.

Giorgio Capogna

General anesthesia is associated with substantially greater maternal risk than regional anesthesia due to difficult airway management or aspiration related deaths. Spinal and epidural anesthesia have therefore become more widely utilized for cesarean section. Spinal anesthesia is simple to institute, rapid in its effect, and produces excellent operating conditions. Continuous epidural analgesia is more titratable, may produce less hemodynamic changes, and can be topped up if surgery is prolonged or postoperative pain relief is required. Spinal anesthesia is the most commonly used technique for elective cesarean section where epidural is most used to convert labor epidural analgesia to surgical anesthesia. The introduction of combined spinal-epidural anesthesia (CSEA) may offer benefits of both spinal and epidural anesthesia.

3.1 Introduction

Selection of the method of anesthesia is traditionally mainly based on the classification of the cesarean section according to the level of urgency since, usually, the risks and morbidity of the procedure basically depend on the level of urgency itself [1].

However, in addition to the time available, factors that may influence the anesthetic choice decision may also include the presence of a working epidural analgesia, maternal preference, expectation or previous experience, the likely duration of surgery, and the presence of maternal pathology, especially cardiac, neurological, or previous back surgery. Local, institutional, anesthetic practice, and the expertise of the physician may also play an important role.

In all cases, prior to cesarean delivery, every patient should undergo an evaluation by an anesthesiologist to give correct information to the patient and determine

G. Capogna
Department of Anesthesiology, Città di Roma Hospital, Rome, Italy
e-mail: dipartimento.anestesia@gruppogarofalo.com

© Springer International Publishing Switzerland 2017
G. Capogna (ed.), *Anesthesia for Cesarean Section*,
DOI 10.1007/978-3-319-42053-0_3

any comorbidities that would impact the anesthetic plan. Even in an emergent situation, an abbreviated examination and adequate preparation are essential for providing a safe anesthesia.

The elective cesarean delivery is the least time sensitive from decision to incision.

The majority of the elective, planned cesarean sections are typically performed with a single-dose spinal anesthetic technique [2, 3].

In cases where the obstetrician expects a prolonged length of the surgical procedure (approximately more than 2 h), a neuraxial catheter-based technique (epidural or combined spinal-epidural) may be utilized.

In some institutions, such as mine, the combined spinal-epidural technique is the technique of choice for elective cesarean section, using the spinal component of the technique for anesthesia and the epidural catheter for epidural postoperative analgesia.

Epidural dosing of a preexisting epidural catheter is also frequently used in the case of the nonurgent delivery of the baby in a laboring woman.

De novo epidural anesthesia is the less frequent option due to the anesthesiologist's fear of more technical difficulties, inadequate intraoperative analgesia, and possible toxic reactions in the case of inadvertent intravenous administration of a full dose of local anesthetic.

In the absence of contraindication to neuraxial anesthesia, it is rare that general anesthesia is induced for an elective cesarean delivery in most developed countries unless there are major contraindications to a neuraxial block or patient's refusal.

The urgent cesarean delivery requires the more rapid progression from decision to delivery.

Although delivery must be rapid, a neuraxial technique is often preferred if time allows for the placement of a spinal anesthetic or the dosing of an existing epidural catheter. A non-reassuring fetal heart rate pattern in itself does not preclude the use of a neuraxial technique [4].

However, in certain emergent circumstances, induction of general anesthesia is needed. These situations occur when the obstetrician must deliver the baby immediately because of maternal and/or fetal indications and when there is insufficient time to induce neuraxial anesthesia or a concern of neuraxial failure. In these cases, general anesthesia provides the most rapid and reliable form of anesthesia for prompt delivery.

3.2 Neuraxial Anesthetic Techniques

Neuraxial anesthesia has the benefit of a conscious mother at delivery and minimal anesthetic exposure to the neonate. Additionally, it allows for the placement of neuraxial opioids to decrease postoperative pain and avoids the risks of maternal aspiration and difficult airway associated with general anesthesia.

Common neuraxial techniques for cesarean delivery include: (1) single-shot spinal technique, (2) epidural catheter technique, or (3) combined spinal-epidural (CSE) technique. There are advantages and disadvantages to each of these techniques.

3.2.1 Spinal Anesthesia

Spinal anesthesia is commonly believed to be technically easier than an epidural block, more rapid in onset and more reliable in providing surgical anesthesia. Although in a training environment it could be higher, the failure rate with spinal anesthesia is usually very low, approximately less than 1% [5, 6].

The risk of profound hypotension is higher with spinal anesthesia than with epidural anesthesia because the onset of the sympathectomy is more rapid and dosing is not titrated. Maternal hypotension and fetal outcome are improved with avoidance of aortocaval compression (left uterine displacement), hydration, and appropriate use of vasopressors.

Colloid solutions are significantly more effective than crystalloid preload [7], and co-loading with colloid is equally as effective as preloading in the prevention of hypotension [8].

Historically, ephedrine was recommended as the vasopressor of choice for treating hypotension from a neuraxial block. However, more recent data confirms that use of phenylephrine for treatment of spinal hypotension, or using phenylephrine as a prophylactic infusion at the time of spinal placement, is effective in preventing hypotension [9], and is associated with less fetal acidosis compared to ephedrine [10].

Data also suggest that spinal anesthesia can be safely used for patients with preeclampsia [11].

A typical spinal anesthetic includes a local anesthetic for the surgical anesthesia with or without morphine added for postoperative pain control. However, a large variety of combinations of local anesthetics and opioids are frequently used.

Although either isobaric or hyperbaric preparations of local anesthetic can be placed intrathecally for a spinal anesthetic [12], hyperbaric solutions containing 8% dextrose are often used to facilitate anatomic and gravitational control of the block distribution. The duration of a single-shot spinal is variable and depends on the agent and the dose used, but normally provides adequate surgical anesthesia for more than 90 min if a full anesthetic dose is given. Bupivacaine is frequently used in doses between 10 and 15 mg. Although cesarean deliveries have been performed with very low doses, the doses of intrathecal bupivacaine that provided a 95% rate of effective anesthesia (ED_{95}) for cesarean delivery when combined with fentanyl (10 mcg) and morphine (0.2 mg) were 11.2 mg for hyperbaric [13] and 13.0 mg for isobaric bupivacaine [14] (Figs. 3.1 and 3.2).

These doses were however determined in a setting where the mean surgical duration was more than 1 h and the uterus was exteriorized during surgery.

With different surgical conditions, lower doses of bupivacaine (less than 9 mg) with opioids have been used to reduce maternal hypotension, but, although the use of lower bupivacaine doses may provide satisfactory anesthesia, there is an increased risk of intraoperative pain or failed spinal with a need for general anesthesia and this risk might be ethically unacceptable for most practitioners [15].

Continuous spinal anesthesia with a subarachnoid catheter is a very rarely used alternative [16]. Use of an epidural catheter intrathecally is sometimes chosen in cases of accidental dural puncture during attempts to place an epidural, or with a

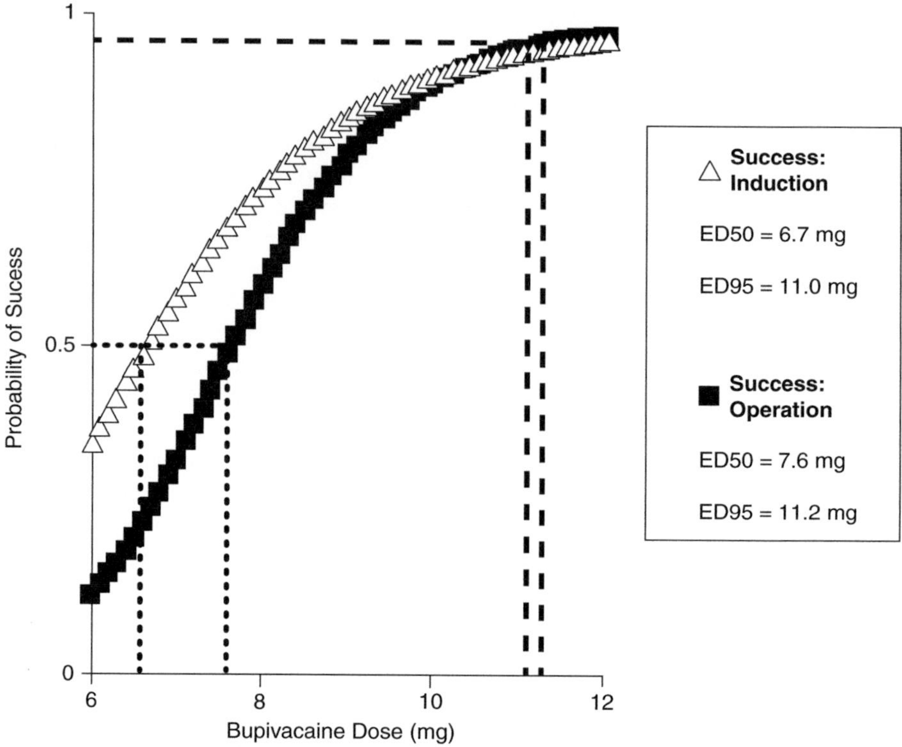

Fig. 3.1 Logistic regression plot of anesthesia success at the induction of anesthesia and throughout surgery (calculation of ED50 and ED95 by using probabilities of 0.5 and 0.95) with hyperbaric bupivacaine. Reproduced with permission from [13]

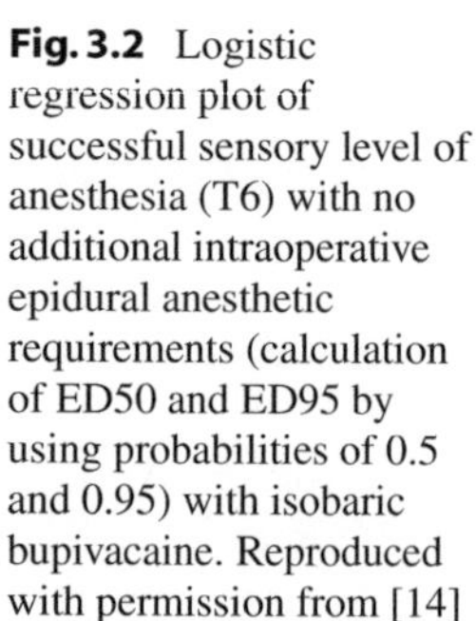

Fig. 3.2 Logistic regression plot of successful sensory level of anesthesia (T6) with no additional intraoperative epidural anesthetic requirements (calculation of ED50 and ED95 by using probabilities of 0.5 and 0.95) with isobaric bupivacaine. Reproduced with permission from [14]

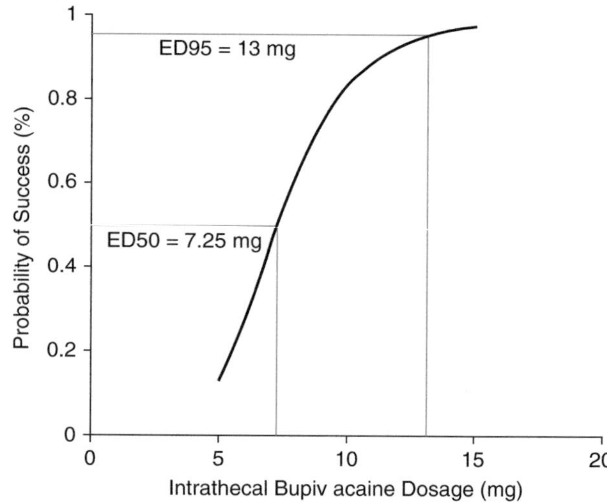

combination of unique circumstances and comorbid conditions (e.g., urgent delivery with severe preeclampsia and morbid obesity). This allows the advantage of a titratable, reliable, dense anesthetic block, but carries the risks of high spinal if the intrathecal catheter is mistaken for an epidural catheter and inappropriately dosed. The rates of rare complications such as meningitis or neurologic impairment from local anesthetic toxicity with the use of a spinal catheter theoretically may be somewhat higher than the other neuraxial techniques; however, currently there are no data to determine the rates of these rare complications.

3.2.2   Epidural Anesthesia

Epidural anesthesia gained its greater popularity among obstetric anesthesiologists between the 1970s and the 1980s [17, 18].

Nowadays spinal anesthesia, on average, has substituted epidural block for elective cesarean section due to the ease of performance of the technique, especially in the teaching setting, rapid onset time, and more profound intraoperative block.

Nevertheless, according to a Cochrane review, both spinal and epidural techniques are shown to provide effective anesthesia for cesarean section. Spinal anesthesia has a shorter onset time, but treatment for hypotension is more likely if spinal anesthesia is used [19].

Converting labor epidural analgesia to surgical anesthesia for cesarean section is instead a common procedure. A large audit from UK reported that 26% of emergency cesarean sections were carried out using an epidural anesthesia [20] and, actually, extending a preexisting epidural block previously used for labor analgesia is a routine practice worldwide in Europe. In my Institution, which has an epidural analgesia rate of 97%, almost all the conversions to anesthesia are performed using the preexisting epidural catheter.

In those cases, the local anesthetic is changed to one that provides more rapid onset and a denser anesthetic block for surgical anesthesia. Extension of a preexisting epidural labor analgesia to the appropriate level of surgical anesthesia can reliably and very rapidly be accomplished with a pH adjusted solution of 2% lidocaine with adrenaline and fentanyl [21].

3.2.3   Combined Spinal-Epidural Anesthesia (CSEA)

The introduction of combined spinal-epidural anesthesia (CSEA) offers the benefits of both spinal and epidural anesthesia. The use of a CSEA technique offers the advantage of a spinal anesthetic with rapid onset of a dense block, as well as the ability to administer additional anesthetics through the epidural catheter.

With this technique, a success rate of 99.4% has been reported [22] and this confirms my personal view (CSEA is the standard technique for elective cesarean section in my Institution) that CSEA is superior to either single-shot spinal or continuous epidural anesthesia alone when used as the routine for cesarean section.

In addition the epidural catheter may be used for routine postoperative epidural analgesia which is highly effective and breastfeeding safe.

In selected circumstances, this technique can be used when the total operative time is expected to take longer than allowed for with a typical spinal anesthetic dose, for example, third or fourth cesarean delivery or combined with an additional procedure.

Similarly, the presence of the epidural catheter as a back-up to supplement a spinal that is too low, gives the anesthesiologist the opportunity to perform a "modified CSEA" by titrating both the spinal and epidural components of the technique when the patient has severe pregnancy-induced hypertension or other disorders that make the prospect of dramatic hemodynamic changes particularly concerning.

3.3 General Anesthesia

General anesthesia is used for cesarean delivery when neuraxial anesthesia is contraindicated or for emergent situations because of its rapid and predictable effect.

However, even in some developed countries it may represent the most common choice of anesthetic technique [23].

Conditions that contraindicate neuraxial procedures include patient refusal, infection at the needle insertion site, significant coagulopathy, hypovolemic shock, and increased intracranial pressure from mass lesions. Inadequate caregivers' expertise might also represent a possible contraindication. Other conditions such as systemic infection, some neurologic diseases and mild coagulopathies should be evaluated on a case-by-case basis. HIV infection is not a contraindication to neuraxial technique [24].

Often many parturients are given for many and different reasons, anticoagulant and antithrombotic drugs during their pregnancy and this may influence the choice of anesthesia in the case of cesarean section. A summary of current guidelines from different international anesthetic societies for neuraxial anesthetic practice in patients receiving anticoagulant and antithrombotic drugs has been published [25].

As with neuraxial techniques, appropriate preparation and a working knowledge of difficult airway techniques and algorithms are essential for providing a safe general anesthesia.

Anesthetic goals during the cesarean delivery include an appropriate anesthetic level to optimize surgical conditions and minimize maternal recall; an adequate perfusion and oxygenation of the mother and neonate; and a minimal transfer of anesthetic agents to the neonate and minimization of uterine atony following delivery.

If a significantly prolonged length of time occurs between induction of general anesthesia and delivery, cardiorespiratory depression and decreased tone of the infant should be anticipated. These are short-lived and easily overcome results of greater transfer of anesthetic agents rather than asphyxia, and respond easily to assisted ventilation of the anesthetized infant to favor excretion of the anesthetic agents.

Spinal anesthesia is commonly believed to be both more practical and safer than other techniques for the mother, and is therefore widely used. It is also often assumed, similarly, that neuraxial techniques must be better for the baby than general anesthesia. However, a Cochrane review stated that there is not enough evidence to show that either regional or general anesthesia is superior to the other in terms of major maternal or neonatal outcomes, except the estimated blood loss which appears to be reduced with the use of regional anesthesia [26].

Spinal anesthesia for cesarean section is associated with a greater degree of fetal metabolic acidosis than in either general or epidural anesthesia [27]; however, spinal anesthesia is not associated with lower umbilical artery pH compared to other types of anesthesia when phenylephrine is used as the vasopressor agent [28].

Furthermore, the differences in acid-base status are not large and most likely not clinically significant, and certainly there are so many good reasons to use spinal anesthesia, which in most circumstances outweigh these disadvantages.

There may be many reasons why general anesthesia should be avoided if possible, but should a mother need to be given it, she can be reassured about its effects on the acid-base status of the baby.

3.4 Maternal Medical Diseases Affecting the Anesthetic Choice

The list of comorbid diseases during pregnancy is endless, and their presence can significantly affect the choice of the anesthetic technique. Morbidities during pregnancy can be treated and managed on an individual basis simultaneously by adequate preanesthetic evaluation, careful multidisciplinary planning of anesthetic technique, and postoperative care. The anesthesiologist requires a complete knowledge of the type, severity, and prognosis of maternal diseases. This paragraph briefly describes the most common comorbidities encountered during pregnancy and their suggested anesthetic management just as an example of how challenging the anesthetic choice in these cases could be: please refer to textbooks for detailed information on this topic [29, 30].

3.4.1 Rheumatic Disease

Rheumatic heart disease is the most frequent of the heart diseases. The goals for the anesthetic management of patients with mitral stenosis are: (1) maintenance of an acceptable slow heart rate, (2) immediate treatment of acute atrial fibrillation and reversion to sinus rhythm, (3) avoidance of aortocaval compression, (4) maintenance of adequate venous return, (5) maintenance of adequate SVR, and (6) prevention of pain, hypoxemia, hypercarbia, and acidosis, which may increase pulmonary vascular resistance.

Epidural and continuous spinal anesthesia techniques are attractive options. With these techniques the anesthetic drug can be administered in incremental doses and the total dose could be titrated to the desired sensory level. This, coupled with the slower onset of anesthesia, allows the maternal cardiovascular system to compensate for the occurrence of sympathetic blockade, resulting in a lower risk of hypotension. Moreover, the segmental blockade spares the lower extremity "muscle pump," aiding in venous return [31, 32].

General anesthesia has the disadvantage of increased pulmonary arterial pressure and tachycardia during laryngoscopy and tracheal intubation. Moreover, the adverse effects of positive-pressure ventilation on the venous return may ultimately lead to cardiac failure [33].

3.4.2 Diabetes

One of the most important aspects in diabetic parturients involves the adequate control of blood sugar so as to prevent the occurrence of neonatal hypoglycemia. As such, the perioperative status has to be optimized with an appropriate insulin regimen taking care not to induce hypoglycemia with aggressive control of hyperglycemia.

General anesthesia can be problematic because of delayed gastric emptying, limited atlanto-occipital joint extension, increased hemodynamic response to intubation [34], and impaired counterregulatory hormone responses to hypoglycemia during sleep [35]. Regional anesthesia is positively indicated as compared to general and there is no specific concern related to the spinal over the epidural group. Either spinal or epidural anesthesia may be appropriate for the diabetic parturient provided maternal glycemic control is satisfactory and the patient receives intra/preanesthetic volume expansion with a non-dextrose containing balanced salt solution. The presence of autonomic neuropathy makes a diabetic parturient highly vulnerable to hemodynamic instability [36]; therefore, in severe diabetics epidural anesthesia may be preferred because of the slower onset of sympathetic blockade.

3.4.3 Asthma

The incidence of pregnancy-induced hypertension (PIH), prematurity, antepartum and postpartum hemorrhage, low birth weight, neonatal hypoxia, and perinatal mortality are much higher in patients with asthma as compared to normal pregnant patients.

Regional anesthesia is preferable since it avoids airway stimulation. Epidural anesthesia may allow slow incremental titration which may lessen the risk of respiratory discomfort from a sudden high sensory level. Unclear etiology acute broncospasm has been precipitated by spinal anesthesia in pregnancy [37].

If the parturient's condition is too poor to tolerate a neuraxial technique because she does not tolerate the supine position, general anesthesia may be provided. Light anesthesia must be avoided since it may aggravate bronchospasm. In the case of uterine atony, prostaglandin agents are contraindicated in asthmatic parturients.

3.4.4 Neurological, Neuromuscular, and Musculoskeletal Disorders

Neurological diseases (seizure disorders, multiple sclerosis, spina bifida, hemiplegia, migraine, any infective infection, trauma, tumors), neuromuscular disorders (myasthenia gravis, poliomyelitis), and musculoskeletal disorders (scoliosis, kyphoscoliosis) can influence the choice of delivery as well as of anesthetic technique, as the involvement of the nervous and musculoskeletal system can be highly variable [30].

Regional anesthesia is preferred in the majority of patients with these disorders except in the case of some strong contraindications such as increased intracranial pressure and tethered spinal cord. Patients who are at high risk of developing intraoperative respiratory insufficiency (kyphoscoliosis) should preferably be administered neuraxial anesthesia in an incremental manner.

Myasthenia gravis should be adequately treated preoperatively with anticholinesterases and regional anesthesia is preferable if respiratory functions are not impaired.

Multiple sclerosis cannot be considered a contraindication for epidural or for spinal anesthesia [38].

3.4.5 Renal Diseases

Regional anesthesia is considered safe if coagulation parameters are normal. In the case of general anesthesia, anesthetic drugs which are primarily excreted through the kidneys, which can enhance the incidence of renal toxicity and renal failure, should be avoided.

Atracurium is preferred as it is not dependent upon hepatic or renal metabolism for its elimination while succinylcholine can cause severe arrhythmias if any evidence of hyperkalemia is present.

3.4.6 Hematological Disorders

In the case of severe anemia the main anesthetic goals during cesarean section are: (1) avoidance of hypoxemia and adequate oxygenation, (2) minimal time in securing the airway in the case of general anesthesia, (3) maintenance of stable hemodynamics, (4) avoidance of hypothermia, and (5) avoidance of hyperventilation. As far as possible, regional anesthesia should be the preferred choice wherever feasible as it is associated with decreased blood loss [26].

There are concerns about spinal hematoma in patients receiving anticoagulants during neuraxial anesthesia for cesarean section. The administration of neuraxial anesthesia in parturients receiving anticoagulant drugs should be individualized in accordance with the published guidelines [25] and a risk-benefit analysis is essential depending upon the urgency of the cesarean section.

3.4.7 Obesity

When compared to normal weight parturients morbidly obese patients are at an increased risk of having either concurrent medical problems or superimposed antenatal diseases including preeclampsia and gestational diabetes. In addition there is an increased incidence of deep vein thrombosis, hypoxemia, and wound infections [39].

The major goals during anesthetic management of the obese parturient include the following: (1) careful titration of anesthetic drugs (especially opioids and sedatives); (2) aspiration prophylaxis; (3) difficult airway management; and (4) maintenance of stable hemodynamics.

Morbidly obese women undergoing scheduled cesarean delivery have greater overall anesthesia-related complications, more complicated placement of regional anesthesia, and a more frequent requirement of general anesthesia than women with lower weight [40].

Women with a BMI more than 45 kg/m^2 are particularly at risk of complications from regional anesthesia. Unfortunately, morbidly obese women have a higher epidural anesthesia failure rate and are likely to have difficult intubations. Inability to identify landmarks, difficulty in placing the regional block, and the unpredictable spread of the anesthetic solution contribute to the failure rate [40].

The use of a continuous lumbar spinal catheter and a low thoracic epidural, respectively, for intraoperative anesthesia and postoperative analgesia, has been reported to have several advantages in the anesthetic management of super-morbidly obese parturients undergoing cesarean delivery [41].

Typically in morbidly obese patients the hypotension is profound and may be refractory to measures like intravenous pressors and intravenous fluids and may require intensive care admission, resuscitation, and monitoring.

Most of the anesthesia-related morbidity and mortality encountered during cesarean section is due to complications of general anesthesia, especially as a consequence of failed intubation and aspiration. These are taken into account when a decision is made for cesarean section.

3.5 Maternal Obstetric Diseases Affecting Anesthetic Choice

3.5.1 Preeclampsia

Neuraxial anesthesia is the preferred anesthetic technique for delivery by cesarean section. Single-shot spinal, combined spinal-epidural, and epidural anesthesia may be used effectively and there is no evidence that one technique has an advantage over the other [42].

Typically hypotension requiring vasopressors during neuraxial anesthesia is less frequent in women with preeclampsia.

General anesthesia may sometimes be necessary in the case of severe coagulopathy, pulmonary edema, or eclampsia. However, if the woman is stable with a normal level of consciousness and no neurological deficits, in the absence of other contraindications, neuraxial anesthesia is a reasonable choice [43].

If general anesthesia is used, extreme attention should be given to control the hypertensive response to intubation, as this has been identified as a cause of direct maternal mortality [44].

3.5.2 HELLP (Hemolysis, Elevated Liver Enzymes, Low Platelets)

Traditionally general anesthesia has been considered to be the technique of choice in the case of the HELLP (hemolysis, elevated liver enzymes, low platelets) syndrome due to the typical coexistence of a very low platelet count in these patients. In selected cases of patients, combined spinal-epidural has been reported to be feasible and safe if the platelet count is above $80,000/mm^3$ [45]. In all cases, the rapid deterioration of the platelet count requires their close monitoring by serial determinations immediately before and during the course of anesthetic management.

3.5.3 Placenta Accreta

General anesthesia is usually considered as the technique of choice for patients with placenta accreta due to the significant risk of massive bleeding, complicated by intense hypotension and coagulopathy and high probability of hysterectomy during cesarean delivery.

In the case of a minimal degree of invasion of the placenta accreta and therefore with a reasonable chance of a conservative management, regional anesthesia may be an alternative. In this case epidural or combined spinal-epidural anesthesia would be preferable [46].

General and regional anesthesia may also be combined, allowing the mother to be awake during the delivery of the baby and eventually converting the block to general anesthesia, required in half of the cases [47], during hysterectomy, if necessary.

References

1. Kinsella SM, Walton B, Sashidharan R, et al. Category-1 caesarean section: a survey of anaesthetic and peri-operative management in the UK. Anaesthesia. 2010;65:362–8.
2. Bucklin BA, Hawkins JL, Anderson JR, et al. Obstetric anesthesia workforce survey: twenty-year update. Anesthesiology. 2005;103:645–53.
3. Staiku C, Paraskeva A, Karmaniolou I, et al. Current practice in obstetric anesthesia: a 2012 European survey. Minerva Anestesiol. 2014;80:347–35.

4. Committee on Obstetric Practice, American College of Obstetricians and Gynecologists. ACOG Committee opinion. Number 326, December 2005. Inappropriate use of the terms fetal distress and birth asphyxia. Obstet Gynecol. 2005;106:1469–70.

5. Riley ET, Cohen SE, Macario A, et al. Spinal versus epidural anesthesia for cesarean section: a comparison of time efficiency, costs, charges, and complications. Anesth Analg. 1995;80:709–12.

6. Fettes PD, Jansson JR, Wildsmith JA. Failed spinal anaesthesia: mechanisms, management, and prevention. Br J Anaesth. 2009;102:739–48.

7. Ko JS, Kim CS, Cho HS, et al. A randomized trial of crystalloid versus colloid solution for prevention of hypotension during spinal or low-dose combined spinal-epidural anesthesia for elective cesarean delivery. Int J Obstet Anesth. 2007;16:8–12.

8. Carvalho B, Mercier FJ, Riley ET, et al. Hetastarch co-loading is as effective as pre-loading for the prevention of hypotension following spinal anesthesia for cesarean delivery. Int J Obstet Anesth. 2009;18:150–5.

9. Allen TK, George RB, White WD, et al. A double-blind, placebo-controlled trial of four fixed rate infusion regimens of phenylephrine for hemodynamic support during spinal anesthesia for cesarean delivery. Anesth Analg. 2010;111:1221–9.

10. Ngan Kee WD, Khaw KS, Tan PE, et al. Placental transfer and fetal metabolic effects of phenylephrine and ephedrine during spinal anesthesia for cesarean delivery. Anesthesiology. 2009;111:506–12.

11. Hood DD, Curry R. Spinal versus epidural anesthesia for cesarean section in severely pre-eclamptic patients: a retrospective survey. Anesthesiology. 1999;90:1276–82.

12. Sia A, Tiong A, Hian K, et al. Hyperbaric versus plain bupivacaine for spinal anesthesia for cesarean delivery. Anesth Analg. 2015;120:132–40.

13. Ginosar Y, Mirikatani E, Drover DR, et al. ED50 and ED95 of intrathecal hyperbaric bupivacaine coadministered with opioids for cesarean delivery. Anesthesiology. 2004;100:676–82.

14. Carvalho B, Durbin M, Drover DR, et al. The ED50 and ED95 of intrathecal isobaric bupivacaine with opioids for cesarean delivery. Anesthesiology. 2005;103:606–12.

15. Rucklidge MWM, Paech MJ. Limiting the dose of local anaesthetic for caesarean section under spinal anaesthesia—has the limbo bar been set too low? Anaesthesia. 2012;67:347–51.

16. Palmer CM. Continuous spinal anesthesia and analgesia in obstetrics. Anesth Analg. 2010;111:1476–9.

17. Js C, Davies P, Lewis M. Some aspects of epidural block provided for caesarean section. Anaesthesia. 1986;41:1039–46.

18. Capogna G, Celleno D, Zangrillo A. Analgesia e anestesia epidurale per il parto. Mosby Year Book Italia; 1995.

19. Ng K, Parson J, Cyna AM, Middelton P. Spinal versus epidural anaesthesia for caesarean section. Cochrane Database Syst Rev. 2004;2:CD003765.

20. Kinsella SM. A prospective audit of regional anaesthesia failure in5080 caesarean sections. Anaesthesia. 2008;63:822–32.

21. Hilliyard SG, Bate TE, Corcoran TB, et al. Extending epidural analgesia for emergency caesarean section: a meta analysis. Br J Anaesth. 2011;107:668–78.

22. Ranasinghe JS, Steadman J, Toyama T, et al. Combined spinal epidural anaesthesia is better than spinal or epidural alone for caesarean delivery. Br J Anaesth. 2003;91:299–300.

23. Sumikura H. When was the last time you induced general anesthesia for cesarean section? J Anesth. 2015;29:819–20.

24. Hignett R, Fernando R. Anesthesia for the pregnant HIV patient. Anesthesiol Clin. 2008;26:127–43.

25. Butwick AJ, Carvalho B. Neuraxial anesthesia in obstetric patients receiving anticoagulant and antithrombotic drugs. Int J Obstet Anesth. 2010;19:193–201.

26. Afolabi BB, Lesi FE, Merah NA. Regional versus general anaesthesia for caesarean section. Cochrane Database Syst Rev. 2006;10:CD004350.

27. Reynolds F, Seed PT. Anaesthesia for caesarean section and neonatal acid-base status: a meta-analysis. Anaesthesia. 2005;60:636–53.

28. Strouch ZY, Dakik CG, Wd W, et al. Anesthetic technique for cesarean delivery and neonatal acid–base status: a retrospective database analysis. Int J Obstet Anesth. 2015;24:22–9.
29. Datta S, editor. Anesthetic and obstetric management of high-risk pregnancy. 3rd ed. New York: Springer-Verlag; 2004.
30. Gambling DR, Douglas MJ, McKey RSF. Obstetric anesthesia and uncommon disorders. 3rd ed. Cambridge: Cambridge University Press; 2008.
31. Langesaeter E, Dragsund M, Rosseland LA. Regional anaesthesia for a caesarean section in women with cardiac disease: a prospective study. Acta Anaesthesiol Scand. 2010;54:46–54.
32. Dresner M, Pinder A. Anaesthesia for caesarean section in women with complex cardiac disease: 34 cases using the Braun Spinocath spinal catheter. Int J Obstet Anesth. 2009;18:131–6.
33. Blaise G, Langleben D, Hubert B. Pulmonary arterial hypertension: pathophysiology and anesthetic approach. Anesthesiology. 2003;99:1415–32.
34. Vohra A, Kumar S, Charlton AJ, Olukoga AO, Boulton AJ, McLeod D. Effect of diabetes mellitus on the cardiovascular responses to induction of anesthesia and tracheal intubation. Br J Anaesth. 1993;71:258–61.
35. Lev-Ran A. Sharp temporary drop in insulin requirement after caesarean section in diabetic patients. Am J Obstet Gynecol. 1974;120:905–8.
36. Hoeldtke RD, Boden G, Shuman CR, et al. Reduced epinephrine secretion and hypoglycemia unawareness in diabetic autonomic neuropathy. Ann Intern Med. 1982;96:459–62.
37. Kawabata KM. Two cases of asthmatic attack caused by spinal anesthesia. Masui. 1996;45:102–6.
38. Drake E, Drake M, Bird J, et al. Obstetric regional blocks for women with multiple sclerosis: a survey of UK experience. Int J Obstet Anesth. 2006;15:115–23.
39. Leykin Y. Which anesthetic (general or regional) is safest for a caesarean section in a morbidly obese parturient? In: Leykin Y, Brodski JB, editors. Controversies in the anesthetic management of the obese surgical patient. Milan: Springer; 2013.
40. Whitty RJ, Maxwell CV, Carvalho JC. Complications of neuraxial anesthesia in an extreme morbidly obese patient for cesarean section. Int J Obstet Anesth. 2007;16:139–44.
41. Polin CM, Hale B, Mauritz AA, et al. Anesthetic management of super-morbidly obese parturients for cesarean delivery with a double neuraxial catheter technique: a case series. Int J Obstet Anesth. 2015;24:276–80.
42. Dennis AT. Management of pre-eclampsia: issues for anaesthetists. Anaesthesia. 2012;67:1009–20.
43. Dyer RA, Piercy JL, Reed AR. The role of the anaesthetist in the management of the pre-eclamptic patient. Curr Opin Anesthesiol. 2007;20:168–74.
44. Lewis G, editor. The confidential enquiry into maternal and child health (CEMACH). Saving mothers' lives: reviewing maternal deaths to make motherhood safer 2003–2005. The seventh report on confidential enquiries into maternal deaths in the United Kingdom. London: CEMACH; 2007.
45. Palit S, Palit G, Vercauteren M, et al. Regional anaesthesia for primary caesarean section in patients with preterm HELLP syndrome: a review of 102 cases. Clin Exp Obstet Gynecol. 2009;36:230–4.
46. Chestnut DH, Dewan DM, Redick LF, et al. Anesthetic management for obstetric hysterectomy: a multiinstitutional study. Anesthesiology. 1989;70:607–10.
47. Munoz LA, Mendoza GA, Gomez M, et al. Anesthetic management of placenta accreta in a low-resource setting: a case series. Int J Obstet Anesth. 2015;29:329–34.

Spinal Anesthesia for Cesarean Section

4

Sarah Armstrong

4.1 Introduction

As the rates of cesarean delivery have escalated, so have the rates of neuraxial anesthesia for cesarean delivery. Pregnant women are known to be at increased risk of morbidity and mortality from the complications of general anesthesia including awareness, failed intubation and/or ventilation, hypoxia and aspiration of gastric contents [1–3]. Neuraxial techniques (spinal, epidural and combined spinal-epidural) are well established as the preferred and safest methods of anesthesia for both planned and emergency cesarean section. The Royal College of Anaesthetists currently recommends that 95% of elective cesarean sections and 85% of emergency cesarean sections are performed under neuraxial anesthesia [3]. Neuraxial anesthesia for cesarean delivery can be provided using a range of techniques as listed below:

- Single-shot spinal anesthesia (SSS)
- Continuous spinal anesthesia
- Combined spinal-epidural anesthesia (CSE)
- Low-dose or sequential CSE anesthesia
- Epidural anesthesia

In this chapter, we will focus on the first two—single-shot spinal and continuous spinal anesthesia.

S. Armstrong
Frimley Health NHS Foundation Trust, Surrey, UK
e-mail: drsaraharmstrong@gmail.com

© Springer International Publishing Switzerland 2017
G. Capogna (ed.), *Anesthesia for Cesarean Section*,
DOI 10.1007/978-3-319-42053-0_4

4.2   Advantages of Neuraxial Anesthesia

As stated previously, neuraxial anesthesia not only reduces the risk of potential complications of general anesthesia but also has independent advantages over and above general anesthesia and these are listed in Table 4.1.

The choice of specific neuraxial anesthetic technique will depend on a multitude of factors including local institutional guidelines, anesthetic and surgical experience and preference, clinical judgement and individual patient requirements. The block must provide adequate anesthesia and analgesia for the duration of the surgery and minimize perioperative discomfort [4].

In addition there are specific advantages of single-shot spinal and continuous spinal anesthesia. Both techniques allow a rapid onset of dense anesthesia. Riley et al. evaluated spinal versus epidural anesthesia for cesarean section and found that spinal anesthesia was associated with significantly shorter operating room times, with supplemental intraoperative intravenous (IV) analgesics and anxiolytics required more often in the epidural group (38%) than in the spinal group (17%) (p <0.05) [5].

Spinal anesthesia is associated with less breakthrough pain and a lower conversion rate to general anesthesia at cesarean section when compared to epidural anesthesia. Garry and Davies examined the quality of regional blockade for cesarean section in a four-year retrospective study [6]. Of 1610 patients who received a spinal anesthesia for cesarean section, 12 (0.75%) received general anesthesia while 175 (10.9%) required some analgesic supplementation. Of the 827 patients in whom epidural analgesia was in progress for labor and a decision was made to proceed to cesarean section, a total of 87 patients (10.5%) needed general anesthesia. Of those (763) in whom cesarean section was started under epidural, only 17 (2.2%) were given general anesthesia because of intraoperative pain. In addition spinal anesthesia is associated with a predictable and relatively prompt recovery, which may be associated with a faster transition through recovery units [7]. It has been suggested that in some institutions this may result in cost savings [5].

Table 4.1 Advantages of neuraxial anesthesia for cesarean delivery [4]

Reduced risk of:
• Dental damage, failed intubation and hypoxia
• Pulmonary aspiration of gastric contents
• Awareness
Improved postoperative pain relief
Reduced incidence of:
• Vomiting and postoperative ileus
• Thromboembolism
Ability to have birth partner present
Alert mother and baby, improved bonding and breastfeeding Increased patient satisfaction

Spinal anesthetic techniques use relatively low doses of both local anesthetic and opioid. This means there is a significantly reduced risk of systemic local anesthetic toxicity and minimal transfer of drugs to the fetus when compared to epidural techniques. Kuhrnet et al. measured both lidocaine and bupivacaine levels in maternal and neonatal blood after spinal anesthesia and epidural anesthesia and found that local anesthetic transfer was perhaps predictably much lower in the spinal group [8, 9]. However, it should be noted that even with spinal anesthesia there is still a small but significant transfer to both maternal and neonatal systemic circulations with neonatal urine containing the local anesthetic or their metabolites for up to 36 h after delivery [8, 9]. The SSS technique has the additional advantage of being technically simple to perform but has a limited duration of anesthesia and no ability to extend the duration or intensity of sensory blockade. Continuous spinal anesthesia however can be used to extend intraoperative anesthesia and also to titrate the extent of sensory blockade, which may be of benefit in those situations where hemodynamic instability should be avoided (e.g., women with congenital or acquired cardiac disease). However continuous spinal anesthesia necessitates a greater diameter of dural sac puncture, increasing the risk of post-dural puncture headache. Unfamiliarity with the continuous spinal technique may also lead to the possibility of total spinal anesthesia or overdose using opioids if the catheter is mistaken for an epidural catheter. With both techniques, the operator is facilitated by a clear visual confirmation that the needle is correctly placed via the aspiration of cerebrospinal fluid from the needle hub.

4.3   Technique

4.3.1   Consent

As with all procedures a discussion with the parturient with regard to the options for neuraxial anesthesia as well as the potential benefits and complications is essential. The preoperative assessment should include a focused obstetric and anesthetic history as well as any relevant physical examination and review of investigations. Potential complications from spinal anesthesia may include the following (Table 4.2):

4.3.2   Preparation

Following consent of the patient there should be communication with all team members, and equipment and medications should be checked. Full resuscitation facilities should be available as well as standard patient monitoring (ECG, noninvasive blood pressure and SpO_2 as a minimum). The worldwide implementation of the WHO surgical safety checklist has been shown to reduce death rates and complications in surgery [11]. Following an alert from the National Patient Safety Agency in 2009, the WHO checklist is now an established part of safe theatre practice in the United Kingdom and has been successfully adapted for maternity theatre cases [12].

Table 4.2 Complications associated with spinal anesthesia

Related to needle insertion	• Post-dural puncture headache • Block failure • Permanent injury from nerve damage 1:166,000 [10] • Backache • Spinal hematoma 1:220,000 • Meningitis/arachnoiditis
Related to exaggerated physiological response	• Hypotension • Shivering • High block • Urinary retention • Cardiac arrest
Related to intrathecal drugs	• Pruritus • Nausea and vomiting • Systemic toxicity • Transient neurological symptoms

4.3.3 Aseptic Technique

Although serious central nervous system infections (meningitis and vertebral canal abscess) following spinal anesthesia are rare in the obstetric population, their occurrence can have potentially devastating consequence in terms of maternal morbidity and mortality [10]. An aseptic technique should be used involving pre-procedural handwashing, skin disinfection and maintenance of a sterile field. In the United Kingdom and Australia, it is recommended that the operator should wear single-use sterile gloves, sterile surgical gown, hat and face mask but this is not standard practice worldwide [13, 14]. Chlorhexidine has been shown to be more effective than iodine solution in terms of onset time, duration of action and ability to eradicate skin flora [15]. Malhotra et al. showed that a single spray of 0.5% chlorhexidine rendered the skin sterile as long as the application was thorough and allowed to dry properly [16]. Chlorhexidine is however neurotoxic and has been implicated in causing severe adhesive arachnoiditis following accidental contamination of neuraxial block equipment or epidural injection of chlorhexidine, so caution must be taken when preparing equipment for these procedures [17].

4.3.4 Needle Selection

Spinal anesthesia may be initiated as either a single-shot technique or a continuous technique using a spinal catheter. A continuous technique where the spinal catheter is sited through an epidural catheter once the intrathecal space has been located is useful after an accidental dural puncture with an epidural needle. In addition, in the morbidly obese population, it may be easier to locate the epidural space and hence the dural sac with a rigid epidural needle so this technique may be employed in this patient population, particularly when there is clinical urgency [7]. For most parturients undergoing cesarean section where a spinal technique is preferred, the decision is usually between a single-shot spinal and a CSE technique (see Chap. 5). Larger needles have the advantage of improved tactile feedback, and they may be technically easier to use to locate the CSF, particularly in an emergency situation. However they are also associated with increased morbidity and this must be balanced against the benefits. Smaller needles (24 gauge or less) are used with an introducer needle to aid skin puncture and facilitate placement within the interspinous ligament through which the small-gauge spinal needle can then pass.

Post-dural puncture headache (PDPH) is a significant cause of maternal morbidity for obstetric patients. In most cases it is moderate and self-limiting but in some situations it may be severe and debilitating [18]. The incidence of post-dural puncture headache varies depending on the size and design of the needle used. Rates of PDPH are increased where cutting needles (such as Quincke or Tuohy needles) are used. In a large meta-analysis, Choi et al. showed that parturients have approximately a 1.5% (95% confidence interval [CI] 1.5% to 1.5%) risk of accidental dural puncture with epidural insertion and of those, approximately 50% developed PDPH [19]. Studies since then have shown that after dural puncture with a Tuohy needle, up to 80% may experience PDPH [20]. As the fibers of the dura are cut, they retract under tension leaving behind a larger deficit. This is significantly reduced when using a pencil-point needle (Sprotte, Whitacre or Gertie Marx).

Dural puncture with a 22G Quincke cutting needle has been shown to have a PDPH incidence of 36% compared to a 22G Whitacre needle in which the incidence is 0.6–4% [21–23]. Choi's meta-analysis showed that the risk of PDPH from spinal needles diminishes with small diameter, atraumatic needles, but was still appreciable (Whitacre 27-gauge needle 1.7%; 95% CI, 1.6% to 1.8%) [19]. The convention is to use a non-cutting atraumatic needle that is 24-gauge or smaller. Interestingly Van de Velde et al. showed that using 29-gauge rather than 27-gauge pencil-point spinal needles conferred no additional benefit [20].

4.3.5 Positioning of the Patient

The spinal should ideally be performed at L3/4 or lower [24]. The rationale behind this is that in most subjects the spinal cord ends at the level of the L1/2 interspace, but that in a small but significant proportion of the population the conus medullaris may extend down to L3. Accidental damage and permanent neurological injury may occur above this level [24]. Tuffier's line is a radiological and anatomical landmark using a virtual line drawn between the superior border of the iliac crests. In general this line bisects the fourth lumbar vertebra at the level of the spinous process and therefore the intervertebral space above this is presumed to be L3/4. However Broadbent et al. demonstrated using magnetic resonance imaging (MRI) that the correct space was identified by only 50% of anesthetists using the landmark technique, even when those anesthetists were experienced [25]. Only a third of the anesthetists correctly identified a specific vertebral level and in general MRI showed that the interspace identified was actually at least one vertebral level higher than expected, especially in obese patients [25]. Lee et al. showed similar results using ultrasound scans, where only clinical estimates of the spinal level of Tuffier's line agreed with the ultrasound measurement only 14% of the time [26]. Shaikh et al. performed a systematic review and meta-analysis of 14 randomized trials that compared ultrasound imaging with standard methods (no imaging) in the performance of a lumbar puncture or epidural catheterization [27]. They concluded that ultrasound imaging can reduce the risk of failed or traumatic lumbar punctures and epidural catheterizations, as well as the number of needle insertions and redirections. As a result there is increasing interest in the use of ultrasound to aid the insertion of spinals and epidurals in obstetrics, particularly in the morbidly obese or those with significant spinal problems.

Patients may have spinal anesthesia sited in either the sitting or the lateral decubitus position. The choice of which position depends on many factors—the baricity of the local anesthetic solution, the anesthetist's or patient's preferences, and the clinical situation encountered including whether the fetal heart can be adequately monitored. Anesthetists should be proficient siting neuraxial blocks in both positions. Often the sitting position may be considered preferable as the iliac crests and midline may be easier to palpate, especially in obese patients. There is evidence to suggest that maternal cardiac output, and therefore uteroplacental blood flow, may be increased in the lateral position and that the lateral decubitus position may be preferable in situations where there is fetal distress [28, 29]. However this must be balanced against the sitting position being technically easier and therefore quicker in some patients in an emergency situation [30].

Patient position relative to the baricity of the solution to be used should be considered. Hallworth et al. performed a double-blinded prospective study where 150 parturients were randomized to receive hyperbaric, isobaric, or hypobaric intrathecal solution of bupivacaine during spinal anesthesia induced in either the sitting or right lateral position [31]. In the lateral position, baricity had no effect on the spread of sensory levels for bupivacaine compared to the sitting position, whereas there was a statistically significant difference in spread with the hypobaric solution producing higher levels of analgesia than the hyperbaric solution ($p = 0.002$). However, the overall differences in maximal spread only differed by one dermatome. Motor block was significantly ($p = 0.029$) reduced with increasing baricity, and this trend was significant ($p = 0.033$) for the lateral position only. Sia et al. reviewed all randomized controlled trials involving patients undergoing spinal anesthesia for elective cesarean delivery that compared the use of hyperbaric bupivacaine with plain bupivacaine [32]. They found the studies of varying quality and methodology and a lack of clear evidence regarding the superiority of hyperbaric compared with plain bupivacaine for spinal anesthesia for cesarean delivery.

4.4 Spinal Technique

To reach the subarachnoid space, the spinal needle should pass through the skin and subcutaneous tissue, the supraspinous ligament, interspinous ligament, ligamentum flavum and dura mater which is closely adherent to the subarachnoid membrane, into the CSF. In the UK a fully aseptic technique is employed with the use of a surgical gown, gloves, mask and hat with full sterile surgical drapes whereas in other areas of the world such as the United States sterile gloves and drapes suffice. The skin and subcutaneous tissues are infiltrated with local anesthetic, such as 1% lidocaine. The most common approach is via the midline where the needle or introducer is placed centrally perpendicular to the spinous processes and aiming slightly cephalad although some anesthetic providers may choose to use the paramedian approach. When using smaller gauge needles (such as 25- or 27-gauge), it will be necessary to use an introducer needle to aid skin puncture and to more accurately guide the trajectory of the needle. After local anesthetic has been infiltrated, the introducer needle is inserted in the midline until it has entered the interspinous ligament and is "gripped" by this ligament. Subsequently the spinal needle is inserted through the introducer needle and advanced through the tissue layers. Sometimes it is difficult to appreciate the tactile feedback with a smaller spinal needle but usually an appreciable "pop" is felt as the needle passes through the ligamentum flavum and dura into the subarachnoid space. The stylet of the spinal needle is removed and if a successful dural tap has been performed, free flowing clear cerebrospinal fluid should be seen at the hub of the needle. Once clear cerebrospinal fluid has reached the end of the needle hub, the syringe containing the local anesthetic dose with or without opioids is attached and cerebrospinal fluid aspirated. Once aspiration has been confirmed, the local anesthetic dose is slowly injected. Some providers confirm at the end of the injection that the needle remains in the subarachnoid space by aspirating a small amount of cerebrospinal fluid and reinjecting it. Pain on inserting the needle may be due to inadequate infiltration of local anesthetic into the soft tissues and may be resolved by removing the spinal needle and reinfiltrating with further local anesthetic. The anesthetist should never inject the local anesthetic spinal mixture whilst there is lancinating pain or paresthesia as this could indicate intraneural injection or injection into the spinal cord itself.

4.5   Intravenous Fluids

Prior to the initiation of spinal anesthesia, every parturient should have large-bore IV access sited to allow administration of fluids, medications and, if necessary, blood products. The rapid onset sympathetic block associated with spinal anesthesia may lead to profound hypotension due to vasodilation for which rapid fluid administration (to maintain the venous return) and vasoconstrictors, such as phenylephrine, may be required. There has been much debate in the literature over the past few years regarding the most appropriate vasopressor to use at cesarean section. Animal and in vitro studies have shown that uteroplacental blood flow is better preserved using ephedrine versus alpha-adrenergic agonists such as phenylephrine [33]. However in many clinical studies since, including a systemic review and meta-analysis of trials, alpha-adrenergic agonists were favored over ephedrine for the preservation of maternal blood pressure at cesarean section in terms of additionally preserving umbilical arterial blood pH and base excess [34]. This topic is covered in depth in other areas of this book.

There has been also much debate about fluid regimes with spinal anesthesia at cesarean section. Preloading was first described by Wollman and Marx, leading to the common practice of the patient being preloaded with 10–20 ml/kg of intravenous fluids prior to the administration of spinal anesthesia [35]. However, the efficacy of this technique, particularly with crystalloids was questioned due to the rapid redistribution of the fluid into the extravascular compartment and that this may lead to the secretion of atrial natriuretic peptide (ANP) causing peripheral vasodilation increasing the rate of excretion of the preload fluid [36, 37]. Colloids appear to be more efficient in preloading in prevention of hypotension following spinal anesthesia, but the decision to use them depends on the clinician's assessment of benefits when compared to the disadvantages of colloids, namely cost, effect on coagulation and hypersensitivity reactions [38, 39]. Chanimov et al. examined the effect of two different preload solutions, Ringer's lactate or saline on the neonatal acid-base status of newborn infants [40]. They found that there was no difference between the two in terms of effects on fetal well-being.

Tawfik et al. looked at 1000 mL crystalloid co-load compared to 500 mL colloid preload in reducing the incidence of hypotension after spinal anesthesia for elective cesarean delivery [41]. They found that both solutions had similar hemodynamic effects. The authors concluded that neither technique was able to prevent hypotension and that any regimes should be combined with vasopressor use.

4.6 Local Anesthetics

Most anesthesia for cesarean delivery under spinal is performed using a hyperbaric solution of local anesthetic. In comparison to isobaric solutions, hyperbaric solutions result in a faster onset of block with higher maximum sensory level achieved and a shorter overall duration [42]. The choice of local anesthetic will very much depend on the expected duration of surgery and the individual anesthetist's preference. In Europe and the United States, the usual choice is to use hyperbaric "heavy" bupivacaine (0.5% solution in dextrose 8% in the UK, 0.75% solution in dextrose 8.25% in the USA), which usually results in a reliable and dense block with a lower incidence of spinal-induced hypotension when compared with isobaric or hypobaric solutions [43]. Another advantage of hyperbaric solutions is their ability to manipulate the block height using gravity. Ropivacaine and levobupivacaine use in spinal anesthesia for cesarean section has been studied given the theoretical advantage of a reduction in risk of systemic toxicity. However given that the doses are small, this advantage is minimal. There is also concern that ropivacaine and levobupivacaine may not provide spinal anesthesia of similar quality to that of bupivacaine. In a study by Gautier et al. 90 parturients were randomized to receive either bupivacaine 8 mg, levobupivacaine 8 mg or ropivacaine 12 mg (all with sufentanil) and they observed effective anesthesia in 97%, 80% and 87% of patients respectively [44]. This data in combination with the fact that the FDA has not approved either levobupivacaine or ropivacaine for intrathecal use means both are not currently used in routine practice [42, 45].

As anesthesia obtained is dose dependent in Europe, relatively larger volumes are used and this has been shown in studies not to affect the height or density of the block [46, 47]. In order to achieve a pain-free experience at cesarean section, it has been suggested that a block to pin-prick to T4 and light touch to T6 are required [48]. The dose ranges of intrathecal bupivacaine that have been successfully used at cesarean section range from 4.5 to 15 mg [7]. Conventionally, 10–12.5 mg is used and less than 8 mg would be considered "low dose". Teoh et al. have reported cesarean deliveries being successfully carried out using "ultra-low" doses (3.75 mg) of bupivacaine with significantly less hypotension in these women [49]. Parturients have a smaller CSF volume and greater sensitivity of the nerve fibers to local anesthetic in pregnancy [50]. There is additionally increased cephalad movement of hyperbaric bupivacaine in the supine position due to the increased lumbar lordosis. As a result pregnant patients generally require smaller doses of intrathecal local anesthetic than the general population. Studies using hyperbaric bupivacaine (12–15 mg) have established that the height of the block is **not** affected by the patient's age, weight, height, vertebral column height, or intra-abdominal pressure [51–53]. Larger doses may result in a longer duration of anesthesia but at the risk of increased incidence of cervical block [7]. Carvalho et al. aimed to determine the effective dose (ED[50]/ED[95]) of intrathecal bupivacaine for cesarean delivery in morbidly obese patients (BMI more than 40). They found that obese and nonobese patients undergoing cesarean delivery do not appear to respond differently to modest alterations in doses of intrathecal bupivacaine [54].

There have been a number of studies examining both hyperbaric and isobaric bupivacaine at cesarean section. Ginosaur et al. determined the effective dose (ED95) of intrathecal hyperbaric bupivacaine with 10 µg fentanyl and 200 µg morphine for planned cesarean section using logistic regression analysis [55]. Sensory levels (pinprick) were evaluated every 2 min until a T6 level was achieved. The dose was a success (induction) if a bilateral T6 block occurred in 10 min; otherwise, it was a failure (no induction). ED50 for success (induction) and success (operation) were 6.7 and 7.6 mg, respectively, whereas the ED95 for success (induction) and success (operation) were 11.0 and 11.2 mg. The same group subsequently established ED50 and ED95 values for overall anesthetic success with isobaric bupivacaine finding them to be 7.25 and 13.0 mg, respectively [56]. No advantages for low doses could be demonstrated with regard to hypotension, nausea, vomiting, pruritus, or maternal satisfaction, although the authors recognized the study was underpowered to detect significant differences in secondary outcome variables.

Comparing hyperbaric or plain bupivacaine in combination with fentanyl, Sarvela et al. found they both provided similar onset, depth, and duration of sensory anesthesia for cesarean delivery with good maternal satisfaction. Motor block developed and diminished faster with the hyperbaric solution. In both groups more than 50% required vasopressor support. Bryson et al. randomly assigned 52 women to either isobaric bupivacaine 4.5 mg or hyperbaric bupivacaine 12 mg in addition to 50 µg fentanyl and 0.2 mg morphine. Median cephalad sensory block was C8 in both groups but the intensity of motor block was significantly less (p <0.001) and of shorter duration (p <0.001) with bupivacaine 4.5 mg. Incidence of hypotension (as defined by use of ephedrine), supplemental analgesia, side effects and patient satisfaction were similar in both groups, provoking debate as to whether low doses should really be used given the risk of requiring supplemental analgesia or conversion to general anesthesia compared to minimum additional benefit [7, 57].

The results of these "low doses" studies should be applied cautiously in the routine clinical practice everywhere. The total number of patients enrolled in all published studies is still too small to suggest a routine change in the dose of local anesthetic to be used for spinal anesthesia for cesarean section.

In addition, usually these studies are not powered to evaluate the analgesic efficacy of such a low doses.

The awareness of the clinical context where a study has been performed is also very important. The surgical technique used, uterine exteriorization maneuver if performed during surgery, the intensity of peritoneal manipulation, and the duration of surgery may significantly affect the density of anesthesia required in order to obtain a pain-free surgery.

4.7 Opioids

Opioids are added to the local anesthetic solution to improve the quality of intraoperative anesthesia (particularly relating to visceral stimulation) and to enhance postoperative analgesia [58, 59]. They have the great advantage of producing analgesia without motor or sympathetic blockade. Other advantages include a low level of maternal sedation compared to systemic opioids, minimal accumulation in the breast milk and facilitation of early ambulation. They are thought to exert their action principally on MOP receptors in the substantia gelatinosa of the dorsal horn by suppressing the release of excitatory neuropeptides from C fibers [60]. Lipid-soluble drugs like fentanyl or sufentanil have better direct diffusion into neural tissue as well as greater delivery to the dorsal horn by spinal segmental arteries. As a result they have rapid onset of action but also short duration, which limits their use postoperatively. Lipid-insoluble opioids such as morphine and diamorphine are retained in the CSF providing an opioid supply to the spinal cord for longer and a prolonged duration of action [61]. The dose and type is variable however and polymorphism in the μ-opioid receptor may cause populations of different genetic populations to respond differently [4]. Scrutton and Kinsella described the "rapid sequence spinal" in order to minimize the anesthetic time in the situation of a category 1 cesarean section [62]. (see Chap. 8) In this technique opioids may be omitted but with the operator prepared for conversion to general anesthetic if required.

4.7.1 Intrathecal Fentanyl

Intrathecal fentanyl is one of the most commonly administered neuraxial opioids worldwide. It has been shown to improve intraoperative analgesia at cesarean section (particularly discomfort associated with uterine exteriorization) and provides a better transition to postoperative pain medications during recovery from neuraxial blockade [63]. It is commonly used in doses of 10–25 µg. Dahl et al. performed a systematic review of randomized controlled trials examining the intraoperative and postoperative analgesic efficacy of intrathecal opioids at cesarean section [64]. Studies were pooled into two groups dependent on spinal fentanyl dose—15–35 µg and 40–60 µg. They established that there was no difference between groups in the need for supplemental intraoperative analgesia and that in the lower dose group postoperative pruritus and nausea and vomiting were significantly reduced.

In addition, in two studies, intrathecal fentanyl when added to bupivacaine or lidocaine at cesarean section has shown to decrease the incidence of intraoperative nausea and/or vomiting [59, 65]. Manullang et al. compared intrathecal fentanyl with IV ondansetron for preventing intraoperative nausea and vomiting during cesarean deliveries performed under spinal anesthesia. They found no difference in the incidence of vomiting and treatment for vomiting was not different ($p = 0.7$). The intrathecal fentanyl group had a lower cumulative perioperative pain score than the IV ondansetron group and required less supplementary intraoperative analgesia [66].

4.7.2 Intrathecal Sufentanil

Intrathecal sufentanil is a thienyl derivative of fentanyl but has higher potency due to greater lipid solubility. It offers some theoretical advantages over fentanyl including faster onset, reduced rostral spread and a lower level of placental transfer. The short duration of action of sufentanil prevents its use as an effective postoperative neuraxial analgesic in this setting. Courtney et al. examined sufentanil 0, 10, 15 or 20 µg added to hyperbaric bupivacaine 10.5 mg [67]. They found the duration of analgesia was prolonged significantly in all patient groups receiving sufentanil as compared to the control group. Pruritus was significantly increased in the sufentanil groups. Respiratory depression was not observed in any patient studied. Apgar scores, umbilical cord gases and Early Neonatal Neurobehavioral Scale scores were not significantly different among the groups. There have been several studies looking at sufentanil use in cesarean section compared to fentanyl. However these studies used arbitrarily chosen doses and the spinal fentanyl:sufentanil potency ratio for cesarean section is currently unknown [59, 68, 69].

4.7.3 Intrathecal Morphine

Preservative free morphine is used intrathecally primarily for the postoperative analgesic benefit it confers. It requires 45–60 min to achieve peak effect as it remains within the CSF for a prolonged period of time, spreading rostrally to reach the trigeminal nerve distribution 3 h after intrathecal injection [70]. The duration of analgesia is 14–36 h, which may be dose dependent.

There have been a number of studies looking at intrathecal morphine doses for cesarean section. In Palmer's original dose-finding study, 108 parturients were randomized to receive a single dose of intrathecal morphine in the dose range 0.0–0.5 mg [71]. Rescue PCA morphine use, incidence and severity of side effects, and need for treatment interventions were recorded for 24 hours. They found a ceiling effect with doses greater than 75 μg with no clear analgesic dose-response relationship demonstrated above 100 μg. There was no difference between control and treatment groups or among treatment groups with respect to nausea and vomiting. Pruritus and the need for treatment interventions increased in direct proportion to the dose of intrathecal morphine. The authors suggested from this data that there was no evidence to suggest intrathecal morphine doses above 0.1 mg were justified for post-cesarean analgesia. Dahl et al. performed a systematic review of randomized controlled trials examining the intraoperative and postoperative analgesic efficacy and adverse effects of intrathecal opioids and again recommended an intrathecal dose of 100 μg morphine [64]. More recently Wong et al. conducted a retrospective chart review of elective cesarean deliveries in patients who had received either 100 or 200 μg of intrathecal morphine. They found that women receiving 200 μg had better analgesia postoperatively but more nausea (mean number of episodes of nausea 1.9 ± 1.3 versus 1.6 ± 1.3, $p = 0.037$) and used more antiemetics (52% versus 24%, $p < 0.0001$). The authors suggested that their results could be used to guide morphine dosing based on patient preference for analgesia versus side effects [72].

Adverse effects of intrathecal morphine use are well documented including pruritus, nausea and vomiting, urinary retention and early (at 6 h) or delayed (up to 18 h) respiratory depression. Of the potential side effects of neuraxial opioids, respiratory depression is the most concerning, with many cases of life-threatening respiratory depression reported [63, 73, 74]. Lipophilic opioids such as fentanyl are more likely to cause early-onset respiratory depression due to significant vascular uptake and rostral spread within the CSF [75, 76]. With morphine, systemic vascular absorption may lead to early-onset respiratory depression within 30–90 min of administration followed by rostral spread in the CSF and slow penetration into the brainstem causing delayed respiratory depression up to 18 h after administration [60, 70]. The ASA has formulated guidelines for the detection, prevention and management of respiratory depression associated with neuraxial opioids but there are no specific guidelines for the parturient [77]. In obstetrics it would seem prudent to identify women at high risk of respiratory depression (the morbidly obese, those on magnesium therapy or those with comorbidities such as sleep apnea) and increase vigilance when monitoring these women. Pruritus increases in severity as the morphine dose increases. It has been estimated that 43% of women receiving 100 μg of intrathecal morphine will experience pruritus [64].

4.7.4 Intrathecal Diamorphine

Diamorphine is a semisynthetic opioid produced by acetylation of morphine. It has intermediate lipid solubility, which increases its permeability to both hydrophobic and hydrophilic tissue compartments when compared with either fentanyl or morphine [63]. It is more lipophilic than morphine so has a faster onset (6–9 min). It undergoes metabolism to active compounds (6-acetyl morphine and morphine), increasing their analgesic effects. In addition these metabolites are less lipid soluble than the parent drug limiting their back diffusion into the CSF. Diamorphine has low protein binding and a high ionized fraction (27%) that increases the bioavailability for opioid receptors within the spinal cord and increases CSF clearance, decreasing the potential for more serious side effects such as respiratory depression [78]. As a result of these physicochemical properties, diamorphine is effective for both intraoperative and postoperative analgesia. Although neuraxial diamorphine is commonly used for postoperative pain relief after cesarean section in the United Kingdom, it should be noted that it is not actually licensed for intrathecal use [79].

There have been a number of studies looking at neuraxial diamorphine for intraoperative and postoperative pain relief in cesarean section. Both Skilton et al. and Kelly et al. examined dose-response relationships (up to 0.375 mg of diamorphine) and found improved analgesia (as determined by the need for rescue analgesia) without a ceiling effect [80, 81]. Stacey et al. studied doses up to 1 mg intrathecally and again found 24-h morphine consumption was significantly lower in the 1 mg group (45% requiring no morphine at all) [82]. Saravanan et al. examined 200 women undergoing cesarean section under spinal with bupivacaine and diamorphine and concluded that the ED95 to prevent intraoperative supplementation was 400 µg providing a mean time interval to first request for analgesia of 601 min. However the incidence of nausea and vomiting was 56% and the incidence of pruritus was 80% [83]. Finally Cowan et al. randomized 74 patients undergoing elective cesarean section to receive intrathecally either 300 µg of diamorphine or 20 µg fentanyl with hyperbaric bupivacaine [84]. There was no difference in intraoperative analgesia requirements and they demonstrated reduced pain scores in the diamorphine group at 12 h postoperatively as compared to only 1 h in the fentanyl group.

4.7.5 Intrathecal Opioid Tolerance

It is commonplace for anesthetists to use both a short-acting, lipid-soluble opioid such as fentanyl or sufentanil in combination with a long-acting, lipid-insoluble opioid such as morphine (but not diamorphine) at cesarean section in order to maximize both intraoperative and postoperative analgesia. There is some debate in the literature however, as the administration of both together leads to acute opioid tolerance and a reduced response to the longer acting opioid. Carvalho et al. randomized 40 women having elective cesarean delivery to receive spinal anesthesia with hyperbaric bupivacaine 12 mg, morphine 200 µg, and fentanyl 0, 5, 10 or 25 µg. Each patient received intravenous patient-controlled analgesia morphine for 24 h postoperatively. They found postoperative pain scores were higher in patients receiving fentanyl 5, 10 and 25 µg compared to fentanyl 0 µg control group ($p = 0.003$), but there was no difference in postoperative analgesia requirements [85]. This followed on from a study by

Cooper et al. comparing fentanyl 25 µg with normal saline in combination with 10 mg heavy bupivacaine [86]. They found no difference in intravenous PCA morphine consumption in the first 6 h after cesarean section but found a 63% increase in morphine consumption between 6 and 23 h. More research is required in this area before any specific recommendations can be made regarding neuraxial opioid tolerance.

4.8 Adjuvants

A number of drugs have been suggested as adjuvants to opioids and bupivacaine in spinal anesthesia for cesarean section in order to improve the block. Clonidine has been shown to improve intraoperative analgesia, decrease shivering and reduce peri-incisional hyperalgesia in cesarean section [87]. However it has also been associated with hypotension and sedation and the FDA has issued a "black box" warning against its use in obstetric patients because of concerns about hemodynamic instability [7]. Cossu et al. performed a systematic review and meta-analysis to assess the efficacy and incidence of adverse events related to the use of neostigmine in obstetric anesthesia [88]. They concluded that neuraxial administration of neostigmine significantly reduces local anesthetic consumption without serious adverse side effects to the mother or fetus. However, neostigmine is only recommended for epidural administration as intrathecal use was found to significantly increase the incidence of maternal nausea and vomiting.

4.9 Continuous Spinal Analgesia

Continuous spinal analgesia involves the use of a microcatheter (28-gauge) or small catheter into the intrathecal space. Theoretically this technique should offer many advantages—producing a rapid onset, accurate, titratable, continuous dense spinal block with the ability to use low doses of local anesthetic and as a result minimize hemodynamic instability [4]. It may be of use in women in whom the siting of an epidural would be difficult—those who have had previous spinal surgery and a scarred epidural space or morbidly obese women. However, the technique is under-utilized due to unavailability and unfamiliarity with the necessary equipment, high failure rates and an increase in post-dural puncture headache rates [89, 90]. There remains a paucity of randomized controlled trials in the literature and a lack of consensus regarding dose of local anesthetic for cesarean section.

Microcatheters were used to provide obstetric anesthesia and analgesia in the 1980s, but in the early 1990s there was a small case series reported of cauda equina syndrome and permanent neurological injury following the use of 28–32G spinal microcatheters and 5% lidocaine solution in the general surgical and orthopedic populations [91]. The food and drug administration authority subsequently withdrew the licensing of catheters below 24 gauge.

Although in theory the intrathecal catheter may be used for delivery at cesarean section, there are often more complications than initially anticipated. The epidural catheter and filter has a dead space of approximately 1 ml or more. In addition the epidural catheter has a number of orifices spaced from the tip. The orifice from which the injectate exits, and thus the spread of the local anesthetic, will depend on the pressure with which it is injected which cannot reasonably be predicted or controlled for between operators. All of these factors may make estimating the correct dose of local anesthetic to use difficult and the use of these catheters unreliable at cesarean section.

References

 1. Mhyre JM, Riesner MN, Polley LS, Naughton NN. A series of anesthesia-related maternal deaths in Michigan, 1985–2003. Anesthesiology. 2007;106(6):1096–104.
 2. Paech MJ, Scott KL, Clavisi O, Chua S, McDonnell N. ANZCA trials group. A prospective study of awareness and recall associated with general anaesthesia for caesarean section. Int J Obstet Anesth. 2008;17(4):298–303.
 3. Purva M, Russell IF, Kinsella M. Caesarean section anaesthesia: a technique and failure rate. In: Raising the Standard: a compendium of audit recipes. Royal College of Anaesthetists; 2012. p. 220–1.
 4. Armstrong S, Walters M, Cheesman K. Neuraxial anaesthesia for caesarean delivery. In: Clarke V, Fernando R, Van de Velde M, editors. Oxford textbook of obstetric anaesthesia. Oxford: Oxford University Press; 2016.
 5. Riley ET, Cohen SE, Macario A, Desai JB, Ratner EF. Spinal versus epidural anesthesia for cesarean section: a comparison of time efficiency, costs, charges, and complications. Anesth Analg. 1995;80(4):709–12.
 6. Garry M, Davies S. Failure of regional blockade for caesarean section. Int J Obstet Anesth. 2002;11(1):9–12.
 7. Tsen L.. Anaesthesia for cesarean delivery. In: Chestnut DH, editors. Chestnut's obstetric anesthesia: principles and practice. 2014.
 8. Kuhnert BR, Philipson EH, Pimental R, Kuhnert PM, Zuspan KJ, Syracuse CD. Lidocaine disposition in mother, fetus, and neonate after spinal anesthesia. Anesth Analg. 1986;65(2):139–44.
 9. Kuhnert BR, Zuspan KJ, Kuhnert PM, Syracuse CD, Brown DE. Bupivacaine disposition in mother, fetus, and neonate after spinal anesthesia for cesarean section. Anesth Analg. 1987;66(5):407–12.
10. Cook TM, Counsell D, Wildsmith JAW. Major complications of central neuraxial block: report on the third national audit project of the royal college of anaesthetists. Br J Anaesth. 2009;102(2):179–90.
11. WHO guidelines for safe surgery 2009: Safe surgery saves lives. World Health Organisation. 2009.
12. de Vries EN, Prins HA, Crolla RMPH, den Outer AJ, van Andel G, van Helden SH, et al. Effect of a comprehensive surgical safety system on patient outcomes. N Engl J Med. 2010;363(20):1928–37.
13. Department of health (DOH). Uniforms and workwear: An evidence base for developing local policy. DOH 2007. Accessed Mar 2014.
14. Benhamou D, Bouaziz H, Chassard D, Ducloy J-C, Fuzier V, Laffon M, et al. Anaesthetic practices for scheduled caesarean delivery: a 2005 french national survey. Eur J Anaesthesiol. 2009;26(8):694–700.
15. Checketts MR. Wash & go—but with what? Skin antiseptic solutions for central neuraxial block. Anaesthesia. 2012;67(8):819–22.
16. Malhotra S, Dharmadasa A, Yentis SM. One vs two applications of chlorhexidine/ethanol for disinfecting the skin: implications for regional anaesthesia. Anaesthesia. 2011;66(7):574–8.

17. Killeen T, Kamat A, Walsh D, Parker A, Aliashkevich A. Severe adhesive arachnoiditis resulting in progressive paraplegia following obstetric spinal anaesthesia: a case report and review. Anaesthesia. 2012;67(12):1386–94.
18. Armstrong S, Fernando R, Tamilselvan P, Stewart A, Columb M. The effect of serial in vitro haemodilution with maternal cerebrospinal fluid and crystalloid on thromboelastographic (TEG(®)) blood coagulation parameters, and the implications for epidural blood patching. Anaesthesia. 2015;70(2):135–41.
19. Choi PT, Galinski SE, Takeuchi L, Lucas S, Tamayo C, Jadad AR. PDPH is a common complication of neuraxial blockade in parturients: a meta-analysis of obstetrical studies. Can J Anaesth. 2003;50(5):460–9.
20. Van de Velde M, Schepers R, Berends N, Vandermeersch E, De Buck F. Ten years of experience with accidental dural puncture and post-dural puncture headache in a tertiary obstetric anaesthesia department. Int J Obstet Anesth. 2008;17(4):329–35.
21. Stocks GM, Wooller DJ, Young JM, Fernando R. Postpartum headache after epidural blood patch: investigation and diagnosis. Br J Anaesth. 2000;84(3):407–10.
22. Tourtellotte WW, Henderson WG, Tucker RP, Walker JE, Kokman E. A randomized, double-blind clinical trial comparing the 22 versus 26 gauge needle in the production of the post-lumbar puncture syndrome in normal individuals. Headache: J Head Face Pain. 1972;12(2): 73–8.
23. Turnbull DK, Shepherd DB. Post-dural puncture headache: pathogenesis, prevention and treatment. Br J Anaesth. 2003;91(5):718–29.
24. Reynolds F. Damage to the conus medullaris following spinal anaesthesia. Anaesthesia. 2001;56(3):238–47.
25. Broadbent CR, Maxwell WB, Ferrie R, Wilson DJ, Gawne-Cain M. Ability of anaesthetists to identify a marked lumbar interspace. (Nuffield department of anaesthetics, john Radcliffe hospital, oxford, United Kingdom). Anaesthesia. 2000;55:1122–6. Pain Practice 2001;1(2): 199–200
26. Lee AJ, Ranasinghe JS, Chehade JM, Arheart K, Saltzman BS, Penning DH, Birnbach DJ. Ultrasound assessment of the vertebral level of the intercristal line in pregnancy. Anesth Analg. 2011;113(3):559–64.
27. Shaikh F, Brzezinski J, Alexander S, Arzola C, Carvalho JCA, Beyene J, Sung L. Ultrasound imaging for lumbar punctures and epidural catheterisations: systematic review and meta-analysis. BMJ. 2013;346:f1720.
28. Armstrong S, Fernando R, Columb M, Jones T. Cardiac index in term pregnant women in the sitting, lateral, and supine positions: an observational, crossover study. Anesth Analg. 2011;113(2):318–22.
29. Yun EM, Marx GF, Santos AC. The effects of maternal position during induction of combined spinal-epidural anesthesia for cesarean delivery. Anesth Analg. 1998;87(3):614–8.
30. Inglis A, Daniel M, McGrady E. Maternal position during induction of spinal anaesthesia for caesarean section. A comparison of right lateral and sitting positions. Anaesthesia. 1995;50(4): 363–5.
31. Hallworth SP, Fernando R, Columb MO, Stocks GM. The effect of posture and baricity on the spread of intrathecal bupivacaine for elective cesarean delivery. Anesth Analg. 2005;100(4): 1159–65.
32. Heng Sia AT, Tan KH, Sng BL, Lim Y, Chan ESY, Siddiqui FJ. Hyperbaric versus plain bupivacaine for spinal anesthesia for cesarean delivery. Anesth Analg. 2015;120(1):132–40.
33. Ralston DH, Shnider SM, DeLorimier AA. Effects of equipotent ephedrine, metaraminol, mephentermine, and methoxamine on uterine blood flow in the pregnant ewe. Anesthesiology. 1974;40(4):354–70.
34. Lee A, Ngan Kee WD, Gin T. A quantitative, systematic review of randomized controlled trials of ephedrine versus phenylephrine for the management of hypotension during spinal anesthesia for cesarean delivery. Anesth Analg. 2002;94(4):920–6. table of contents
35. Wollman SB, Marx GF. Acute hydration for prevention of hypotension of spinal anesthesia in parturients. Anesthesiology. 1968;29(2):374–80.

36. Pouta AM, Karinen J, Vuolteenaho OJ, Laatikainen TJ. Effect of intravenous fluid preload on vasoactive peptide secretion during caesarean section under spinal anaesthesia. Anaesthesia. 1996;51(2):128–32.
37. Ueyama H, He YL, Tanigami H, Mashimo T, Yoshiya I. Effects of crystalloid and colloid preload on blood volume in the parturient undergoing spinal anesthesia for elective cesarean section. Anesthesiology. 1999;91(6):1571–6.
38. Cyna AM, Andrew M, Emmett RS, Middleton P, Simmons SW. Techniques for preventing hypotension during spinal anaesthesia for caesarean section. Cochrane Database Syst Rev. 2006;4:CD002251.
39. Bajwa SJS, Kulshrestha A, Jindal R. Co-loading or pre-loading for prevention of hypotension after spinal anaesthesia! A therapeutic dilemma. Anesth Essays Res. 2013;7(2):155–9.
40. Chanimov M, Gershfeld S, Cohen ML, Sherman D, Bahar M. Fluid preload before spinal anaesthesia in caesarean section: the effect on neonatal acid-base status. Eur J Anaesthesiol. 2006;23(8):676–9.
41. Tawfik MM, Hayes SM, Jacoub FY, Badran BA, Gohar FM, Shabana AM, et al. Comparison between colloid preload and crystalloid co-load in cesarean section under spinal anesthesia: a randomized controlled trial. Int J Obstet Anesth. 2014;23(4):317–23.
42. Khaw KS, Ngan Kee WD, Wong M, Ng F, Lee A. Spinal ropivacaine for cesarean delivery: a comparison of hyperbaric and plain solutions. Anesth Analg. 2002;94(3):680–5. table of contents
43. Vercauteren MP, Coppejans HC, Hoffmann VL, Saldien V, Adriaensen HA. Small-dose hyperbaric versus plain bupivacaine during spinal anesthesia for cesarean section. Anesth Analg. 1998;86(5):989–93.
44. Gautier P, De Kock M, Huberty L, Demir T, Izydorczic M, Vanderick B. Comparison of the effects of intrathecal ropivacaine, levobupivacaine, and bupivacaine for caesarean section. Br J Anaesth. 2003;91(5):684–9.
45. Oğün CO, Kirgiz EN, Duman A, Okesli S, Akyürek C. Comparison of intrathecal isobaric bupivacaine-morphine and ropivacaine-morphine for caesarean delivery. Br J Anaesth. 2003;90(5):659–64.
46. Lanz E, Schmitz D. No effect of injection volume on sensory and motor blockade in isobaric spinal anesthesia. Reg Anaesth. 1990;13(7):153–8.
47. Russell IF. Spinal anesthesia for cesarean delivery with dilute solutions of plain bupivacaine: the relationship between infused volume and spread. Reg Anesth. 1991;16(3):130–6.
48. Russell IF. At caesarean section under regional anaesthesia, it is essential to test sensory block with light touch before allowing surgery to start. Int J Obstet Anesth. 2006;15(4):294–7.
49. Teoh WHL, Thomas E, Tan HM. Ultra-low dose combined spinal-epidural anesthesia with intrathecal bupivacaine 3.75 mg for cesarean delivery: a randomized controlled trial. Int J Obstet Anesth. 2006;15(4):273–8.
50. Kestin IG. Spinal anaesthesia in obstetrics. Br J Anaesth. 1991;66(5):596–607.
51. Hartwell BL, Aglio LS, Hauch MA, Datta S. Vertebral column length and spread of hyperbaric subarachnoid bupivacaine in the term parturient. Reg Anesth. 1991;16(1):17–9.
52. Norris MC. Height, weight, and the spread of subarachnoid hyperbaric bupivacaine in the term parturient. Anesth Analg. 1988;67(6):555–8.
53. Ozkan Seyhan T, Orhan-Sungur M, Basaran B, Savran Karadeniz M, Demircan F, Xu Z, Sessler DI. The effect of intra-abdominal pressure on sensory block level of single-shot spinal anesthesia for cesarean section: an observational study. Int J Obstet Anesth. 2015;24(1):35–40.
54. Carvalho B, Collins J, Drover DR, Atkinson Ralls L, Riley ET. ED(50) and ED(95) of intrathecal bupivacaine in morbidly obese patients undergoing cesarean delivery. Anesthesiology. 2011;114(3):529–35.
55. Ginosar Y, Mirikatani E, Drover DR, Cohen SE, Riley ET. ED50 and ED95 of intrathecal hyperbaric bupivacaine coadministered with opioids for cesarean delivery. Anesthesiology. 2004;100(3):676–82.
56. Carvalho B, Durbin M, Drover DR, Cohen SE, Ginosar Y, Riley ET. The ED50 and ED95 of intrathecal isobaric bupivacaine with opioids for cesarean delivery. Anesthesiology. 2005;103(3):606–12.

57. Bryson GL, Macneil R, Jeyaraj LM, Rosaeg OP. Small dose spinal bupivacaine for cesarean delivery does not reduce hypotension but accelerates motor recovery. Can J Anaesth. 2007;54(7):531–7.
58. Choi DH, Ahn HJ, Kim MH. Bupivacaine-sparing effect of fentanyl in spinal anesthesia for cesarean delivery. Reg Anesth Pain Med. 2000;25(3):240–5.
59. Dahlgren G, Hultstrand C, Jakobsson J, Norman M, Eriksson EW, Martin H. Intrathecal sufentanil, fentanyl, or placebo added to bupivacaine for cesarean section. Anesth Analg. 1997;85(6):1288–93.
60. Cousins MJ, Mather LE. Intrathecal and epidural administration of opioids. Anesthesiology. 1984;61(3):276–310.
61. Bernards CM, Hill HF. Physical and chemical properties of drug molecules governing their diffusion through the spinal meninges. Anesthesiology. 1992;77(4):750–6.
62. Scrutton M, Kinsella SM. The immediate caesarean section: rapid-sequence spinal and risk of infection. Int J Obstet Anesth. 2003;12(2):144.
63. Armstrong S, Stocks G. Postoperative analgesia after caesarean delivery. In: Clarke V, Fernando R, Van de Velde M, editors. Oxford textbook of obstetric anaesthesia. Oxford: Oxford University Press; 2016.
64. Dahl JB, Jeppesen IS, Jørgensen H, Wetterslev J, Møiniche S. Intraoperative and postoperative analgesic efficacy and adverse effects of intrathecal opioids in patients undergoing cesarean section with spinal anesthesia: a qualitative and quantitative systematic review of randomized controlled trials. Anesthesiology. 1999;91(6):1919–27.
65. Palmer CM, Voulgaropoulos D, Alves D. Subarachnoid fentanyl augments lidocaine spinal anesthesia for cesarean delivery. Reg Anesth. 1995;20(5):389–94.
66. Manullang TR, Viscomi CM, Pace NL. Intrathecal fentanyl is superior to intravenous ondansetron for the prevention of perioperative nausea during cesarean delivery with spinal anesthesia. Anesth Analg. 2000;90(5):1162–6.
67. Courtney MA, Bader AM, Hartwell B, Hauch M, Grennan MJ, Datta S. Perioperative analgesia with subarachnoid sufentanil administration. Reg Anesth. 1992;17(5):274–8.
68. Lee JH, Chung KH, Lee JY, Chun DH, Yang HJ, Ko TK, Yun WS. Comparison of fentanyl and sufentanil added to 0.5% hyperbaric bupivacaine for spinal anesthesia in patients undergoing cesarean section. Korean J Anesthesiol. 2011;60(2):103–8.
69. Ngiam SK, Chong JL. The addition of intrathecal sufentanil and fentanyl to bupivacaine for caesarean section. Singap Med J. 1998;39(7):290–4.
70. Bromage PR, Camporesi EM, Durant PA, Nielsen CH. Rostral spread of epidural morphine. Anesthesiology. 1982;56(6):431–6.
71. Palmer CM, Emerson S, Volgoropolous D, Alves D. Dose-response relationship of intrathecal morphine for postcesarean analgesia. Anesthesiology. 1999;90(2):437–44.
72. Wong JY, Carvalho B, Riley ET. Intrathecal morphine 100 and 200 µg for post-cesarean delivery analgesia: a trade-off between analgesic efficacy and side effects. Int J Obstet Anesth. 2013;22(1):36–41.
73. Glynn CJ, Mather LE, Cousins MJ, Wilson PR, Graham JR. Spinal narcotics and respiratory depression. Lancet. 1979;2(8138):356–7.
74. Scott DB, McClure J. Selective epidural analgesia. Lancet. 1979;1(8131):1410–1.
75. Cohen SE, Labaille T, Benhamou D, Levron JC. Respiratory effects of epidural sufentanil after cesarean section. Anesth Analg. 1992;74(5):677–82.
76. Negre I, Gueneron JP, Ecoffey C, Penon C, Gross JB, Levron JC, Samii K. Ventilatory response to carbon dioxide after intramuscular and epidural fentanyl. Anesth Analg. 1987;66(8):707–10.
77. Practice guidelines for the prevention, detection, and management of respiratory depression associated with neuraxial opioid administration: An updated report by the American Society of Anesthesiologists task force on neuraxial opioids and the American Society of Regional Anesthesia and Pain Medicine. Anesthesiology 2015, Dec 2011.
78. Hallworth SP, Fernando R, Bell R, Parry MG, Lim GH. Comparison of intrathecal and epidural diamorphine for elective caesarean section using a combined spinal-epidural technique. Br J Anaesth. 1999;82(2):228–32.

79. Giovannelli M, Bedforth N, Aitkenhead A. Survey of intrathecal opioid usage in the UK. Eur J Anaesthesiol. 2008;25(2):118–22.
80. Skilton RW, Kinsella SM, Smith A, Thomas TA. Dose response study of subarachnoid diamorphine for analgesia after elective caesarean section. Int J Obstet Anesth. 1999;8(4):231–5.
81. Kelly MC, Carabine UA, Mirakhur RK. Intrathecal diamorphine for analgesia after caesarean section. A dose finding study and assessment of side-effects. Anaesthesia. 1998;53(3):231–7.
82. Stacey R, Jones R, Kar G, Poon A. High-dose intrathecal diamorphine for analgesia after caesarean section. Anaesthesia. 2001;56(1):54–60.
83. Saravanan S, Robinson APC, Qayoum Dar A, Columb MO, Lyons GR. Minimum dose of intrathecal diamorphine required to prevent intraoperative supplementation of spinal anaesthesia for caesarean section. Br J Anaesth. 2003;91(3):368–72.
84. Cowan CM, Kendall JB, Barclay PM, Wilkes RG. Comparison of intrathecal fentanyl and diamorphine in addition to bupivacaine for caesarean section under spinal anaesthesia. Br J Anaesth. 2002;89(3):452–8.
85. Carvalho B, Drover DR, Ginosar Y, Cohen SE, Riley ET. Intrathecal fentanyl added to bupivacaine and morphine for cesarean delivery may induce a subtle acute opioid tolerance. Int J Obstet Anesth. 2012;21(1):29–34.
86. Cooper DW, Lindsay SL, Ryall DM, Kokri MS, Eldabe SS, Lear GA. Does intrathecal fentanyl produce acute cross-tolerance to i.V. Morphine? Br J Anaesth. 1997;78(3):311–3.
87. Lavand'homme PM, Roelants F, Waterloos H, Collet V, De Kock MF. An evaluation of the postoperative antihyperalgesic and analgesic effects of intrathecal clonidine administered during elective cesarean delivery. Anesth Analg. 2008;107(3):948–55.
88. Cossu AP, De Giudici LM, Piras D, Mura P, Scanu M, Cossu M, et al. A systematic review of the effects of adding neostigmine to local anesthetics for neuraxial administration in obstetric anesthesia and analgesia. Int J Obstet Anesth. 2015;24(3):237–46.
89. Alonso E, Gilsanz F, Gredilla E, Martínez B, Canser E, Alsina E. Observational study of continuous spinal anesthesia with the catheter-over-needle technique for cesarean delivery. Int J Obstet Anesth. 2009, Apr;18(2):137–41.
90. Arkoosh VA, Palmer CM, Yun EM, Sharma SK, Bates JN, Wissler RN, et al. A randomized, double-masked, multicenter comparison of the safety of continuous intrathecal labor analgesia using a 28-gauge catheter versus continuous epidural labor analgesia. Anesthesiology. 2008;108(2):286–98.
91. Rigler ML, Drasner K, Krejcie TC, Yelich SJ, Scholnick FT, DeFontes J, Bohner D. Cauda equina syndrome after continuous spinal anesthesia. Anesth Analg. 1991;72(3):275–81.

Epidural and CSE Anesthesia (Technique–Drugs)

5

Giorgio Capogna

"Last November, whilst giving a spinal anaesthetic, it occurred to me to block the nerves between the intervertebral spaces and the meninges rather than pierce the dura." This is the first description on the intentional injection of anesthetic drugs in the lumbar epidural space, as described by the Spanish surgeon Fidel Pages in 1921 [1].

Ten years later, the Italian surgeon Achille Mario Dogliotti described, published, and popularized the loss of resistance technique to identify the epidural space, which remains in use at present and is commonly referred to as the loss of resistance to saline (LORS) technique or its variation [2].

A few years later, Graffagnino and Seyler published one of the first reports on the use of epidural block in obstetrics, which included ten cesarean sections: "in the Charity Hospital of New Orleans, we have attempted to add to the anesthetic armamentarium of the obstetrician another procedure, epidural anesthesia, which we have thus far administered to 76 patients [3]."

5.1 Epidural Technique

The following description of the epidural technique is that used for 30 years by the author, and it is consistent with the original one described by Dogliotti in 1935 and with the subsequent modifications adapted for the obstetric patient by Bromage, Moore, and Bonica [4–7].

G. Capogna
Department of Anesthesiology, Città di Roma Hospital, Rome, Italy
e-mail: dipartimento.anestesia@gruppogarofalo.com

© Springer International Publishing Switzerland 2017
G. Capogna (ed.), *Anesthesia for Cesarean Section*,
DOI 10.1007/978-3-319-42053-0_5

5.1.1 Preparation and Position of the Patient

Epidural block may be performed in a lateral or in a sitting position. The favorite, routine position of the author is the lateral one. Aortocaval compression is minimized in the lateral position and uteroplacental blood flow is optimized; in addition, there is a lower incidence of epidural vein cannulation compared to the sitting position [8].

However, since the ability to identify the midline of the back and iliac crests may be easier and the distance to the epidural space is reduced [9, 10], the sitting position may be preferred particularly for trainees or for obese women [11].

The parturient is placed in the lateral position with her back at the edge of the bed, legs drawn up to her abdomen, upper arm lying across her chest and the lower arm lying tight on the bed, with the head resting on a pillow, flexed on the abdomen. Every effort is made to keep the spinous process of the vertebral column parallel to the table and the patient well flexed, so as to open the interspaces. In order to do that the shoulders and the iliac crest should be perpendicular to the table plane.

However, parturients may not flex their back very well, due to the gravid uterus.

Repeated or inappropriate efforts to improve dorsal flexion may result in bringing the upper shoulder forward toward the abdomen which rotates the spinous process of the vertebral column out of the parallel alignment with the bed surface and thus favoring the contact of the epidural needle on the vertebral bony arch during the attempt to reach the epidural space.

The epidural anesthesia tray and all the material necessary for the procedure should have been previously placed on a cart at the disposal of the operator. The cart is placed conveniently close to the back of the patient and to the right side of the operator (unless he/she is left handed, and in this case it will be placed on the left side).

The anesthesiologist wearing cap, facial mask, and sterile gloves applies the antiseptic solution, usually more than once, over a wide area, including the iliac crest region down to the surface of the bed. While the applied antiseptic solution is drying, the anesthesia tray is checked for proper materials.

5.1.2 Landmarks

It is commonly believed that Tuffier's line (the transverse line connecting the tops of the iliac crests) intersects the spine at the L4 spinous process or at the L4-L5 intervertebral space. However, full-term parturient women undergo various physical changes and determining the vertebral level with Tuffier's line based on palpation may not be very accurate. Vertebral levels are more cephalad in the parturient women compared to the non-parturient women and this should be taken into account when performing an epidural block in term pregnant women [12].

Several spinous processes and interspaces should be palpated to determine the widest interspace and the possible presence of scoliosis or vertebral column deviations.

Since the epidural space is widest at L2-L3 and the spinal cord usually ends at L1 but may extend to L2, midlumbar interspaces are usually selected.

5.1.3 Procedure

The index finger and the middle finger of the nondominant hand are placed parallel to the spine, indicating the interspace chosen ("landmark fingers") (Fig. 5.1). They facilitate the proper placement of the needle in the center of the interspinous space, indicate the landmark for the Tuohy needle insertion, and should be kept in place until the Tuohy needle reaches the next landmark, which is the ligamentum flavum.

A small gauge needle attached to a 5 mL disposable syringe containing the local anesthetic solution (such as 1 or 2% lidocaine) is inserted through the skin to make a wheal over the selected interspace and eventually gently inserted into the underlying tissues until the interspinous ligament, while the local anesthetic solution is slowly injected.

The angle of penetration should be the same as planned for the epidural needle.

Without moving the "landmark fingers," the epidural Tuohy needle is inserted through the skin wheal previously made exactly in the middle of the interspace.

The epidural needle is held with the palm of the hand resting on the hub, and the shaft of the needle between the fingers of the dominant hand (Fig. 5.2).

Once inserted into the skin, the epidural needle should be advanced with the bevel directed cephalad, taking care to remain in the midline. The needle must be

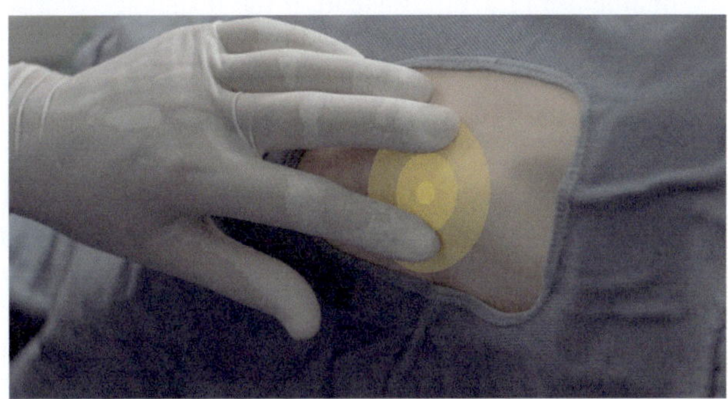

Fig. 5.1 Choice of lumbar interspace

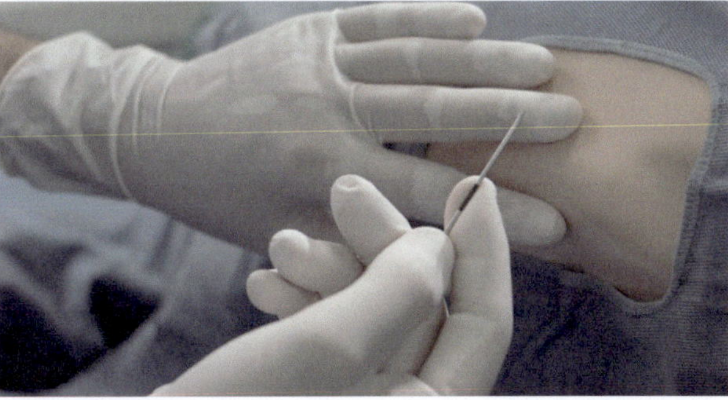

Fig. 5.2 Introduction of the needle

Fig. 5.3 Loss of resistance

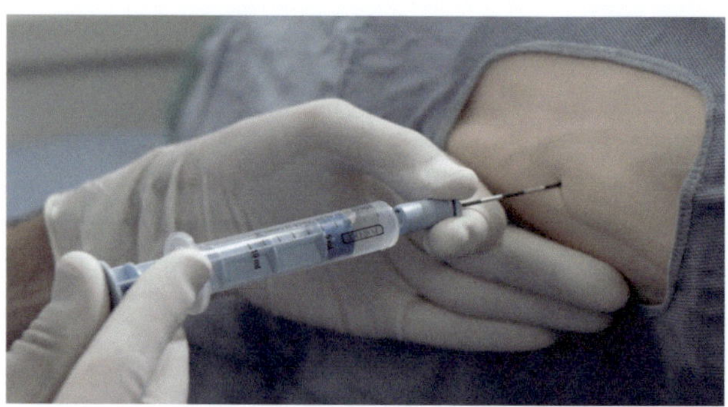

advanced very slowly but constantly, without any interruption, in order to be able to recognize the different densities of the underlying tissues (subcutaneous tissue, supraspinous and interspinous ligaments) during its advancement. As soon as it reaches the supraspinous ligament, a resistance is encountered due to the nature of the bevel and the density of the ligament. The needle is then advanced through the loose interspinous ligament which offers much less resistance than the supraspinous ligament (often felt as a "no resistance feeling" in the obstetric patient), until the point of the needle is felt to meet the third, and greater, point of resistance, the ligamentum flavum. This feeling of a greater increase of resistance is often associated with a "crunch" that indicates the initial penetration of the needle in the rear wall of the ligamentum flavum. Instead, if the resistance is absolute the bevel of the needle may be against the bony vertebral arch and any attempt to force the needle may result in pain for the patient due to periostium stimulation. In this case, the needle should be withdrawn, its angle of inclination checked, and the direction changed accordingly.

As soon as the point of the needle has engaged the ligamentum flavum, the advancement of the needle is immediately stopped, and the hands of the operator must change their initial position. The back of the nondominant hand (usually the left hand) rests firmly against the patient's back to prevent advancement as the needle enters the epidural space with the hub of the needle grasped between the thumb and index fingers. The dominant hand (usually the right hand) removes the stylet and gently attaches to the needle a disposable 10 mL loss of resistance syringe containing a few milliliters (5–7 mL) of sterile saline solution.

Constant, unremitting, pressure is now exerted on the plunger of the syringe by the thumb of the dominant hand and since the content of the syringe (saline) is incompressible, the syringe and needle advance together solely by means of the pressure exerted by the operator on the plunger of the syringe (Fig. 5.3).

As long as the needle point is in the ligamentum flavum there is a great resistance to injection and the pressure exerted by the thumb on the plunger causes the advancement of the needle.

As the point of the needle emerges from the ligamentum flavum into the epidural space, the resistance suddenly disappears and the advancement of the needle immediately stops, since the driving force exerted on the piston is discharged by the sudden entering of the liquid in the epidural space.

When the epidural needle is positioned in the epidural space, the syringe is removed and the needle observed for the appearance of spinal fluid (a few drops of syringe solution may leak from the needle).

5.1.4 Air or Rebound Test

After negative aspiration for blood or cerebrospinal fluid, proper placement of the needle may be further checked with the air or rebound test. A very small amount of air (1–1.5 mL) is drawn in the loss of resistance syringe and attached to the needle and the plunger of the syringe is tapped sharply. A positive test results when the syringe collapses and does not refill at all, or only refills 0.1–0.2 mL.

This rapid injection of a very few millimeters of air, mixed with the previously injected liquid already in the epidural space, may occasionally result in small air-water bubbles escaping from the hub of the needle. If this occurs, it may be considered another indirect sign of confirmation that the epidural needle is in the right place.

When the plunger rebounds, a partially inserted bevel of the needle in the epidural space could be suspected.

5.1.5 Catheter Placement and Needle Removal

Once the needle is in place, the epidural catheter is advanced through the needle by the dominant hand while the back of the nondominant hand (usually the left hand) keeps resting firmly against the patient's back with the hub of the needle grasped between the thumb and index fingers.

The parturient should be warned that she might feel an "intense tingle" in her hip or legs when the catheter is advanced a few centimeters beyond the bevel. Such paresthesia may occur when the epidural catheter contacts a spinal nerve root, depending on the type and material of the catheter, on the needle position (midline, paramedian), and on the epidural anatomy of the patient. It may be interpreted as an indirect sign that the catheter is in the epidural space.

Before removing the needle, the catheter should be aspirated with a 2 or 5 mL empty syringe in order to detect blood or cerebrospinal fluid which are, respectively, signs of accidental intravascular or subarachnoid placement of the catheter.

If the aspiration test is negative, the needle is removed. This is an important maneuver since the catheter may be dislodged from the epidural space while removing the needle. The catheter is grasped 1–2 cm distal to the hub of the needle by the thumb and the index finger of the dominant hand while the thumb and the index finger of the other hand pull the needle out of the back of the patient. The dominant hand should attempt to advance the catheter while the nondominant is pulling out the catheter. At the end of the procedure, the catheter distance marks are checked and the catheter properly positioned. Placement of the catheter more than 5 cm in the lumbar epidural space may be associated with a higher incidence of unilateral block and a greater likelihood of the tip entering an epidural blood vessel, while too little catheter length predisposes the catheter to falling out [13].

The catheter is then secured with tape and adhesive dressings, and used for the intended purpose.

Once the catheter is placed, after a test dose, anesthesia for cesarean delivery is achieved by administration of local anesthetics with or without opioids.

Box 1 Dogliotti's Loss of Resistance to Saline Technique

"When the needle has penetrated the ligamentum interspinosum for a certain distance and before it has gone through the ligamenta subflava into the spinal canal one removes the trocar and attaches a syringe filled with physiological saline. When an attempt is made to inject this fluid a very great resistance is met with since the ligamentum interspinosum and the ligamenta subflava are so dense. If they can be injected at all, it will be only after the employment of considerable force. This resistance is most certain evidence that the needle is still in the posterior fibers of these tissues. The following manoeuvres are then carried out: the syringe is held in one hand the thumb of which applies a continued and uniform pressure to the piston. The other hand slowly advances the needle into the tissues and when it has traversed a few millimetres the hand which is holding it will suddenly note a diminution in the resistance to its passage which has previously been due to the tissues of the ligamenta subflava. At the same instant the injection fluid enters freely. This is certain, practical, and unequivocal evidence that the point of the needle has pierced the ligamenta subflava and is in the peridural space which offers no resistance to the flow of the injected fluid. As soon as this position has been recognized the needle should be left in the position which it now occupies for its point is in the peridural space; any attempt to advance it farther would entail the risk of penetrating the dura." (Reprinted from [14] with the permission of the Publisher)

5.1.6   Ultrasound Assisted Identification of the Epidural Space

Evidence on ultrasound-guided identification of the epidural space in pregnancy is still limited and this technique is not commonly used as a routine tool to detect the epidural space in obstetrics.

In addition, the visibility of the ligamentum flavum, the dura mater, and of the epidural space decreases significantly during pregnancy [15]. However, preliminary evidence suggests that it is safe and may be helpful in achieving correct placement, especially for teaching purposes and in the obese parturient [16, 17].

Ultrasound can be used in two different ways to ease the performance of an epidural block [18]. One method is to use real-time ultrasound imaging, under sterile conditions, to observe the passage of the needle on the way to the epidural space. In the second method (prepuncture ultrasound), an initial ultrasound scan of the patient's lumbar area is performed to find the midline and the interspinous space in order to mark on the skin the position of each. The depth of the epidural space may also be determined by using the ultrasound scan. Epidural block is eventually performed in the usual way with the skin markings as an additional guide.

5.2 Epidural Anesthesia

One of the main advantages of epidural anesthesia is that the local anesthetic can be administered in incremental doses and that the total dose can be titrated to the desired sensory level.

This, with the slower onset of anesthesia, allows the maternal cardiovascular system to compensate for the occurrence of sympathetic block reducing the risk of severe hypotension and reduced uteroplacental perfusion.

The use of the epidural catheter, and therefore of a continuous technique, allows the anesthesiologist to give additional local anesthetic to maintain anesthesia, regardless of the duration of surgery and the intensity of surgical stimulation. Usually epidural anesthesia results in less intense motor block than dose spinal anesthesia, especially at the beginning of the block. This may be advantageous for patients in which a high level of motor block may impair ventilation, such as multiple gestation or pulmonary diseases. The epidural catheter may also be used for postoperative analgesia either with exclusive epidural opiods or with an analgesic ultra low concentration solution of local anesthetic and opioids.

5.2.1 Test Dose

The aim of the epidural test dose is to detect the inadvertent intravenous or subarachnoid placement of the epidural catheter in order to avoid, respectively, a too high or a total spinal block or local anesthetic toxicity. The test dose must be formulated to produce a rapid, reliable, and easily detected result when in one of these two situations, without compromising the safety of the mother and the fetus.

In all cases, careful aspiration of the epidural catheter before administering any dose of anesthetic solution is the first extremely important step.

Subarachnoid placement is relatively easy to detect. For practical reasons, the same local anesthetic that is used for producing the anesthetic block is usually chosen. Lidocaine 20–60 mg or bupivacaine (or levobupivacaine or ropivacaine) 7.5–12.5 mg are commonly used. Signs of sensory block in the lower lumbar segments and, most importantly, motor block of the legs should be sought after 3–5 min and this is considered to be specific and sensitive in almost 100% of cases. When the test dose is performed with a relatively "high dose" of local anesthetic, such as 40–60 mg of lidocaine or 12 mg of bupivacaine, in the case of accidental intrathecal injection, a safe but complete sensory and motor block accompanied by maternal hypotension may be observed [19].

Inadvertent intravascular placement of the epidural catheter usually relies on the use of a dose of epinephrine (15 µg) capable of producing detectable changes in heart rate and blood pressure but unfortunately, in obstetrics, intravenous injection of epinephrine has been shown to have a low positive predictive value and may be associated with side effects [20].

Therefore, detection of intravascular multiorifice epidural catheter placement relies on repeated catheter aspiration, observation of gravity-induced fluid efflux within an open-ended catheter, failure of local anesthetic to produce the anticipated effect, and detection of early signs of toxicity by means of slow and incremental injection.

It is therefore vital to aspirate the catheter before giving each dose and fraction-ate the whole anesthetic dose in small boluses given intermittently, always.

5.2.2 Anesthetic Solution

Approximately 3–5 min after a negative aspiration test and a negative test dose, the therapeutic dose is then administered, in fractionated boluses of 5 mL each.

Although the nerve supply to the uterus extends no higher than the eighth to tenth thoracic nerve roots, it is generally agreed among anesthesiologists that anesthesia for cesarean section should extend to the level of the fourth thoracic dermatome to include afferent fibers running in the greater splanchic nerve. However in some cases, peritoneal stimulation may require a sensory block up to the first thoracic dermatome. An adequate sacral anesthesia level is also required to prevent pain from bladder retraction or uterosacral ligaments traction.

An inadequate sensory assessment prior to surgery or an unrecognized sensory block regression during surgery is a common cause of intraoperative pain. It is therefore most important to check the sensory block with an appropriate and reli-able method, such as the loss of sensation to pinprick or to light touch and by using an appropriate evaluation scale [21].

A bilateral, adequately, dense sensory level to T4 is required for cesarean surgery and this could be reached in the majority of cases with 20–25 mL of local anesthetic.

A frequent assessment of the sensory block allows a careful titration of the anes-thetic dose at the desired level.

Most anesthesiologists use lidocaine 2%, bupivacaine 0.5%, levobupivacaine 0.5 or 0.75%, or ropivacaine 0.75–1%. 2-chlorprocaine is also used where available (not in Europe).

Epinephrine may be added at the concentration of 1:200,000 or 1:400,000 to decrease vascular absorption of the local anesthetic and to prolong the duration of the block. Due to the well-known pharmacological characteristics of the different local anesthetics, the addition of epinephrine appears to have a rationale only with lidocaine. The addition of sodium bicarbonate to lidocaine hastens the onset of anesthesia and may also improve the quality of analgesia [22].

Opioids are frequently given epidurally to enhance intraoperative analgesia and to provide postoperative pain relief. Fentanyl 50–100 µg or sufentanil 10 µg may be added to the therapeutic dose or given separately at some point during the administration of the epidural boluses without adversely affecting the neonate.

The choice of the drug depends on the desired onset of action and the expected duration of surgery and may vary with the local clinical practice. The most effective solution is 2% lidocaine with epinephrine with a liposoluble opioid, the least is 0.5% plain bupivacaine.

The local anesthetic solution used by the author is a pH adjusted solution of 2% lidocaine with epinephrine 1:400,000 with the addition of 10 µg of sufentanil.

5.2.3 Fluid Preloading and Control of Maternal Hypotension

The incidence and the degree of maternal hypotension after epidural block are dependent on the speed of onset of the sympathetic block, being less with fractioned incremental boluses.

Maternal hypotension may be prevented and/or treated with fluid preloading and vasopressor drugs.

Unfortunately, almost all the recent studies on this topic investigated exclusively spinal rather than epidural anesthesia.

Current literature highlights that prevention of hypotension during spinal anesthesia for cesarean section is mainly based on the use of vasopressor drugs prophylaxis. However, fluid administration remains helpful to further decrease the incidence and severity of maternal hypotension and vasopressor requirement. Hydroxyethyl starch (HES) solution preloading or coloading is the best acknowledged and the more consistent method [23].

With regard to vasopressor use, ephedrine seemed initially to be the logical vasopressor for obstetrics, with both α- and β-sympathomimetic effects, the ideal protection for placental intervillous blood flow. Most likely ephedrine is still the most commonly used vasopressor to prevent and treat maternal hypotension after a spinal block for cesarean section.

Now numerous studies have compared this agent with pure α stimulants, usually phenylephrine, with confusing results, but meta-analysis has shown convincingly that ephedrine is associated with lower pH and BE of the neonate and with a higher risk for fetal acidosis when compared with phenylephrine. Comparing the maternal effects, phenylephrine is associated with an increased risk of maternal bradycardia. Unfortunately, a number of not controlled factors that may also influence fetal blood gases such as the total amount of vasopressor given before delivery, timing of administration, duration, and severity of maternal hypotension and, in addition, a clear definition of hypotension is often not reported in these studies [24, 25].

However, these findings concern spinal rather than epidural anesthesia, and a comparison between vasopressors during epidural anesthesia has not been performed.

Placental intervillous blood flow is not exclusively dependent on maternal blood pressure but also on maternal cardiac output and its distribution. It has been shown that spinal but not epidural anesthesia is associated with a reduction in cardiac output even in the presence of a normal blood pressure [26] and this must be taken into account when interpreting the results of the spinal studies.

5.2.4 Intraoperative Discomfort and Pain

One of the major concerns about epidural anesthesia along with the more technical difficulty in performing the block and the relatively slow onset time is the frequent occurrence of intraoperative discomfort or pain when compared to spinal anesthesia. This problem may require additional measures and, depending on the severity of pain, conversion to general anesthesia may be occasionally necessary.

However, the percentage of patients experiencing intraoperative pain requiring additional medications during surgery is extremely variable, and has been reported to be up to 50% [27], depending on a number of factors, such as the expertise of the operator, the epidural technique, the local anesthetic solution, the method of sensory block assessment, and the type of surgery [28].

The best analgesic success, comparable to that obtained with spinal anesthesia, is usually achieved when the block is performed by an experienced anesthesiologist, with loss of resistance to saline, with 2% lidocaine with epinephrine and opioids or 2-chlorprocaine, with a complete loss of sensations from S5 to at least T4 assessed by pinprick or light touch, and with a surgery without the uterine exteriorization maneuver. The least successful rate is associated with physicians in training, loss of resistance with air, 0.5% bupivacaine, assessment of the sensory block with cold, and uterine exteriorization. I have used for 20 years, in a teaching hospital, a pH adjusted solution of 2% lidocaine with epinephrine 1:400,000 with the addition of 10 µg of sufentanil and the incidence of inadequate intraoperative anesthesia was as low as 3% [22].

Among the causes of maternal intraoperative discomfort is the sensation of pressure on the chest and on the abdomen, shivering, nausea and vomiting, and discomfort due to the position on the operating table is worth mentioning.

The sensation of pressure on the chest is usually associated with a sensory block above T2 and this may generate anxiety in the unprepared patient. This sensation may be prevented by carefully titrating the individual dose of local anesthetic solution, extending the block incrementally and frequently checking the block. If it is necessary to obtain a block above T2 to eliminate the occurrence of visceral pain, the patient should be informed to consider this as a "normal effect" of anesthesia.

The sensation of pressure on the abdomen is typically due to the excessive pressure of the obstetric maneuvers during fetal extraction, especially if they are difficult or prolonged. Mothers should always be advised of this possible sensation of pressure during the extraction of the baby and surgeons should always consider the condition of the mother and be as gentle as possible. This sensation is more frequent with epidural rather than with spinal anesthesia, due to a denser sensory block with the latter.

Shivering remains a common symptom after the delivery. It may be a compensatory mechanism for heat loss from increased cutaneous blood flow but its etiology is not well known. If severe, it may lead to significant discomfort for the mother. A force air warmer before and during surgery may be used to reduce this phenomenon [29].

Nausea and vomiting are unpleasant, disturbing symptoms occurring with different frequency during cesarean section under epidural or spinal anesthesia, depending on the technique used and thus on the rapidity of onset of the block, the depth and duration of hypotension (more frequent with spinal), the occurrence of visceral surgical stimuli (such as uterine exteriorization or peritoneal tractions), the patient's position (the Trendelenburg position may favor gastric reflux), and the drug used (opioids, oxytocin, or ergometrine).

Nausea and vomiting, due to relative cerebral hypoxia, are very often the very first symptom of hypotension, especially if they occur immediately after the performance of the anesthetic block.

Causes of intraoperative pain include inadequate block, visceral pain, and shoulder and precordial pain.

Even in the presence of an adequate sensory block provided by a sufficient local anesthetic dose to produce a complete sensory block to T4, sometimes, if peritoneal structures are vigorously stimulated or the uterus is exteriorized, visceral pain may occur. Pain is often preceded by vague symptoms of nausea and discomfort which are indicators of subliminal visceral pain. In these cases, the sensory block should be immediately rechecked and the epidural catheter redosed as necessary. According to the intensity and duration of intraoperative visceral pain a wide range of drugs have been proposed and used, according to local anesthetic practice (such as ev fentanyl, ketamine, propofol, nitrous oxide) but it should be remembered that profound sedation may put the mother at risk if her airways are not secured.

The incidence of visceral pain may be reduced using epidural opioids in the anesthetic mixture.

Another kind of visceral pain that may occur during cesarean section is shoulder pain due to the presence of amniotic fluid or blood in the subdiaphragmatic region. This region is innervated by the phrenic nerve (C3–C5) and therefore this pain cannot be abolished by any safe anesthetic block. It may be prevented by elevating the mother's head by 10 degrees to reduce the cephalad spread of the fluids [30].

Precordial pain, mostly due to venous air embolism (VAE), has also been reported during cesarean section under regional anesthesia. A negative pressure gradient between the uterus and the heart due to the Trendelenburg position or to the exteriorization of the uterus may predispose to VAE and therefore the simultaneous performance of these two maneuvers should be banned [31].

5.2.5 Epidural Postoperative Analgesia

For this topic, please refer to Chap. 11.

5.3   Extension of a Preexisting Epidural Analgesia

The use of epidural analgesia during labor offers the possibility of rapid extension of the block in the case of emergency cesarean section by the injection through the catheter of a dose of a local anesthetic of a suitable concentration for surgical anesthesia. This is most important considering the consequences of possible complications during an urgent induction of general anesthesia, including a difficult or failed intubation combined with a significantly reduced maternal oxygen reserve and a high risk of regurgitation and aspiration.

The conversion of epidural labor analgesia to surgical anesthesia for cesarean section was first reported by Milne and Lawson in 1973 [32] who reported that 93% of parturients underwent successful epidural extension using 2% lidocaine with 1:200,000 epinephrine.

The current literature does not strongly support one particular epidural top-up solution when converting labor epidural analgesia to epidural anesthesia for surgery. Meta-analysis of the few trials investigating this topic although limited by both small numbers of studies and methodological variance [33] indicates that bupivacaine or levobupivacaine 0.5% is the least efficacious solution with respect to both the speed of onset and quality of block, while lidocaine 2% with epinephrine, with or without fentanyl, produces the fastest onset of surgical block. Establishment of a sensory block is more rapid with chloroprocaine [34], but the difference is clinically small and this agent is not available in Europe.

At our institution, we only use a pH adjusted solution of lidocaine 2% with epinephrine solution to augment labor epidurals for emergency cesarean section and this practice is similar to that of other European colleagues [35–37].

The success rate of epidural conversion to anesthesia is usually high [38], however, even a small percentage of failures or inadequacies in extending the block for an emergency cesarean section may not be tolerable and therefore the importance of maintaining effective epidural labor analgesia should be highlighted, frequently checking the efficiency of the block during labor, not solely for the purpose of providing analgesia, but, more importantly, to increase the success rate of conversion to epidural surgical anesthesia should an emergency or unplanned cesarean section become necessary.

Inadequate labor epidural is associated with inadequate epidural extension for cesarean [38] and there are some factors, such as obesity [39] that may be associated with a higher failure rate.

Whether the top-up should be administered in the delivery room or in the surgical theater is controversial and depends on the local hospital organization. Extending the block in the delivery room might save time, but maternal monitoring may be suboptimal when the risk of high block or systemic local anesthetic toxicity is greatest. Waiting until arrival in theater before starting to extend the block can facilitate obstetrician impatience and a call for general anesthesia. A compromise may be to administer a small initial dose in the delivery room (such as the test dose) and to proceed to the full extension of the block in the surgical theater by using 5 mL increments as needed.

5.4 Combined Spinal Epidural Anesthesia (CSEA)

"By combining the two methods many of the disadvantages of both methods are eliminated and their advantages are enhanced to an almost incredible degree" with these words Angelo Luigi Soresi, an Italian surgeon settled in the USA, introduced the "episubdural anesthesia" in 1937 [40]. This procedure involved use of the same needle for both the epidural and the subarachnoid injection.

In theory, the combination of two different routes of anesthesia administration on the same patient improves effectiveness and reduces side effects. The spinal anesthesia component provides fast and reliable segmental anesthesia with minimal risk of toxicity, while the epidural anesthesia component may contribute, if necessary, to intraoperative anesthesia, may be used to maintain anesthesia in the case of prolonged surgery and may be used for excellent analgesia in the postoperative period.

5.5 Technique

5.5.1 Needle-Through-Needle

This is the most widely used CSEA technique. An epidural needle is used to identify the epidural space according to the previously described technique. A long spinal needle is then passed through the epidural needle into the subarachnoid space and the subarachnoid block performed. After the removal of the spinal needle, an epidural catheter is placed and can be used subsequently.

The spinal needle must be long enough to extend beyond the tip of the epidural needle to reliably puncture the dura and therefore special needles have been designed specifically for this technique. A minimum of 13 mm length of the spinal needle protrusion beyond the epidural needle tip is recommended for the CSEA sets for a reasonably high success rate [41].

During the needle-through-needle technique, the epidural needle acts as the spinal needle introducer and therefore the spinal needle is poorly anchored and inadvertent spinal needle displacement during injection may occur. For this reason some commercial kits include spinal needles with Luer-locks or other devices to allow fixation to the epidural needle to reduce the risk of spinal needle displacement during intrathecal injection with the subsequent risk of failure of spinal anesthesia.

The epidural needle can also be modified to facilitate the procedure with the addition of a small hole at the tip to minimize damage of the spinal needle or with the addition of "backeyes" or holes in the greater curvature to allow the epidural catheter to be inserted away from the dural puncture site.

The addition of a separate conduit for the spinal needle has also been described. These needles have been designed with two barrels: one for the performance of the spinal component and the other for the passage of the epidural catheter, allowing the separation of the sites of dural puncture and epidural catheter placement. However, they are not commonly used.

Once having injected the spinal anesthetic dose, in the case of difficulties in placing or replacing the epidural catheter, the spinal block inevitably starts developing before the completion of the procedure.

Parturients undergoing cesarean section are at particular risk as onset of subarachnoid block is fast and hypotension may occur rapidly. Hyperbaric local anesthetic solutions are frequently used and any delay in positioning the patient can potentially lead to unilateral or too low a block depending on the patient's position. In my practice this problem is easily overcome by rolling the patient onto the other side immediately after the end of the procedure in the case of the block being performed in the lateral position. If the performance of the block is carried out in the sitting position, the patient can be positioned in the Trendelenburg position to extend the block until an adequate anesthetic spread occurs.

5.5.2 Separate Needle

This technique uses two separate needles to perform the spinal and epidural components of the CSEA. Both needles can be inserted at the same vertebral interspace or at two separate interspaces. The spinal and epidural components of the CSEA can be performed in either order.

The major advantage of performing the epidural component first is the chance to test the epidural catheter before the occurrence of the spinal block, since the location of the epidural catheter cannot be tested with the needle-through-needle technique after the injection of the spinal anesthetic dose. The advantage of performing the spinal component first may also be that the rapid onset of analgesia reduces the risk of the patient moving during the subsequent insertion of the epidural needle.

Although a higher rate of failure of the spinal component with the needle-through-needle technique has been reported [42], in experienced hands, there are most likely no differences between the two techniques even if the needle-through-needle technique is associated with greater patient satisfaction (only one puncture) and may be quicker to perform.

5.5.3 Epidural Test Dose After CSEA

When spinal block is established before placing an epidural catheter, a conventional epidural 'test dose' cannot be interpreted and may be potentially dangerous by extending subarachnoid block. In theory, the test dose could be delayed until subarachnoid block is regressing but this interrupts analgesia and correct interpretation remains difficult if residual block persists.

The problem cannot be avoided using needle-through-needle technique but may be if the separate-needle technique is used and the epidural catheter is placed and tested before subarachnoid block. However, this may often be impractical and time consuming.

Problems with test doses may lead to greater reliance on negative aspiration tests to confirm epidural catheter placement. It is self-evident, therefore, that all boluses injected into an epidural catheter after CSEA should be regarded as a test dose and of such a nature that unintentional subarachnoid administration will not be dangerous and neural blockade should be monitored rigorously after boluses.

5.5.4   Anesthetic Solution

CSEA may be used in two different ways:

(1) Surgical anesthesia is provided exclusively by the spinal component of the block and the epidural catheter is eventually used for postoperative analgesia or in the case of insufficient spinal block or prolonged surgery ("parachute" usage). In this case the local anesthetic solution used for the spinal component is equal to that used for the single shot spinal technique and the prevention and treatment of maternal hypotension is also similar (see also Chap. 4).

(2) A small spinal dose is administered to develop a low block, and this is eventually extended by using the epidural catheter to gradually achieve an adequate level of surgical anesthesia ("sequential CSE") [43].

In this case a dense sacral anesthesia associated to a slow onset of the anesthetic block is obtained. This technique may be particularly suitable for patients with cardiac disease or to avoid maternal hypotension since it minimizes sympathetic blockade.

The disadvantage of the sequential technique is that adequate block takes longer to be produced than with full doses, making it unsuitable for urgent surgery.

5.6   CSEA vs. Epidural or Spinal Block

Neither epidural nor subarachnoid blockade are able to totally abolish neural transmission in the anesthetized regions. One study compared the two techniques [44] using a double catheter technique to evaluate electrical sensory thresholds with epidural, subarachnoid, or CSEA blocks. CSEA raised sensory thresholds more than spinal or epidural block suggesting that CSEA may produce a physiologically denser block than either technique alone, but whether this may be of any clinical benefit is not known.

References

1. Pages MF. Segmental anestesia. Rev Sanid Mil. 1921;11:351–65.
2. Dogliotti AM. Research and clinical observations on spinal anesthesia: with special reference to the peridural technique. Anesth Analg. 1933;12:59–65.
3. Graffagnino P, Seyler LW. Anesth Analg. 1939;18:48–51.
4. Dogliotti AM. Trattato di anestesia. Torino: UTET; 1935.
5. Moore DC. Regional block. Springfield: CH Thomas Publisher; 1953.
6. Bonica JJ. The management of pain. Philadelphia: Lea & Febiger; 1953.
7. Bromage PR. Epidural analgesia. 2nd ed. Philadelphia: WB Saunders Company; 1978.
8. Tsen LC. Neuraxial techniques for labor analgesia should be placed in the lateral position. Int J Obstet Anesth. 2008;17:146–52.
9. Hamilton CL, Riley ET, Cohen SE. Changes in the position of epidural catheters associated with patient movement. Anesthesiology. 1997;86:778–84.
10. Hamza J, Smida M, Benhamou D, et al. Parturient's posture during epidural puncture affects the distance from skin to epidural space. J Clin Anesth. 1995;7:1–4.
11. Vincent RD, Chestnut DH. Which position is more comfortable for the parturient during identification of the epidural space? Int J Obstet Anesth. 1991;1:9–11.
12. Kim SH, Kim DY, Han JI, et al. Vertebral level of Tuffier's line measured by ultrasonography in parturients in the lateral decubitus position. Korean J Anesthesiol. 2014;67:181–5.
13. Beilin Y, Bernstein HH, Zucker-Pinchoff B. The optimal distance that a multiorifice epidural catheter should be threaded into the epidural space. Anesth Analg. 1995;81:301–3.
14. Dogliotti AM. Segmental peridural spinal anesthesia. A new method of block anesthesia. Am J Surg. 1933. April, 04
15. Grau T, Leipold RW, Horter J, et al. The lumbar epidural space in pregnancy : visualization by ultrasonography. Br J Anaesth. 2001;86:798–804.
16. Grau T, Bartusseck E, Conradi R, et al. Ultrasound imaging improves learning curves in obstetric epidural anesthesia: a preliminary study. Can J Anaesth. 2003;50:1047–50.
17. Balki M, Lee Y, Halpern S, et al. Ultrasound imaging of the lumbar spine in the transverse plane: the correlation between estimated and actual depth to the epidural space in obese parturients. Anesth Analg. 2009;108:1876–81.
18. Carvalho JC. Ultrasound-facilitated epidurals and spinals in obstetrics. Anesthesiol Clin. 2008;26:145–58.
19. Carmocia M. Testing the epidural catheter. Curr Opin Anaesthesiol. 2009;22:336–40.
20. Guay J. The epidural test dose: a review. Anesth Analg. 2006;102:921–9.
21. Camorcia M, Capogna G. Sensory assessment of epidural block for caesarean section: a systematic comparison of pinprick, cold and touch sensation. Eur J Anaesthesiol. 2006;23:611–7.
22. Capogna G, Celleno D, Costantino P. Alkalinization improves the quality of lidocaine-fentanyl epidural anaesthesia for caesarean section. Can J Anaesth. 1993;40:425–30.
23. Mercier F. Cesarean delivery fluid management. Curr Opin Anesthesiol. 2012;25:286–91.
24. Veeser M, Hofman T, Toth R, et al. Vasopressors for the management of hypotension after spinal anesthesia for elective caesarean section. Systematic review and cumulative meta-analysis. Acta Anaesthesiol Scand. 2012;56:810–6.
25. Lee A, Ngan Kee WD, Gin T. A quantitative, systematic review of randomized controlled trials of ephedrine versus phenylephrine for the management of hypotension during spinal anesthesia for cesarean delivery. Anesth Analg. 2002;94:920–6.
26. Robson SC, Boys RJ, Rodeck C, Morgan B. Maternal and fetal haemodynamic effects of spinal and extradural anaesthesia for elective caesarean section. Br J Anaesth. 1992;68:54–9.
27. Alahuhta S, Kangas-Saarela T, Hollmén AI, et al. Visceral pain during caesarean section under spinal and epidural anaesthesia with bupivacaine. Acta Anaesthesiol Scand. 1990;34:95–9.
28. Capogna G, Celleno D. Improving epidural anesthesia during cesarean section: causes of maternal discomfort or pain during surgery. Int J Obstet Anesth. 1994;3:149–52.

29. Horn EP, Schroeder F, Gottschalk A, et al. Active warming during cesarean delivery. Anesth Analg. 2002;94:409–15.
30. Skikuchi C, Tonozaki S, Gi E, et al. Shoulder-tip pain during cesarean section under combined spinal-epidural anesthesia. Masui. 2014;63:149–52.
31. Kim CS, Liu J, Know JY, et al. Venous air embolism during surgery, especially cesarean delivery. J Korean Med Sci. 2008;23:753–61.
32. Milne MK, Lawson JI. Epidural analgesia for caesarean section. A review of 182 cases. Br J Anaesth. 1973;45:1206–10.
33. Hillyard SG, Bate TE, Corcoran TB, et al. Extending epidural analgesia for emergency caesarean section: a meta-analysis. Br J Anaesth. 2011;107:668–78.
34. Gaiser RR, Cheek TG, Gutsche BB. Epidural lidocaine versus 2-chloroprocaine for fetal distress requiring urgent cesarean section. Int J Obstet Anesth. 1994;3:208–10.
35. Malhotra S, Yentis S, Lucas N. Extending epidural analgesia for emergency caesarean section. Br J Anaesth. 2012;108:879–80.
36. Allam J, Malhotra S, Hemingway C, et al. Epidural lidocaine–bicarbonate–adrenaline vs levobupivacaine for emergency caesarean section: a randomized controlled trial. Anaesthesia. 2008;63(243-9):37.
37. Tortosa JC, Parry NS, Mercier FJ. Efficacy of augmentation of epidural analgesia for caesarean section. Br J Anaesth. 2003;91:532–5.
38. Dc C, Tan T. Conversion of epidural labour analgesia to epidural anesthesia for intrapartum cesarean delivery. Can J Anaesth. 2009;56:19–26.
39. Eley V, Van Zundert A, Callaway L. What is the failure rate in extending labour analgesia in patients with a body mass index $\geq$ 40 kg/m^{2}compared with patients with a body mass index $<$ 30 kg/m^2? A retrospective pilot study. BMC Anesthesiol. 2015;15:115.
40. Soresi AL. Episubdural anesthesia. Anesth Analg. 1937;16:306–10.
41. Joshi GP, McCaroll MC. Evaluation of combined spinal-epidural anesthesia using two different techniques. Reg Anesth. 1994;19:169–74.
42. Lyons G, Macdonald R, Mikl B. Combined epidural-spinal anaesthesia for caesarean section. Through the needle or in separate spaces? Anaesthesia. 1992;47:199–201.
43. Rawal N, Schollin J, Wesstrom G. Epidural versus spinal epidural block for caesarean section. Acta Anaesthesiol Scand. 1988;32:61–6.
44. Dirkes WE, Rosenberg J, Lund C, Kehlet H. The effect of subarachnoid lidocaine and combined subarachnoid lidocaine and epidural bupivacaine on electrical sensory thresholds. Reg Anesth. 1991;16:262–4.

General Anaesthesia for Caesarean Section

6

Pierre Diemunsch and Eric Noll

6.1 Introduction

Caesarean section delivery consists of birth after surgical laparotomy and hysterotomy. Originally only used as a life-saving procedure for the mother and child, its use has increased with the progression of both obstetrical and anesthesiological arts [1]. It is a common procedure for many anaesthesiologists as part of their daily or on call activities because of its high frequency in most developed countries. In the United States, the rate of birth through caesarean delivery has constantly increased, over the last decade [2]. Additionally, the rate of caesarean delivery in the United States was 32.9% [2] in 2009, corresponding to an absolute number of approximately one million births per year. In England, NHS trusts reports the rate of caesarean section delivery for singleton pregnancies at 24% in 2008 [3], corresponding to more than 147,000 interventions. Numerous reasons are involved in the increasing proportion of caesarean section delivery, including maternal, obstetrical, foetal, and environmental aspects [4], but a clearly defined reason for the underlying pattern remains a challenge [5, 6].

In developed countries, caesarean indications can be divided into two main categories: scheduled caesarean section and emergency caesarean section. Scheduled caesarean sections are indicated in cases of anticipated maternal, foetal, or obstetrician reasons, such as a prior uterine incision, prior dystocia, suspected macrosomia, or maternal request. Emergency caesarean sections are performed in acutely evolving situations, for example, foetal intolerance of labour or impairment of maternal status.

Despite being a major factor of improvement for neonatal, maternal, and foetal morbidity and mortality [1], caesarean section delivery, as a rescue therapy in many

P. Diemunsch (✉) • E. Noll
Service d'Anesthésie—Réanimation Chirurgicale, Hôpitaux de Hautepierre,
CCOM-Illkirch et CMCO-Schiltigheim, Strasbourg, France
e-mail: pierre.diemunsch@chru-strasbourg.fr

© Springer International Publishing Switzerland 2017
G. Capogna (ed.), *Anesthesia for Cesarean Section*,
DOI 10.1007/978-3-319-42053-0_6

85

pathological cases, is associated with higher morbidity and mortality than vaginal delivery [7, 8].

Anaesthesia for caesarean section can involve neuraxial (spinal/epidural) analgesia or general anaesthesia. Neuraxial techniques are predominantly used for caesarean section delivery [9] because of the several advantages compared to general anaesthesia, which include limited systemic drug exposure for both the mother and child, limited airway management issues, and allowance of the mother to actively experience her child's birth. However, general anaesthesia may be the preferred choice in certain situations like profound foetal bradycardia, ruptured uterus, severe haemorrhage, placental abruption, umbilical cord prolapse, and preterm footling breech [10].

Considering the overwhelming majority of neuraxial-based anaesthesia for caesarean section in the actual clinical setting, it is challenging to broadly gain and maintain skills in performing general anaesthesia-based caesarean delivery.

6.2   Preanaesthesia Assessment for General Anaesthesia Caesarean Section

As standard of care for every anesthesiological case, a focused history and physical examination should be conducted prior to any procedure initiation [10, 11]. Particularly in the comfortable setting of scheduled caesarean section delivery, preanaesthesia assessment should include maternal health and anaesthetic history, baseline blood pressure measurement, and an airway, heart, and lung examination.

Airway management issues should be meticulously anticipated. Unfortunately, pregnant women have several criteria for intubation-related morbidity. Pregnancy-induced anatomical changes on the airway increase the Mallampati class and the likelihood of airway bleeding or swelling [12–15]. Breast hypertrophy can alter the laryngoscope's insertion. Apnoea tolerance time is decreased due to the reduced functional residual capacity [15]. Gastric reflux can occur due to a reduced lower oesophageal sphincter tone and horizontalization of the stomach since gastric emptying can be delayed during labour. All these factors lead to an increased risk for pulmonary aspiration of the gastric content which is of higher volume and lower pH due to the placental gastrine-like activity.

The Obstetric Anaesthetists Association and the Difficult Airway Society developed guidelines for the management of difficult and failed tracheal intubation in obstetrics [15]. They recommend a thorough airway assessment for any possible criteria of difficult tracheal intubation, mask ventilation, and supraglottic airway device insertion. Oral piercing and haircut support devices should be removed before the initiation of anaesthesia. Concerning fasting for elective caesarean delivery, food should be withheld for at least 6 h before anaesthesia and clear liquids 2 h before surgery (in the absence of any risk factors for delayed gastric clearance). In case of doubt, an US evaluation of the stomach will provide information about the volume and the type of the gastric content.

Strategies for bleeding management should also be clearly anticipated by evaluating particularly the obstetrical risk factors for perioperative bleeding, the ease of venous access, preoperative blood type and screen, the blood product availability, and transfusion equipment availability. Caesarean delivery comes with an increased bleeding risk compared with vaginal delivery [16]. The precise criteria for preoperative assessment of blood type and screen or cross-match are not consensual. In our institution, however, it is done for every caesarean section delivery.

In the case of general anaesthesia for caesarean section, the risk–benefit assessment and discussion should be clearly documented. The reasons for avoiding neuraxial anaesthesia should be especially listed and explained to the patient. The patient should also be informed the procedural implications (e.g. preoperative fasting, operative day timeline, and postoperative recovery) and risks of general anaesthesia prior to obtaining consent. Particularly, the risk ratio of general versus neuraxial anaesthesia (i.e., 1.7) should be mentioned and explained in the context of the actual situation. Additionally, the anaesthesiology strategy should be communicated early to the obstetrical team.

In case of emergency caesarean delivery, whatever the indication, the preanaesthesia assessment should not be disregarded in order to gain a few seconds, but rather be pragmatically conducted to promptly ensure that all key safety points are gathered prior to anaesthesia initiation.

6.3 Procedural Aspects of Caesarean Delivery Under General Anaesthesia

6.3.1 Premedication

The goal of maternal premedication is to reduce the gastric content and increase gastric pH to minimize the potential damage in cases of pulmonary aspiration. H_2 receptor antagonists can be administered the night before and 2 h before anaesthesia [15]. Prokinetic drugs like metoclopramide [17] may be considered to improve gastric emptying. Ingestion of a clear, non-particulate solution of sodium citrate may help buffer gastric contents.

6.3.2 Preoperative Setup

Patients should be preferably laid in the left lateral decubitus position until placed supine on the operating table with a left uterine displacement.

When possible, some procedures should be anticipated in a warm and comfortable setting. These include bladder catheterization, peripheral venous access, and compression stockings placement. Though historically administered after umbilical cord clamping to minimize foetal exposure, the UK National Institute for Health and Clinical Excellence guidelines for caesarean section now recommend "appropriate prophylactic antibiotics before skin incision" in accordance with evidence showing reduced maternal infectious morbidity without negative foetal consequences [18–23]. Also, in cases of scheduled caesarean section, the foetal heart rate should be monitored before anaesthesia initiation.

6.3.3 Intraoperative Positioning

Patients should be placed supine on the operating table with left uterine displacement. If possible, the operating table should have a left lateral tilt of 15° [18].

In order to facilitate the laryngoscope introduction, and improve laryngoscopic view [24], functional residual capacity [25], and apnoea tolerance time [26, 27], the patient may be placed in a 20–30° head-up position.

6.3.4 Patient Monitoring

Standard general monitoring should be used, including ECG, non-invasive blood pressure, pulse oximetry, and capnography. The use of an EEG-derived depth of anaesthesia monitoring device to prevent awareness and recollection during caesarean delivery under general anaesthesia is still a topic of debate and investigation [28–30]. Peripheral nerve stimulators should be available and used after induction to assess neuromuscular transmission abolition as well as recovery.

In order to minimize the time between anaesthesia induction and delivery, the patient's abdomen should be prepared and draped prior to initiation of the general anaesthesia. In every situation and particularly in the stressful and complicated context of emergency caesarean sections, the World Health Organization's Surgical Safety Checklist should be completed [31]. In this situation, particular attention is paid to the items concerning difficult airway, aspiration, and blood loss, for strategy planning and assistance availability.

In addition to the preparation and monitoring of the mother, the anaesthesiologist should make sure the neonatal resuscitation team is prepared to receive and care for the newborn.

6.3.5 Anaesthesia Induction

Preoxygenation should be performed to lengthen the time of safe apnoea. Preoxygenation requires that a high fresh high gas flow ($\geq$10 l.min^{-1}) of 100% oxygen be applied to the respiratory circuit [32]. Gas leaks should be minimized with a tight mask-to-face seal. End-tidal oxygen fraction ($F_{ET}O2$) $\geq$0.9 is an optimal endpoint for efficient preoxygenation [15] and should be obtained within 2–3 min. The place of the THRIVE oxygenation method is of the highest interest in difficult situations but is not yet specifically validated in obstetrics.

After the preoxygenation sequence is performed, a rapid sequence induction is initiated to minimize the risk of gastric content aspiration until intubation is secured. To be properly performed, this requires at least two persons. The rapid sequence induction begins with the application of the Sellick's manoeuvre as the induction agents are administered. Induction agents include a hypnotic drug and a myorelaxant. The most commonly used hypnotic agent is thiopental (4–5 mg.kg^{-1}). A survey by the UK Obstetric Anaesthetists Association in 2011 concerning the current choice for induction and inhalation agents [33] found that thiopental was the routine induction agent for 93% of the responders. It has been substituted by propofol (2–3 mg.kg^{-1}) in many US and European institutions due to thiopental shortage. In case of maternal haemodynamic instability, ketamine (1–1.5 mg.kg^{-1}) or etomidate (0.3 mg.kg^{-1}) should be considered for hypnosis. Etomidate may promote neonatal hypoglycemia and the paediatric team should be informed of its use.

The most commonly used myorelaxant for these situations is succinylcholine (1–1.5 mg.kg^{-1}) because of its rapid onset of action and short span of duration. Rocuronium (1–1.2 mg.kg^{-1}) may be an alternate medication for rapid onset of myorelaxation. If needed, this aminosteroid compound can be reversed by sugammadex (16 mg.kg^{-1}).

After loss of consciousness, cricoid pressure should be increased from 10 N to 30 N. The master algorithm guidelines (Fig. 6.1) of the Obstetric Anaesthetists' Association and the Difficult Airway Society state that facemask ventilation with a maximal ventilation pressure <20 cmH$_2$O may be considered [15]. To improve the intubation success rate and to limit trauma, a reduced tracheal size tube (6.0–7.0 mm, inner diameter) should be preferred [15] and a soft intubation stylet is used as a routine in many institutions. A difficult intubation cart and a video laryngoscope should be readily available.

Tracheal intubations should be confirmed successful using capnography trace inspection, thorax inspection, and auscultation. Additionally, the management of

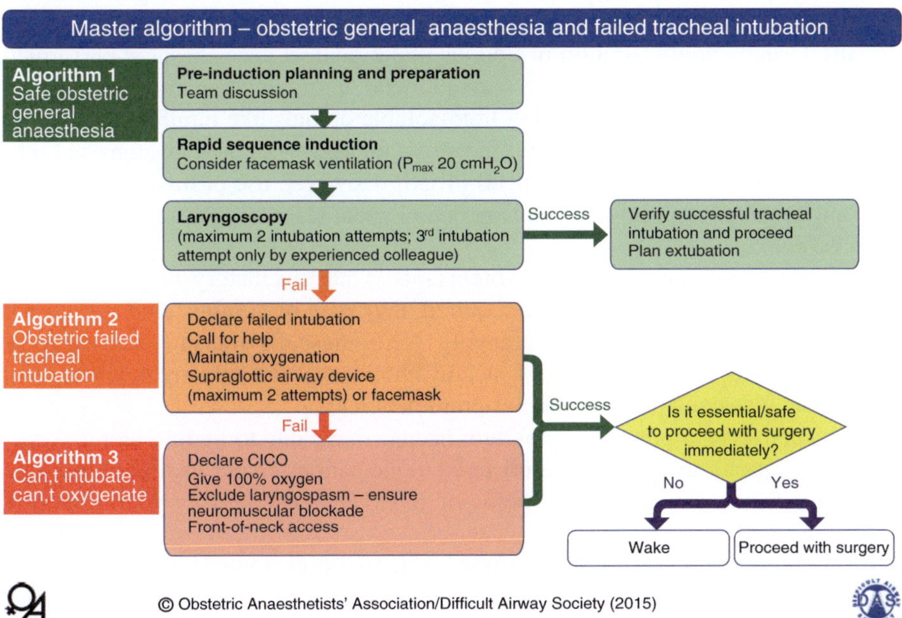

Fig. 6.1 Master algorithm—obstetric general anaesthesia and failed intubation. The *yellow diamond* represents a decision-making step. P$_{max}$, maximal inflation pressure; CICO, "can't intubate, can't oxygenate". The algorithms and tables are reproduced with permission from the OAA and DAS and are available online in pdf and PowerPoint formats

failed tracheal intubation and "can't intubate, can't oxygenate" scenarios are detailed in the Obstetric Anaesthetist Association and the Difficult Airway Society algorithms [15]. There is a strong emphasis on the importance of a supraglottic airway device placement for proper oxygenation after two or at the most three intubation attempts. Once oxygenation is secured, tracheal intubation via the supraglottic airway device is performed, best under bronchoscopic visual control.

6.3.6 Anaesthesia Maintenance

Anaesthetic maintenance requires optimal maternal and foetal oxygenation, normocapnia, avoidance of awareness and recall, optimal surgical conditions, maternal comfort, and unimpaired uterine tone [4]. In our institution, we maintain an FiO_2 of 100% until clamping of the umbilical vessels. Ventilation settings are aimed to maintain normocapnia (corresponding to a $PaCO_2$ of 30 to 32 mmHg at term).

In 2011, a UK Obstetric Anaesthetists Association survey found that volatile halogenated anaesthetics were used in 98.8% of the cases. Experimental [34] and clinical [35] data suggest that volatile halogenated anaesthetic requirements are reduced during pregnancy. Volatile halogenated anaesthetic concentration should not exceed one minimum alveolar concentration (MAC). Higher doses of volatile halogenated anaesthetics may not be given before delivery to avoid significant foetal depression and after delivery to prevent myometrial contraction alteration [4, 36–38]. Usually administration of opioids under general anaesthesia is performed only after umbilical cord clamping to avoid foetal opioid impregnation. Recently, it has been suggested that short-acting lipid-soluble opioids like remifentanil at general anaesthesia induction may limit the stress induced with laryngoscopy in high-risk patients (e.g. severe preeclampsia) [4, 36]. However, use of this strategy must be complemented with informing the neonatological team so as to adjust their neonatal care.

The use of non-depolarizing myorelaxants is not mandatory to proceed with good surgical comfort. However, if required, they may be administered and do not cross the placenta in significant amounts. Neuromuscular transmission recovery should always be monitored, even if succinylcholine was the only myorelaxant used (to rule out plasmatic pseudocholynesterase deficiency).

After delivery, to prevent postpartum haemorrhage due to uterine atony, uterotonic medications are usually administered to the patient. In our institution we routinely administer an initial slow bolus of oxytocin after delivery followed by a continuous perfusion.

Any hypotension should be promptly treated with phenylephrine or in case of low heart rate, with ephedrine titration. The use of fluid therapy is also usually beneficial to treat hypotension. Glucose-free crystalloid solutions are preferred since they do not promote neonatal hypoglycaemia.

It is important to record the anaesthesia induction to umbilical cord clamping time interval and the hysterotomy to extraction time interval. Ideally, these intervals should stay below 30 min and 180 sec, respectively.

6.3.7 Emergence from Anaesthesia

Emergence from anaesthesia must be prepared with the initiation of postoperative analgesia taking any comorbidities into account. Paracetamol, ketoprofene, and rescue therapy with IV morphine titration during the PACU stay, and oral morphine after PACU (Post Anaesthesia Care Unit) discharge can be considered as analgesic strategies.

As part of the "End of Procedure" checklist and before initiating awakening, both the obstetrician and the anaesthesiologist should share critical information, including the absence of residual bleeding and maternal stability status.

After the patient is cleared for awakening, the appropriate reversal of all neuromuscular blocking agents should be assessed.

It must be remembered that a significant part of the anaesthesia-related complications, particularly pulmonary aspiration, may occur during extubation and postoperative care [15, 39, 40]. In case of hypertensive disorder of pregnancy and/or after a difficult intubation with several attempts, a leak test should be performed before considering extubation. Where the risk for a potentially difficult reintubation is present, an airway exchange catheter may be left in place for 2–4 h following removal of the tracheal tube [41].

After a caesarean section under general anaesthesia, the early contact with the baby, with early breast-feeding where appropriate, is an important part of the general enhanced recovery programme.

> **Conclusion**
>
> General anaesthesia for caesarean section is a challenging scenario that the majority of the anaesthesiologists may have to manage although its occurence became rare when compared with spinal or epidural techniques. Two different clinical vignettes can summarize the most frequent cases: the scheduled caesarean delivery for non-favourable vaginal delivery planning and the emergency caesarean procedure for severe altered foetal or maternal status. If the operational procedure for both situations is similar, the environmental system differs dramatically. The holy grail of the emergency caesarean delivery is to combine a very short decision-to-delivery time period and maximizing the safety of every procedure step. To achieve this goal, optimal teaching aims at reducing the risk of cognitive overload by mastering the different technical and non-technical skills involved. Improving the initial teaching and skill retention is particularly important given the low number of general anaesthesia for caesarean section an anesthesiologist has to give in the actual context.

References

1. Gibbons L, Belizan JM, Lauer JA, Betran AP, Merialdi M, Althabe F. Inequitics in the use of cesarean section deliveries in the world. Am J Obstet Gynecol. 2012;206:331. e1–19
2. Kochanek KD, Kirmeyer SE, Martin JA, Strobino DM, Guyer B. Annual summary of vital statistics: 2009. Pediatrics. 2012;129:338–48.

3. Bragg F, Cromwell DA, Edozien LC, Gurol-Urganci I, Mahmood TA, Templeton A, van der Meulen JH. Variation in rates of caesarean section among English NHS trusts after accounting for maternal and clinical risk: cross sectional study. BMJ. 2010;341:c5065.

4. Tsen LC. Anesthesia for ceasarian delivery, Chestnut's Obstetric Anesthesia: Principles and Practice. 5th ed. Elsevier. pp. 545–603.

5. Hanley GE, Janssen PA, Greyson D. Regional variation in the cesarean delivery and assisted vaginal delivery rates. Obstet Gynecol. 2010;115:1201–8.

6. Clark SL, Belfort MA, Hankins GDV, Meyers JA, Houser FM. Variation in the rates of operative delivery in the United States. Am J Obstet Gynecol. 2007;196:526. e1–5

7. Pallasmaa N, Ekblad U, Gissler M. Severe maternal morbidity and the mode of delivery. Acta Obstet Gynecol Scand. 2008;87:662–8.

8. van Dillen J, Zwart JJ, Schutte J, Bloemenkamp KWM, van Roosmalen J. Severe acute maternal morbidity and mode of delivery in the Netherlands. Acta Obstet Gynecol Scand. 2010;89:1460–5.

9. Bucklin BA, Hawkins JL, Anderson JR, Ullrich FA. Obstetric anesthesia workforce survey: twenty-year update. Anesthesiology. 2005;103:645–53.

10. Practice guidelines for obstetric anesthesia: an updated report by the American Society of Anesthesiologists Task Force on obstetric anesthesia and the Society for Obstetric Anesthesia and Perinatology. Anesthesiology. 2016;124:270–300.

11. Committee on Standards and Practice Parameters, Apfelbaum JL, Connis RT, Nickinovich DG, American Society of Anesthesiologists Task Force on Preanesthesia Evaluation, Pasternak LR, Arens JF, Caplan RA, Connis RT, Fleisher LA, Flowerdew R, Gold BS, Mayhew JF, Nickinovich DG, Rice LJ, Roizen MF, Twersky RS. Practice advisory for preanesthesia evaluation: an updated report by the American Society of Anesthesiologists Task Force on preanesthesia evaluation. Anesthesiology. 2012;116:522–38.

12. Pilkington S, Carli F, Dakin MJ, Romney M, De Witt KA, Doré CJ, Cormack RS. Increase in Mallampati score during pregnancy. Br J Anaesth. 1995;74:638–42.

13. Kodali B-S, Chandrasekhar S, Bulich LN, Topulos GP, Datta S. Airway changes during labor and delivery. Anesthesiology. 2008;108:357–62.

14. Leboulanger N, Louvet N, Rigouzzo A, de Mesmay M, Louis B, Farrugia M, Girault L, Ramirez A, Constant I, Jouannic J-M, Fauroux B. Pregnancy is associated with a decrease in pharyngeal but not tracheal or laryngeal cross-sectional area: a pilot study using the acoustic reflection method. Int J Obstet Anesth. 2014;23:35–9.

15. Mushambi MC, Kinsella SM, Popat M, Swales H, Ramaswamy KK, Winton AL, Quinn AC. Obstetric Anaesthetists' association, difficult airway society: obstetric Anaesthetists' association and difficult airway society guidelines for the management of difficult and failed tracheal intubation in obstetrics. Anaesthesia. 2015;70:1286–306.

16. Al-Zirqi I, Vangen S, Forsen L, Stray-Pedersen B. Prevalence and risk factors of severe obstetric haemorrhage. BJOG. 2008;115:1265–72.

17. Murphy DF, Nally B, Gardiner J, Unwin A. Effect of metoclopramide on gastric emptying before elective and emergency caesarean section. Br J Anaesth. 1984;56:1113–6.

18. Soltanifar S, Russell R. The National Institute for health and clinical excellence (NICE) guidelines for caesarean section, 2011 update: implications for the anaesthetist. Int J Obstet Anesth. 2012;21:264–72.

19. Gordon HR, Phelps D, Blanchard K. Prophylactic cesarean section antibiotics: maternal and neonatal morbidity before or after cord clamping. Obstet Gynecol. 1979;53:151–6.

20. Sullivan SA, Smith T, Chang E, Hulsey T, Vandorsten JP, Soper D. Administration of cefazolin prior to skin incision is superior to cefazolin at cord clamping in preventing postcesarean infectious morbidity: a randomized, controlled trial. Am J Obstet Gynecol. 2007;196:455. e1–5

21. Thigpen BD, Hood WA, Chauhan S, Bufkin L, Bofill J, Magann E, Morrison JC. Timing of prophylactic antibiotic administration in the uninfected laboring gravida: a randomized clinical trial. Am J Obstet Gynecol. 2005;192:1864–8. discussion 1868–71

22. Wax JR, Hersey K, Philput C, Wright MS, Nichols KV, Eggleston MK, Smith JF. Single dose cefazolin prophylaxis for postcesarean infections: before vs. after cord clamping. J Matern Fetal Med. 1997;6:61–5.

23. Yildirim G, Gungorduk K, Guven HZ, Aslan H, Celikkol O, Sudolmus S, Ceylan Y. When should we perform prophylactic antibiotics in elective cesarean cases? Arch Gynecol Obstet. 2009;280:13–8.
24. Lee BJ, Kang JM, Kim DO. Laryngeal exposure during laryngoscopy is better in the 25 degrees back-up position than in the supine position. Br J Anaesth. 2007;99:581–6.
25. Hignett R, Fernando R, McGlennan A, McDonald S, Stewart A, Columb M, Adamou T, Dilworth P. A randomized crossover study to determine the effect of a 30° head-up versus a supine position on the functional residual capacity of term parturients. Anesth Analg. 2011;113:1098–102.
26. Lane S, Saunders D, Schofield A, Padmanabhan R, Hildreth A, Laws D. A prospective, randomised controlled trial comparing the efficacy of pre-oxygenation in the 20 degrees head-up vs supine position. Anaesthesia. 2005;60:1064–7.
27. Ramkumar V, Umesh G, Philip FA. Preoxygenation with 20° head-up tilt provides longer duration of non-hypoxic apnea than conventional preoxygenation in non-obese healthy adults. J Anesth. 2011;25:189–94.
28. Zand F, Hadavi SMR, Chohedri A, Sabetian P. Survey on the adequacy of depth of anaesthesia with bispectral index and isolated forearm technique in elective caesarean section under general anaesthesia with sevoflurane. Br J Anaesth. 2014;112:871–8.
29. Robins K, Lyons G. Intraoperative awareness during general anesthesia for cesarean delivery. Anesth Analg. 2009;109:886–90.
30. Sanders RD, Avidan MS. Evidence is lacking for interventions proposed to prevent unintended awareness during general anesthesia for cesarean delivery. Anesth Analg. 2010;110:972–3. author reply 973–4
31. Haynes AB, Weiser TG, Berry WR, Lipsitz SR, Breizat A-HS, Dellinger EP, Herbosa T, Joseph S, Kibatala PL, Lapitan MCM, Merry AF, Moorthy K, Reznick RK, Taylor B, Gawande AA. Safe surgery saves lives study group: a surgical safety checklist to reduce morbidity and mortality in a global population. N Engl J Med. 2009;360:491–9.
32. Russell EC, Wrench I, Feast M, Mohammed F. Pre-oxygenation in pregnancy: the effect of fresh gas flow rates within a circle breathing system. Anaesthesia. 2008;63:833–6.
33. Murdoch H, Scrutton M, Laxton CH. Choice of anaesthetic agents for caesarean section: a UK survey of current practice. Int J Obstet Anesth. 2013;22:31–5.
34. Palahniuk RJ, Shnider SM, Eger EI. Pregnancy decreases the requirement for inhaled anesthetic agents. Anesthesiology. 1974;41:82–3.
35. Erden V, Erkalp K, Yangin Z, Delatioglu H, Kiroglu S, Ortaküz S, Ozdemir B. The effect of labor on sevoflurane requirements during cesarean delivery. Int J Obstet Anesth. 2011;20:17–21.
36. Devroe S, Van de Velde M, Rex S. General anesthesia for caesarean section. Curr Opin Anaesthesiol. 2015;28:240–6.
37. Gultekin H, Yildiz K, Sezer Z, Dogru K. Comparing the relaxing effects of desflurane and sevoflurane on oxytocin-induced contractions of isolated myometrium in both pregnant and nonpregnant rats. Adv Ther. 2006;23:39–46.
38. Dogru K, Yildiz K, Dalgiç H, Sezer Z, Yaba G, Madenoglu H. Inhibitory effects of desflurane and sevoflurane on contractions of isolated gravid rat myometrium under oxytocin stimulation. Acta Anaesthesiol Scand. 2003;47:472–4.
39. McDonnell NJ, Paech MJ, Clavisi OM, Scott KL, ANZCA Trials Group. Difficult and failed intubation in obstetric anaesthesia: an observational study of airway management and complications associated with general anaesthesia for caesarean section. Int J Obstet Anesth. 2008;17:292–7.
40. Cook TM, Woodall N, Frerk C. Fourth National Audit Project: major complications of airway management in the UK: results of the fourth National Audit Project of the Royal College of Anaesthetists and the difficult airway society. Part 1: anaesthesia. Br J Anaesth. 2011;106:617–31.
41. Spong AD, Vaughan DJ. Safe extubation of a parturient using an airway exchange technique. Int J Obstet Anesth. 2014;23:282–5.

Anaesthesia for Caesarean Section: Effect on the Foetus, Neonate and Breastfeeding

Sarah Devroe

7.1 Effects on the Foetus and Neonate of Anaesthesia During Caesarean Section

If we want to compare the neonatal effect of different anaesthetic techniques for caesarean section, various markers of neonatal outcome and their clinical relevance should be discussed. This chapter will firstly summarize the most commonly used parameters of neonatal and foetal outcome. Secondly, direct and indirect effects of general and regional anaesthesia on the neonate will be discussed. Finally, neonatal outcomes of both techniques will be compared.

7.1.1 Assessment of Foetal Wellbeing and Neonatal Outcome

7.1.1.1 Foetal Heart Rate Monitoring

The primary goal of intrapartum monitoring of the foetal heart rate (FHR) and analysis of the patterns of the FHR is to identify foetuses at risk for intrapartum asphyxia. Based on baseline heart rate, FHR variability, accelerations and deceleration, in relation to uterine activity, FHR tracings are classified into three categories. Category I tracings are strongly predictive of a healthy non-acidotic foetus; Category III tracings are associated with acidemia and require immediate intervention. Category II tracings are not predictive of asphyxia but need frequent re-evaluation. Anaesthetic interventions can cause FHR changes directly (tachycardia after atropine administration to the mother, decreased FHR variability during general anaesthesia and direct anaesthetic effects due to trans-placental passage) or indirectly (bradycardia due to spinal-induced hypotension and consequent decreased uterine perfusion).

S. Devroe
Department of Anaesthesiology, University Hospital Leuven,
Herestraat 49, 3000 Leuven, Belgium
e-mail: Sarah.devroe@uzleuven.be

© Springer International Publishing Switzerland 2017
G. Capogna (ed.), *Anesthesia for Cesarean Section*,
DOI 10.1007/978-3-319-42053-0_7

Following, FHR patterns should be assessed taking the anaesthetic action into account and prompt identification (e.g. spinal-induced hypotension) and treatment (e.g. vasopressor) of the cause of non-reassuring FHR can prevent an emergency caesarean section [1].

7.1.1.2 Mortality and Resuscitation

Although the most significant adverse outcome, mortality is not a useful parameter to compare the safety of different anaesthetic techniques used for caesarean section, due to its extreme low incidence. The need for a life-saving intervention (bag and mask ventilation or need for intubation) by a paediatrician is another frequently used parameter for adverse neonatal outcome.

7.1.1.3 Neuro-Behaviour Scores: Apgar Score and NASC

In most studies neonatal outcome is assessed using Apgar scores in combination with umbilical cord blood gas with pH analysis. The Apgar score gives us an idea of the condition of the neonate in the first minutes after birth. It is important to underline that the Apgar score does not predict individual neonatal mortality or adverse neurological outcome but Apgar scores of <5 at 5 min may correlate with some degree of cerebral palsy. Many factors may influence the Apgar score, including maternal anaesthesia, resuscitation setting, prematurity and congenital pathology. Apgar scores alone can certainly not be used to determine the diagnosis of asphyxia [2].

The neonatal Neurologic and Adaptive Capacity Score (NASC) is another tool to evaluate neonatal outcome and was designed to assess the effect of labour medication on full-term healthy babies [3]. It scores the adaptation of the newborn by observing and scoring adaptive capacity, passive and active tone, primary reflexes and alertness, and crying and motor activity (Tables 7.1 and 7.2).

7.1.1.4 Umbilical Blood Gas Analysis

Umbilical blood gas and pH analysis reflects more the foetal condition immediately before birth and is considered a crucial outcome measure. Low arterial pH is strongly associated with long-term sequelae. But what pH threshold is significant for long-term outcome? An observational cohort study, in which 51,519 umbilical blood gas samples were related to neonatal outcome, concluded that the threshold pH of adverse neurological outcome was 7.10 and the ideal cord pH was 7.26–7.30. But most neonates with neurological morbidity had normal pH values, suggesting that other variables than acidemia are important in the prediction of neurological outcome [7]. Increasing

Table 7.1 Components of the Apgar score and scoring guidelines [4–6]

Sign	0	1	2
Heart rate	Absent	<100	≥100
Respiratory effort	Absent	Weak cry, hypoventilation	Good, crying
Reflex irritability	No response	Grimace	Cry or active withdrawal
Muscle tone	Limp	Some flexion of extremities	Active motion
Colour	Blue, pale	Body pink, extremities blue	Completely pink

Table 7.2 NASC score [3]

NEUROLOGICAL AND ADAPTIVE CAPACITY SCORES

			0	1	2
Adaptive Capacity	1 Response to Sound		absent:	mild:	Vigorous
	2 Habituation to Sound		absent:	7-12 stimuli:	< 6 stimuli:
	3 Response to Light		absent:	mild:	brisk blink or startle:
	4 Habituation to Light		absent:	7-12 stimuli:	< 6 stimuli:
	5 Consolability		absent:	difficult:	easy:

TOTAL [ ]   ADAPTIVE CAPACITY

			0	1	2
Passive Tone	6 Scarf Sign		encircles the neck	elbow slightly passes midline:	elbow doss not reach midline:
	7 Recoil of Elbows		absent	slow, week	brisk: reproducible:
	8 Popliteal Angle		>110°	100°–110°	<90°
	9 Recoil of Lower Limbs		absent	slow. weak.	brisk: reproducible:
Active Tone	10 Active Contraction of Neck Flexors		absent or abnormal	difficult	good: head is maintained in the axis of the body:
	11 Active Contraction of Neck Extensors (from leaning forward position)		absent or abnormal	difficult	good: head is maintained in the axis of the body:
	12 Palmar Grasp*		absent	weak*	excellent: reproducible:
	13 Response to Traction (following palmar grasp)		absent	Lifts part of the body weight:	Lifts all of the body weight:
	14 supporting Reaction (upright position)		absent	incomplete transitory:	Strong: supports all body weight:
*Primary reflexes	15 Automatic Walking*		absent	difficult to obtain*	Perfect: reproducible:
	16 Moro Reflex*		absent	weak: incomplete.	pertect: complete:
	17 Sucking*		absent	weak:	pertect: synchronous with swallowing:
General Assessment	18 Alertness		coma	lethargy:	normal:
	19 Crying		absent	weak: high pitched: excessive:	normal:
	20 Motor Activity		absent of grossly excessive	diminished or mildly excessive	normal:

TOTAL [ ]   NEUROLOGICAL

TOTAL SCORE [ ] AT   MINUTES OF LIFE

arterial base deficits (base excess [BE]) are associated with higher complication rates. The BE threshold has been quoted as -12 mmol/L. When using umbilical arterial values as an outcome parameter in research in severe acidosis (pH < 7), a low pH is probably sufficient. The metabolic component (BE) does not predict the neonates that are more at risk of adverse outcomes than the ones predicted by the low pH [8].

7.1.2 Effect of Anaesthesia on the Foetus and the Neonate

7.1.2.1 General Anaesthesia

General anaesthesia for caesarean section (CS) is nowadays mostly used in emergency situations or when neuraxial anaesthesia techniques have failed or are contraindicated. Nearly all drugs used for this purpose will have some degree of placental transfer resulting in direct foetal or neonatal effects. Alternatively, maternal haemodynamic effects of anaesthetic drugs will indirectly affect the foetus by interference of uteroplacental blood flow. Moreover, general anaesthesia for CS implies muscle relaxation, intubation and positive pressure ventilation, also resulting in indirect consequences for foetus and neonate.

Direct Effects

Induction Agents

Most textbooks still recommend a single dose of thiopental 4–5 mg/kg as induction agent of choice for GA in CS, arguing that this approach should result in an acceptable depth of anaesthesia for the mother with only limited neonatal depression. Propofol, in a dose sufficient for induction and to prevent maternal awareness (2–2.5 mg/kg), depresses the infant more (lower Apgar and NASC) than thiopental and causes a reduction in maternal blood pressure. Neither the use of propofol in general nor a thiopental dose exceeding 250 mg is licenced for the use in pregnancy. Hence, their use is off-label. Because of the limited global availability of thiopental, propofol becomes increasingly popular for induction. Ketamine crosses the placenta rapidly but an induction dose of 1 mg/ kg appeared not to be associated with lower Apgar scores or more need for resuscitation. Based on current literature, all three induction agents can be used safely.

Opioids

Historically, opioids were administered only after umbilical cord clamping in an attempt to avoid respiratory depression of the neonate. However, in the presence of maternal disease, a judicious use of opioids can provide haemodynamic stability offering protection from an abrupt increase in arterial pressure. Opioids at induction might also increase anaesthetic depth and help to avoid awareness, which is a significant problem in obstetric general anaesthesia. All opioids have a high transplacental passage resulting in dose-dependent neonatal depression. Due to its rapid onset and offset, the use of remifentanil has gained increasing popularity for obstetric GA in high-risk women. A recent meta-analysis on the maternal and foetal effects of remifentanil for GA in parturients undergoing CS found that remifentanil attenuated the maternal circulatory response to intubation and surgery. Less negative base excess and higher pH in the remifentanil group suggested a beneficial neonatal effect. It was concluded that an adequately powered trial addressing neonatal side effects of remifentanil is warranted. Remifentanil doses differed sharply among the included studies and dose–response effects should be further defined to find the optimal dose for both mother and infant [9, 10]. All doses of remifentanil are associated with a transient respiratory depression of the newborn. It is mandatory to anticipate neonatal resuscitation when remifentanil is used, especially in preterm infants.

Muscle Relaxants

Muscle relaxants are used to facilitate endotracheal intubation and to provide optimal surgical conditions. Until recently, 1 mg/kg of succinylcholine was routinely used for RSI because of its rapid onset. Succinylcholine is highly ionized and poorly lipid soluble, and only small amounts undergo trans-placental transfer without clinical relevance for the neonate. Rocuronium was introduced in 1994. Due to its rapid onset in higher doses (1 mg/kg), it soon gained popularity for RSI in the obstetric patient. Rocuronium did not adversely affect neonatal Apgar scores, acid-base measurements, time to sustained respiration or neurobehavioural scores [11].

Volatile Anaesthetics

All volatile anaesthetics cross the placenta and will cause a dose-dependent neurological depression of the neonate. Moreover, high doses of volatile anaesthetic agents have been associated with acute cardiovascular depression of the neonate [12]. Concentrations of volatile anaesthetics higher than 1 minimum alveolar concentration (MAC) should be avoided during caesarean section to avoid inappropriate respiratory adaptation because of neurological depression. Moreover, long-term neurological effects should be considered.

Long-Term Effect of Anaesthetic Drugs on the Developing Brain

When exposed to anaesthetics drugs, the foetal or neonatal brain can be injured, resulting in long-term neurobehavioral deficits. Preclinical studies noted anaesthetic-induced developmental neurotoxicity (AIDN) with all general anaesthetic agents, even the ones approved for paediatric anaesthesia. The degree of which this AIDN occurs in humans has yet to be confirmed in well-designed clinical trials [13].

Indirect Effects

Maternal Haemodynamic Changes

Normal perfusion of the foeto-maternal unit is mandatory for foetal wellbeing. Uterine-placental blood flow is mostly dependent upon maternal cardiac output and blood pressure. Vascular re-modelling of the uterine spiral arteries in a normal pregnancy involves a loss of smooth muscle and the elastic lamina from the vessel wall and a 5–10 fold dilation of the vessel mouth. This loss of smooth muscle makes the arteries less responsive to endogenous or exogenous sympathetic input.

Most anaesthetic drugs used for a general anaesthesia reduce maternal cardiac output, resulting in a lower blood pressure. This reduction in maternal cardiac output may lead to a reduction of uteroplacental blood flow. Since spiral arteries are not responsive to vaso-active drugs, the use of these drugs will correct maternal cardiac output and blood pressure and re-establish placental blood flow. In case of pre-eclampsia, spiral arteries do not manage to develop normally and will still respond to vaso-active drugs. Vasoconstriction of the spiral arteries will reduce the already impaired placental blood flow in pre-eclampsia and can acutely jeopardize the foetuses' life. In pre-eclampsia, the ideal vasopressor is still a field of research.

Due to an inadequate technique of general anaesthesia for caesarean section (light anaesthesia with omission of opioids), a hypertensive response may occur during laryngoscopy and intubation. In healthy parturients, this time-limited rise in blood pressure will probably not cause any harm to the mother but in some patients with co-existing disease (especially pre-eclampsia) a sudden rise in blood pressure can cause intracranial haemorrhage. Though, the increase of catecholamine levels that accompanies the increase in blood pressure can jeopardize the uteroplacental blood flow that is of utmost importance if the foetus is in acute distress (often the case if general anaesthesia for caesarean section is warranted).

Many medications have been used to attenuate this response with varying success. Most of these drugs have been studied in patients with pre-eclampsia. Some authors prefer esmolol (1.5 mg/kg) or NTG (2 µg/kg), in combination with propofol (2 mg/kg) [14] while others will use, for reasons of availability, cost-effectiveness and safety, magnesium for the control of the hypertensive response in pre-eclampsia. The institution of the author of this chapter prefers the use of remifentanil for this purpose. Apart from the fact that remifentanil is a perfect surgical analgesic that in addition to propofol will prevent awareness during caesarean section, it permits to attenuate the maternal response to laryngoscopy with a time-limited neonatal depression [15]. A recent meta-analysis on the maternal and foetal effects of remifentanil for general anaesthesia in parturients undergoing caesarean section found that remifentanil attenuated the maternal circulatory response to intubation and surgery [9]. Less negative base excess and higher pH in the remifentanil group suggested a beneficial neonatal effect. It was concluded that an adequately powered trial addressing neonatal side effects of remifentanil is warranted. Remifentanil doses differed strongly among the included studies and dose–response effects should be further defined to find the optimal dose for both mother and infant [9]. Park et al. demonstrated that a single bolus of remifentanil of 0.5 or 1 mg/kg for induction of anaesthesia in severely pre-eclamptic patients attenuated maternal heart rate and pressor responses, with only minimal and transient neonatal respiratory depression [16]. More recently, Yoo et al. determined the effective dose (ED50/ED95) of remifentanil to prevent the pressor response to intubation in patients with severe pre-eclampsia. Intubation-induced increases of heart rate and blood pressure were attenuated in a dose-dependent manner by remifentanil, with the ED50 and ED95 being 0.59 [95% confidence interval (95% CI) 0.47–0.70] and 1.34 (1.04–2.19) mg/kg, respectively. However, all doses of remifentanil were associated with a transient respiratory depression of the newborn, and higher doses were associated with maternal hypotension (13%) [17]. The anticipation of brief neonatal resuscitation is necessary when remifentanil is used.

Maternal Respiratory Changes

Rapid sequence induction with cricoid pressure, no mask ventilation and tracheal intubation remains the gold standard for a caesarean section under general anaesthesia. Reduced oxygen reserve due to a reduced functional residual capacity and an increased oxygen demand result in a shorter time to desaturation during apnoea. Preoxygenation with 100% oxygen is an effective measurement to prologue the time to desaturation, resulting in a longer time between induction and intubation. Keeping in mind that airway management and difficult intubation in pregnant patients are more frequent than in the routine surgical population, a difficult airway should always be anticipated with the right equipment and algorithms. Oxygenation and ventilator goals should be a PaO_2 above 70 mmHg and a $PaCO_2$ of 28–32 mmHg. Maternal hypoxia results in foetoplacental vasoconstriction, which reduces placental blood flow and foetal oxygen transfer and will compromise the foetus [18]. Maternal hypocarbia and lower bicarbonate are normal adaptations to pregnancy. Further hyperventilation should be avoided to prevent impairment of the uterine blood flow and maternal pH control within normal ranges for pregnancy is essential [18].

During mechanical ventilation, pregnant patients usually need higher peak inspiratory pressures and a positive end-expiratory pressure to overcome the increased chest wall compliance and the higher abdominal pressure due to the pregnant uterus [18]. The increased intrathoracic pressure can result in a reduction of the venous return and cardiac output and thus aggravate the haemodynamic effects of the aortocaval compression.

7.1.2.2 Neuraxial Anaesthesia

Direct Effects

Spinal drug doses of local anaesthetics and opioids used for a caesarean section are usually so small that plasma levels will never reach sufficient height to exert any foetal pharmacological effect [19]. Concerns have been raised about foetal heart rate abnormalities after CSE with opioids during labour. Van de Velde et al. suggested not to use high-dose intrathecal opioids for the induction of labour analgesia in the case of non-reassuring foetal heart rate or indications of uterine hypertonia during labour [20]. No such studies have been performed in the scenario of an urgent caesarean section, so we do not know if we can extrapolate the omission of spinal opioids for C-section. Epidural local anaesthetics will only reach significant plasma concentration when accidently administered intravenously. Maternal-administered epidural opioids can be detected in the umbilical vein and artery suggesting foetal uptake or metabolism [21]. When converting a labour epidural analgesia with a continuous opioid infusion to a surgical epidural for an emergency caesarean section, supplemental epidural opioids should be avoided until after delivery. The opioid in the epidural labour solution has probably already produced its near-maximal effect [22], and an extra dose can result in neonatal neurological depression. More research is needed to evaluate opioid-induced side effects on the neonate after maternal administration of neuraxial opioids [23].

Indirect Effects

Nausea and Vomiting

Nausea and vomiting are common symptoms after anaesthesia (general and loco-regional) for caesarean section with an incidence of 20–60%. Intraoperatively this can be challenging for the obstetrician, and it can be associated with accidental surgical trauma, jeopardizing the mother and the foetus. Moreover, there is a risk for aspiration of gastric content, resulting in bronchospasm, hypoxemia and postoperatively pneumonitis. Maternal hypoxemia can also adversely affect the foetus. Hypotension, reduced cardiac output, surgical stimulation and peri-operatively used drugs (opioids and uterotonics) have all been suggested to contribute to this high incidence. Many agents are efficacious in the prevention of nausea and vomiting, but there are no data on the potential adverse effects on the mother and neonate [24]. Hypotension is probably the most important cause of intraoperative nausea and vomiting (IONV). Hypoperfusion and consequent ischemia of the brainstem may lead to the activation of the vomiting centre. Also, gut hypoperfusion with the release of emetogenic substances has been suggested as possible cause of IONV [25]. Prevention or treatment of hypotension will decrease the incidence of IONV. Phenylephrine may be associated with less IONV compared to ephedrine, and a prophylactic continuous infusion seems more effective than bolus administration [25]. Interestingly, a recent study suggested that prophylactic ondansetron in obstetric patients undergoing spinal anaesthesia not only decreased the incidence of IONV but also improved the degree of hypotension and reduced the required amount of vasopressors [26].

Hypotension

Hypotension remains the most important side effect of spinal anaesthesia for a caesarean section with a reported incidence between 20% and 80%. The sympathetic block will result in a decreased systemic vascular resistance and venous return, impaired cardiac output and eventually decreased uteroplacental perfusion. The risk of foetal acidemia depends on the severity and duration of the hypotensive episode [27]. Active management to prevent spinal-induced hypotension and prompt treatment of spinal-induced haemodynamic changes minimize the adverse effect on foetal outcome.

Several methods have been described to prevent or treat spinal hypotension. Physical methods (e.g. leg wrapping) and the prevention of aortocaval compression (left lateral tilt) have been useful preventive measurements to attenuate the severity of hypotension. Also lowering the dose of spinal anaesthetic drugs can reduce the incidence and the severity of the spinal hypotension. However, the cornerstone of the management of spinal-induced hypotension relies on the use of vasopressors, intravascular fluid therapy or a combination of both. All described preventive interventions have been shown to reduce the incidence but did not eliminate the need for active treatment of hypotension [28].

Physiological Methods

A recent randomized double-blind placebo-controlled study concluded that leg wrapping prevented hypotension compared with no intervention by attenuating spinal anaesthesia-mediated venodilatation. In that same study phenylephrine (bolus followed by low-dose infusion) was superior in preventing hypotension, by correcting the spinal-induced reduction in PVR [29].

Aortocaval Compression

Hypotension during advanced pregnancy can be exacerbated by aortocaval compression. The gravid uterus compresses the inferior vena cava, impending venous return and leading to a decreased cardiac output. Moreover, in severe cases, direct compression of the aorta may reduce the uteroplacental perfusion, even more, possibly resulting in foetal acidosis. In non-labouring women, aortocaval compression is mostly asymptomatic, and the patients manage to maintain normal arterial blood pressure, despite a reduction in cardiac output. Additional sympathetic blockade during neuraxial anaesthesia in these patients will result in severe hypotension. Left uterine displacement by placing a wedge under the right hip of the patient or by tilting the table can prevent the aortocaval component of the hypotension by improving the venous return and cardiac output but will not prevent spinal-induced hypotension. The optimal degree of tilt is unknown, but a recent trial showed that the effect of aortocaval compression on the cardiac output could be minimized by a tilt of at least 15° [30]. Though, magnetic resonance imaging could not confirm that 15° left lateral tilt effectively reduced the compression of the inferior vena cava in term pregnant women [31].

Intravenous Fluids: Choice, Dosage and Timing

Crystalloids and colloids, in different volumes and at different time points, have been used to increase the intravascular volume to overcome hypotension associated with spinal anaesthesia. The higher intravascular volume will increase venous return, cardiac output and systolic blood pressure. The timing of this administration can be before the spinal anaesthesia ('preload') or at the time of the initiation of the spinal anaesthesia ('coload'). Current data show that that preloading with crystalloids is inefficacious, and that coloading with colloids is more efficient than with crystalloids in preventing maternal spinal-induced hypotension. However colloids always carry the risk of an anaphylactic reaction, cannot be used in case of renal impairment and are very costly [32]. Mercier et al. provided the most recent data (CAESAR trial) showing that compared with pure crystalloid preload, a mixed HES–Ringer lactate preload, together with early phenylephrine bolus administration (if blood pressure dropped 5% from the baseline), can improve the prevention of spinal-induced hypotension. Based on this study, a third-generation HES preload in combination with phenylephrine can be considered as efficacious against spinal-induced hypotension and safe for mother and foetus [33].

Vasopressors

Because physical methods, reducing the aortocaval compression and fluid loading are only moderately efficient in preventing hypotension after spinal anaesthesia, vasopressors are considered crucial in the management of spinal-induced hypotension. As with the fluid management, various vasopressors, at different doses and variable timings, have been studied over the last two decades. Ephedrine was considered the vasopressor of choice in obstetric patients undergoing neuraxial anaesthesia, until Lee et al. [34] showed that ephedrine and phenylephrine were equally efficient but that the umbilical cord blood pH of neonates born from mothers who received ephedrine was lower than of those from mothers who received phenylephrine, although the risk of true acidosis (pH < 7.20) was not different in both groups and clinical neonatal outcome, as measured by Apgar scores, was similar. As a consequence of that publication, ephedrine lost its position as 'gold standard' vasopressor and the quest for the optimal vasopressor regime started. From then on a plethora of trials on different vasopressor regimes (ephedrine vs. phenylephrine vs. the combination of both, continuous vs. bolus, prophylactic vs. therapeutic) in different circumstances (healthy vs. compromised mothers and foetuses) have been investigated. In all of these studies neonatal outcome was assessed using Apgar scores and umbilical cord blood gas and pH analysis. As mentioned before, Apgar scores give us an idea of the condition of the neonate in the first minutes after birth, but its role as a predictor of neonatal outcome remains unclear. Umbilical blood gas and pH analysis reflects more the foetal condition immediately before birth and is considered more indicative when assessing the foetal impact of different vasopressor regimes. A systematic review analysing all studies that compared ephedrine and phenylephrine during spinal anaesthesia for elective caesarean section showed that neonates from women given phenylephrine had higher arterial pH values compared to neonates from mothers given ephedrine. Of note, no difference was observed between both groups in the incidence of true acidosis or Apgar score < 7 at 1 and 5 min [34]. The greater placental transfer of ephedrine is probably responsible for an increased foetal metabolism with depression of the foetal pH.

Titrated phenylephrine infusions (starting at 50 µg/min) are currently recommended to keep maternal arterial blood pressure as close as possible to the baseline values (and not within 20% range as advised previously) [35], resulting in better foetal umbilical gas values and lower incidence of postoperative nausea and vomiting [36].

Others

As mentioned previously, the prophylactic use of ondansetron may also reduce spinal hypotension and the consequent consumption of vasopressors [26].

7.1.3 Regional Versus General Anaesthesia for Caesarean Section and Neonatal Outcome

Literature addressing the comparison of neonatal outcome after general or regional anaesthesia for caesarean section must be interpreted with caution. Most studies are retrospective, not randomized or not blinded.

There was heterogeneity in indication for caesarean section (elective or emergency) or the indication for either anaesthetic technique. Choice of anaesthesia technique or mode of delivery can be dependent on maternal and foetal risk factors already independently responsible for an increased risk of adverse outcome. The grade of foetal or maternal compromise has an influence on the choice of anaesthesia. Moreover, general anaesthesia because of failed loco-regional techniques was categorized into the general anaesthesia group in most of the studies. In these cases, the delay in providing anaesthesia had certainly more consequences on the neonatal outcome in emergency caesarean sections than the effects of general anaesthesia.

Some studies used Apgar scores as a surrogate of neonatal outcome. Mancuso et al. found lower Apgar scores at 1 and 5 min in neonates whose mothers had a general anaesthesia compared to infants whose mothers had spinal anaesthesia. Trans-placental passage of anaesthetic drugs was mentioned to contribute to the transient depression of the neonate [37]. Algert et al. found in a major cohort study, involving 50,806 caesarean deliveries, an increased risk of adverse neonatal outcome for caesarean sections under general anaesthesia. Neonatal outcome was assessed by the need for neonatal intubation and Apgar scores of <7 at 5 min. Moreover, this study controlled for confounding by the specification of pregnancy risk (low-moderate or high) and indication (planned-failure to progress-foetal distress). They concluded that the neonate already compromised before the caesarean section suffered the most of the general anaesthesia. They also suggested that based on the effect on the Apgar score at 5 min, the adverse effects of a general anaesthesia lasted longer than previously thought [38].

In a meta-analysis comparing neonatal acid-base status for different techniques of anaesthesia for caesarean section, Reynolds and co-workers found significant lower cord pH after spinal than after both general and epidural anaesthesia. Most data of the analysed studies came from the era in which ephedrine was the first choice vasopressor. They contributed the lower pH to the large doses of ephedrine given to overcome spinal-induced hypotension [39]. Although proven safer for the mothers, spinal anaesthesia for an elective caesarean section is not associated with better neonatal outcome if defined by umbilical cord pH.

Choice of anaesthesia technique will eventually depend on the grade of maternal or foetal compromise, the experience of the anaesthesiologist and the availability of a paediatric team. It is mandatory to anticipate neonatal resuscitation when general anaesthesia is provided.

7.2   Effects on the Breastfeeding

The beneficial health effects of breastfeeding are well recognized and apply to mothers and children in developed nations as well as to those in developing countries. Supported by the international recommendations of the World Health Organization (WHO), there has been a worldwide increase in breastfeeding incidence. Good knowledge of the physiology of breastfeeding and the possible effects of anaesthetic drugs on the suckling infants are mandatory in guiding the decision to permit breastfeeding after maternal anaesthesia [40]. The most up-to-date information can be found in the drugs and lactation database (Lactmed) of the National Library of Medicines Toxicology Data Network (TOXNET). (Drugs and Lactation Database [LactMed] is available at http://toxnet.nlm.nih.gov/cgi-bin/sis/htmlgen?LACT.)

7.2.1 Effect of Caesarean Section on Breastfeeding

Caesarean delivery is believed to affect the rate of breastfeeding adversely. Timely breastfeeding initiation is thought to be the key to a successful breastfeeding and the delay in first breastfeeding was considered to be the principal reason for the lower success in breastfeeding following a caesarean section. In the literature, studies have shown that caesarean delivery was a risk factor for not initiating breastfeeding within the first hour of life and for not initiating breastfeeding at all. Moreover, babies born by caesarean section and exclusively breastfed had less weight gain patterns than infants born by vaginal delivery [41].

But recently, a meta-analysis of the world literature on breastfeeding success after caesarean delivery, including over 500,000 subjects, only showed a negative association between *prelabour* caesarean section and early breastfeeding. Once breastfeeding was initiated, mode of delivery did not affect the long-term continuation (6 months) of breastfeeding. Numbers of prelabour-elective caesarean sections are rising each year, partially explained by an increased preference of pregnant women. Sub-group analysis in that same study showed that early breastfeeding was not different in women who had an emergency caesarean section compared with those who had a vaginal delivery. Since emergency caesarean sections mostly occur during labour, this finding supports the theory that the metabolic and endocrine milieu of labour may also be crucial in the initiation of lactation [42]. The lower breastfeeding rate, together with other minor adverse clinical outcomes in children born by prelabour caesarean sections, is of matter of public health, and indications may need reconsideration. Prospective mothers and health providers involved in perinatal care should be informed about the negative association between elective caesarean sections and breastfeeding success. Women that underwent an elective caesarean delivery could benefit from increased professional breastfeeding support [42].

7.2.2 Mode of Anaesthesia and Its Effect on Breastfeeding

7.2.2.1 Spinal/Epidural Anaesthesia

Very little research has been done on the influence of the anaesthetic technique for caesarean section on breastfeeding. Sener et al. found that breastfeeding was initiated earlier following neuraxial than general anaesthesia for caesarean section [43].

7.2.2.2 General Anaesthesia

Direct effects of drug passage through the placenta can influence the adaptation of neonate and delay early feeding reflexes.

Because of the delay of awakening and recovery of cognitive functions of the mother following general anaesthesia, communication between the mother and the newborn can also be postponed. This interval between birth and the first feeding can negatively affect the success of breastfeeding. Skin-to-skin contact immediately after birth is crucial in this process. If the mother is not able to do this herself during the surgical procedure, a companion present at birth and designated by the mother can perform the skin-to-skin contact [44].

Only tiny concentrations of the frequently used drugs during the anaesthesia for a caesarean section will pass into the colostrum, making them unlikely to affect the neonate. Discarding breast milk after anaesthesia is not considered necessary for the safety of the infant.

References

1. Macones GA, Hankins GDV, Spong CY, et al. The 2008 National Institute of Child Health and Human Development workshop report on electronic fetal monitoring: update on definitions, interpretation, and research guidelines. Obstet Gynecol. 2008;112(3):661–6.
2. American Academy of Pediatrics Committee on Fetus and Newborn, American College of Obstetricians, and Gynecologists Committee on Obstetric Practice. The Apgar score. Pediatrics. 2015;136:819–22. doi:10.1542/peds.2015-2651.
3. Amiel-Tison C, Barrier G, Shnider SM, et al. The neonatal neurologic and adaptive capacity score (NACS). Anesthesiology. 1982;56:492–3.
4. Committee on Obstetric Practice, ACOG, American Academy of Pediatrics, Committee on Fetus and Newborn, ACOG. ACOG Committee Opinion. Number 333, May 2006 (replaces No. 174, 1996): the Apgar score. Obstet Gynecol. 2006;107:1209–12.
5. Ehrenstein V. Association of Apgar scores with death and neurologic disability. Clin Epigenetics. 2009;1:45–53.
6. Apgar V. A proposal for a new method of evaluation of the newborn infant. Originally published in July 1953, volume 32, pages 250-259. Anesth Analg. 2015;120:1056–9. doi:10.1213/ANE.0b013e31829bdc5c.
7. Yeh P, Emary K, Impey L. The relationship between umbilical cord arterial pH and serious adverse neonatal outcome: analysis of 51,519 consecutive validated samples. BJOG. 2012;119:824–31. doi:10.1111/j.1471-0528.2012.03335.x.
8. Knutzen L, Svirko E, Impey L. The significance of base deficit in acidemic term neonates. Am J Obstet Gynecol. 2015;213:373.e1–7. doi:10.1016/j.ajog.2015.03.051.
9. Heesen M, Klöhr S, Hofmann T, et al. Maternal and foetal effects of remifentanil for general anaesthesia in parturients undergoing caesarean section: a systematic review and meta-analysis. Acta Anaesthesiol Scand. 2013;57:29–36. doi:10.1111/j.1399-6576.2012.02723.x.
10. Devroe S, van de Velde M, Rex S. General anesthesia for caesarean section. Curr Opin Anaesthesiol. 2015;28:240–6. doi:10.1097/ACO.0000000000000185.
11. Abouleish E, Abboud T, Lechevalier T, et al. Rocuronium (Org 9426) for caesarean section. Br J Anaesth. 1994;73:336–41. doi:10.1093/bja/73.3.336.
12. Rychik J. Acute cardiovascular effects of fetal surgery in the human. Circulation. 2004;110:1549–56. doi:10.1161/01.CIR.0000142294.95388.C4.
13. Maze M. Preclinical neuroprotective actions of xenon and possible implications for human therapeutics: a narrative review. Can J Anaesth. 2016;63:212–26. doi:10.1007/s12630-015-0507-8.
14. Pant M, Fong R, Scavone B. Prevention of peri-induction hypertension in preeclamptic patients: a focused review. Anesth Analg. 2014;119:1350–6. doi:10.1213/ANE.0000000000000424.
15. van de Velde M, Teunkens A, Kuypers M, et al. General anaesthesia with target controlled infusion of propofol for planned caesarean section: maternal and neonatal effects of a remifentanil-based technique. Int J Obstet Anesth. 2004;13:153–8. doi:10.1016/j.ijoa.2004.01.005.
16. Park BY, Jeong CW, Jang EA, et al. Dose-related attenuation of cardiovascular responses to tracheal intubation by intravenous remifentanil bolus in severe pre-eclamptic patients undergoing caesarean delivery. Br J Anaesth. 2011;106:82–7. doi:10.1093/bja/aeq275.

17. Yoo KY, Kang DH, Jeong H, et al. A dose-response study of remifentanil for attenuation of the hypertensive response to laryngoscopy and tracheal intubation in severely preeclamptic women undergoing caesarean delivery under general anaesthesia. Int J Obstet Anesth. 2013;22:10–8. doi:10.1016/j.ijoa.2012.09.010.

18. Schwaiberger D, Karcz M, Menk M, et al. Respiratory failure and mechanical ventilation in the pregnant patient. Crit Care Clin. 2016;32:85–95. doi:10.1016/j.ccc.2015.08.001.

19. Ginosar Y, Reynolds F, Halpern SH, Weiner C. Anesthesia and the fetus. 2012. doi:10.1002/9781118477076

20. van de Velde M, Teunkens A, Hanssens M, et al. Intrathecal sufentanil and fetal heart rate abnormalities: a double-blind, double placebo-controlled trial comparing two forms of combined spinal epidural analgesia with epidural analgesia in labor. Anesth Analg. 2004;98:1153–1159.

21. Desprats R, Dumas JC, Giroux M, et al. Maternal and umbilical cord concentrations of fentanyl after epidural analgesia for cesarean section. Eur J Obstet Gynecol Reprod Biol. 1991;42:89–94.

22. Hillyard SG, Bate TE, Corcoran TB, et al. Extending epidural analgesia for emergency caesarean section: a meta-analysis. Br J Anaesth. 2011;107:668–78. doi:10.1093/bja/aer300.

23. Armstrong S, Fernando R. Side effects and efficacy of neuraxial opioids in pregnant patients at delivery: a comprehensive review. Drug Saf. 2016;39(5):381–99. doi:10.1007/s40264-015-0386-5.

24. Griffiths JD, Gyte GML, Paranjothy S, et al. Interventions for preventing nausea and vomiting in women undergoing regional anaesthesia for caesarean section. Cochrane Database Syst Rev. 2012;9:CD007579. doi:10.1002/14651858.CD007579.pub2.

25. Habib AS. A review of the impact of phenylephrine administration on maternal hemodynamics and maternal and neonatal outcomes in women undergoing cesarean delivery under spinal anesthesia. Anesth Analg. 2012;114:377–90. doi:10.1213/ANE.0b013e3182373a3e.

26. Gao L, Zheng G, Han J, et al. Effects of prophylactic ondansetron on spinal anesthesia-induced hypotension: a meta-analysis. Int J Obstet Anesth. 2015;24:335–43. doi:10.1016/j.ijoa.2015.08.012.

27. Roofthooft E, van de Velde M. Low-dose spinal anaesthesia for caesarean section to prevent spinal-induced hypotension. Curr Opin Anaesthesiol. 2008;21:259–62. doi:10.1097/ACO.0b013e3282ff5e41.

28. Cyna AM, Andrew M, Emmett RS, et al. Techniques for preventing hypotension during spinal anaesthesia for caesarean section. Cochrane Database Syst Rev. 2006;(18):CD002251. doi:10.1002/14651858.CD002251.pub2.

29. Kuhn JC, Hauge TH, Rosseland LA, et al. Hemodynamics of phenylephrine infusion versus lower extremity compression during spinal anesthesia for cesarean delivery: a randomized, double-blind, placebo-controlled study. Anesth Analg. 2016;122:1120–9. doi:10.1213/ANE.0000000000001174.

30. Lee SWY, Khaw KS, Ngan Kee WD, et al. Haemodynamic effects from aortocaval compression at different angles of lateral tilt in non-labouring term pregnant women. Br J Anaesth. 2012;109:950–6. doi:10.1093/bja/aes349.

31. Higuchi H, Takagi S, Zhang K, et al. Effect of lateral tilt angle on the volume of the abdominal aorta and inferior vena cava in pregnant and nonpregnant women determined by magnetic resonance imaging. Anesthesiology. 2015;122:286–93. doi:10.1097/ALN.0000000000000553.

32. Teoh WHL, Westphal M, Kampmeier TG. Update on volume therapy in obstetrics. Best Pract Res Clin Anaesthesiol. 2014;28:297–303. doi:10.1016/j.bpa.2014.07.004.

33. Mercier FJ, Diemunsch P, Ducloy-Bouthors A-S, et al. 6% Hydroxyethyl starch (130/0.4) vs Ringer's lactate preloading before spinal anaesthesia for caesarean delivery: the randomized, double-blind, multicentre CAESAR trial. Br J Anaesth. 2014;113:459–67. doi:10.1093/bja/aeu103.

34. Lee A, Ngan Kee WD, Gin T. A quantitative, systematic review of randomized controlled trials of ephedrine versus phenylephrine for the management of hypotension during spinal anesthesia for cesarean delivery. Anesth Analg. 2002;94:920–926; table of contents. doi:10.1097/00000539-200204000-00028

35. Butwick AJ, Columb MO, Carvalho B. Preventing spinal hypotension during caesarean delivery: what is the latest? Br J Anaesth. 2015;114:183–6. doi:10.1093/bja/aeu267.
36. Lee AJ, Smiley RM. Phenylephrine infusions during cesarean section under spinal anesthesia. Int Anesthesiol Clin. 2014;52:29–47. doi:10.1097/AIA.0000000000000010.
37. Mancuso A, De Vivo A, Giacobbe A, et al. General versus spinal anaesthesia for elective caesarean sections: effects on neonatal short-term outcome. A prospective randomised study. J Matern Fetal Neonatal Med. 2010;23:1114–8. doi:10.3109/14767050903572158.
38. Algert CS, Bowen JR, Giles WB, et al. Regional block versus general anaesthesia for caesarean section and neonatal outcomes: a population-based study. BMC Med. 2009;7:20. doi:10.1186/1741-7015-7-20.
39. Reynolds F, Seed PT. Anaesthesia for caesarean section and neonatal acid-base status: a meta-analysis. Anaesthesia. 2005;60:636–53. doi:10.1111/j.1365-2044.2005.04223.x.
40. Masho SW. Leadership, expertise, and creativity: the right mix for breastfeeding research. Breastfeed Med. 2015;10(8):397–8. doi:10.1089/bfm.2015.0105.
41. Samayam P, Ranganathan PK, Balasundaram R. Study of weight patterns in exclusively breast fed neonates—does the route of delivery have an impact? J Clin Diagn Res. 2016;10:SC01–3. doi:10.7860/JCDR/2016/17889.7025.
42. Prior E, Santhakumaran S, Gale C, et al. Breastfeeding after cesarean delivery: a systematic review and meta-analysis of world literature. Am J Clin Nutr. 2012;95:1113–35. doi:10.3945/ajcn.111.030254.
43. Sener EB, Guldogus F, Karakaya D, et al. Comparison of neonatal effects of epidural and general anesthesia for cesarean section. Gynecol Obstet Investig. 2003;55:41–5. doi:10.1159/000068956.
44. de Alba-Romero C, Camaño-Gutiérrez I, López-Hernández P, et al. Postcesarean section skin-to-skin contact of mother and child. J Hum Lact. 2014;30:283–6. doi:10.1177/0890334414535506.

Choice of Anaesthesia for Emergency Caesarean Section

Olivia Clancy and Nuala Lucas

The number of caesarean sections performed worldwide has increased over the last two decades. There are many reasons for including: changing demographics, the rising age of first-time mothers, rising levels of obesity, a maternal preference in some countries for caesarean section over vaginal delivery, a rising proportion of multiple births, increasing medico-legal concerns and organizational factors. Many of these factors are interrelated.

Data from the Organisation for Economic Co-operation and Development (OECD) demonstrates that in 2013 caesarean section rates were lowest in Nordic countries (Iceland being the lowest with a rate of 15/100 live births), Israel and the Netherlands. The highest rates were observed in Turkey, Mexico and Chile, with rates ranging from 45 to 50% [1].

Caesarean section is a unique situation where the anaesthetist has to provide care to both the mother and the baby. A team approach is vital to ensure optimal outcome for both while ensuring that the process is a safe and pleasant experience for the parturient.

8.1 Factors Affecting the Choice of Anaesthesia for Emergency Caesarean Section

There are several factors that may affect the choice of anaesthesia in the emergency situation and these may be categorised as patient, anaesthetic and surgical factors (Table 8.1). In addition, the risks and benefits of the anaesthetic options need to be quickly evaluated in the context of these factors. This evaluation can be aided by anticipation and planning, along with good communication with the obstetric team. It is important to remember that many 'emergencies' do not occur entirely de novo

O. Clancy • N. Lucas (✉)
Northwick Park Hospital, Harrow, UK
e-mail: nuala@tuesday5.co.uk

© Springer International Publishing Switzerland 2017
G. Capogna (ed.), *Anesthesia for Cesarean Section*,
DOI 10.1007/978-3-319-42053-0_8

Table 8.1 Factors affecting choice of anaesthesia for emergency CS

Patient factors
• Pre-existing co-morbidities, e.g. obesity, cardiac disease
• Pregnancy-related pathology, e.g. pre-eclampsia, thrombocytopenia
• Acute physiological derangement, e.g. sepsis, major haemorrhage
• Fasting status
Anaesthetic factors
• Anticipated difficulty with either neuraxial or general anaesthesia, e.g. obesity, airway examination
• The presence (or not) of an epidural in situ
• Contraindications to neuraxial block
• Experience of the anaesthetist
Surgical factors
• The urgency of caesarean section
• Nature of emergency, e.g. major haemorrhage

[2] and some anaesthetic planning can take place in advance of the obstetric decision to proceed to emergency caesarean section. When planning has not been possible, it is fundamental that the anaesthetist be quickly familiarized with salient points in the history and perform a rapid airway assessment.

8.2 The Urgency of Caesarean Section

The traditional classification of urgency of caesarean section categorized all-planned operations as 'elective' while all others were 'emergencies'. These definitions were clearly inadequate in terms of communication (between obstetricians, midwives and anaesthetists) with further implications for training and audit/data collection. An agreed classification system would improve communication between obstetricians/anaesthetists and midwives and facilitate prioritization of the most urgent cases, potentially leading to improved maternal and neonatal outcomes. The classification advocated by the UK Royal College of Obstetricians and Gynaecologists is shown in Table 8.2 [3].

The recommendation for this classification was accompanied by additional commentary that highlighted other important considerations. It stresses that in the non-elective caesarean section there is a *continuum of urgency* and that each situation should be assessed on a case-by-case basis; to emphasize this point, the statement includes a colour scale. The adoption of a single classification system leading to improved clarity for the rationale for individual caesarean sections can assist with data collection, which can then be used as part of routine audit of which can in turn improve outcomes.

One of the most contentious aspects in describing emergency caesarean section is the optimal decision-to-delivery interval (DDI). Thirty minutes is the widely cited 'decision-to-delivery' time that should be achieved in emergency caesarean section. However, whether this is a meaningful time to aim for has become increasingly

Table 8.2 Classification of urgency of caesarean section relating the degree of urgency to the presence or absence of maternal or fetal compromise

	Definition	Category
Maternal or fetal compromise	Immediate threat to life of woman or foetus	1
	No immediate threat to life of woman or foetus	2
No maternal or fetal compromise	Requires early delivery	3
	At a time to suit the woman and maternity services	4

controversial. Use of this figure has various inherent problems. Firstly there is no compelling evidence that delivery within 30 min of the decision is meaningful in terms of neonatal outcome. There are no randomized controlled trials demonstrating that the faster a baby is delivered the better the neonatal (or maternal) outcome. Studies suggest that either no difference or reduced neonatal morbidity with longer decision-to-delivery interval. One of the largest studies used data from the National Sentinel Caesarean Section Audit to determine whether decision-to-delivery interval is critical in emergency caesarean section. The National Cross Sectional Survey looked at 17,780 CS performed between over a 3-month period [4]. Maternal and neonatal outcomes were correlated with decision to delivery. Data were categorized into 15 min intervals. No difference in neonatal outcome was found with a decision to delivery of less than 30 min compared to time intervals greater than 30 min. In fact, there was no difference in neonatal outcome with a DDI of less than 15 min compared to all time intervals greater than 15 min up to 75 min at which point neonatal outcomes started to deteriorate. Maternal outcome was similarly unaffected; only women who were delivered after 75 min, compared to women who were delivered within 30 min, had an increase in requirement for post-operative special care although maternal outcome in this context may be affected by the presence of co-morbid disease.

The second problem with the 30 min figure is that it is often used as a response time to a situation that is in itself poorly understood—that is foetal distress. The term 'foetal distress' describes abnormalities of the foetal heart rate detected with cardiotocography or a disturbance in foetal pH assessed using foetal blood sampling, which are in turn deemed to be a sign of hypoxia; both of these tools have limitations [5]. Furthermore, the development of intrapartum hypoxia (and consequent foetal distress) is multifactorial [6]. Factors such as congenital disease and infection may play a part, so that when foetal distress develops in labour it may be difficult to determine whether the abnormalities represent an acute event, such as cord compression or the effect of labour on a chronically compromised foetus [7].

8.3 Modes of Anaesthesia for Caesarean Section

Neuraxial anaesthesia is the preferred mode of anaesthesia for elective or emergency caesarean section and the proportion of caesarean sections performed under neuraxial anaesthesia has increased dramatically over the last 30 years [8]. The main types of regional techniques used for caesarean delivery are single-shot spinal anaesthesia, epidural anaesthesia (as extension of labour epidural analgesia) and combined spinal–epidural anaesthesia (CSE). Recommendations in the United Kingdom have proposed that more than 95% of elective caesarean deliveries and more than 85% of emergency caesarean deliveries should be performed using neuraxial anaesthetic techniques [9].

The relative merits of spinal, epidural, combined spinal anaesthesia and general anaesthesia are summarized in Table 8.3.

Table 8.3 Benefits and risks of different modes of anaesthesia for caesarean section

Anaesthetic technique	Benefit	Risk
General anaesthetic	• Generally considered to be faster option for foetal delivery	• Increased maternal mortality and morbidity
	• Suitable if neuraxial block contraindicated, e.g. the presence of coagulopathy	• Risks associated with airway management (*increased risk of difficult intubation/high risk of pulmonary aspiration of gastric contents*)
	• May be easier to manage an asleep patient in some emergency situations, e.g. major haemorrhage	• Risk of awareness
	• Can modify drugs used for rapid sequence induction if haemodynamic instability present	• Uterine atony with volatile anaesthetic agents
	• Not contraindicated in systemic sepsis	• Maternal transfer of drugs with risk of foetal sedation and respiratory depression
		• Lack of parental presence at delivery
		• Does not provide post-operative analgesia
Spinal	• Generally considered to be the fastest option for neuraxial blockade	• Least suitable for lengthy procedures
	• Low incidence of maternal morbidity including infection and nerve damage	• May require conversion to general anaesthesia if technical failure
	• Avoids risks of general anaesthesia	
	• Can maintain patient in lateral position if situations such as cord prolapse present	
	• Patient remains awake for birth of child	
Epidural extension of labour analgesia	• Relatively fast onset	• Generally considered to take longer than general anaesthesia or spinal techniques
	• Avoids risk of technical failure (e.g. with spinal) in high-risk situation	• Requires adequately working epidural
CSE	• Can be used to provide a more stable induction of neuraxial anaesthesia in cases such as failed top-up of previous epidural, or cardiac disease	• Higher maternal morbidity than spinal or epidural anaesthesia alone
	• Can 'top-up' for longer procedures	

8.3.1 Spinal Anaesthesia

Spinal anaesthesia is the most popular mode of neuraxial anaesthesia used for caesarean section [8, 10]. The incidence of post-dural puncture headache, which for many years made the technique unacceptable, has been dramatically reduced with the evolution in small gauge spinal needles with pencil point tips. Spinal anaesthesia is fast and effective and there is an extremely low risk of systemic toxicity as the doses of drugs used are minimal. The addition of intrathecal opioids (fentanyl, morphine and diamorphine) has been demonstrated to improve the quality of block and reduce intraoperative pain and is recommended [11, 12]. Morphine and diamorphine (though not fentanyl) can contribute to post-operative analgesia between 12 and 24 h.

The most significant acute complication of spinal anaesthesia is maternal hypotension, which occurs in up to three quarters of women without prophylactic measures [13]. This can be associated with maternal nausea and vomiting and impaired uteroplacental perfusion that can lead to foetal acidaemia. Prophylactic measures to avoid/minimize hypotension are mandatory and include the use of an intravenous fluid bolus, given as a pre-load or co-load and the use of vasopressor drugs. For many years ephedrine was the main vasopressor used for the treatment of spinal hypotension. This was based on studies in pregnant ewes that demonstrated it was associated with less reduction in uterine blood flow and thus recommended it over metaraminol and other α-adrenoreceptor agonists [14]. However, subsequent work demonstrated that although blood pressure control was better with ephedrine than without, there was no improvement in neonatal outcome; indeed, the use of ephedrine was associated with a higher incidence of umbilical arterial pH < 7.2 compared to controls [15]. This renewed interest in vasopressors with more α-agonist activity (phenylephrine and metaraminol) and studies with these agents showed there was improved foetal acid-base status compared with ephedrine [16]. Subsequently, phenylephrine has emerged as the vasopressor of choice to minimize hypotension associated with spinal anaesthesia [17]. There has been some debate about whether phenylephrine should be given as an infusion started immediately after initiation of spinal anaesthesia or as a bolus dose (either given only in response to a fall in blood pressure or prophylactically). Prophylactic administration of phenylephrine could potentially cause reactive hypertension and associated bradycardia. A meta-analysis looking at the use of prophylactic phenylephrine for caesarean section under spinal anaesthesia concluded that a continuous infusion started immediately after initiation of spinal anaesthesia significantly reduced the incidence of spinal hypotension compared with bolus doses given only in response to a fall in blood pressure [17]. In addition, a more recent study demonstrated a reduction in anaesthetists' workload by the use of an algorithm adjusting the infusion rate of a prophylactic phenylephrine infusion according to changes in blood pressure and heart rate [18]. The ideal infusion regimen that will control the maternal blood pressure, with minimal maternal side effects, while avoiding maternal hypertension has not yet been identified.

A major reason cited as to why general anaesthesia continues to be used over spinal anaesthesia in cases of extreme urgency is speed, general anaesthesia being perceived as faster and consistently reliable. Although spinal anaesthesia can be almost as fast as general anaesthesia in skilled anaesthetists there are inherent aspects, such as the time required for an adequate surgical block to develop, that will in general make it slower than general anaesthesia [19]. The 'rapid sequence spinal' has been described as an approach for spinal anaesthesia for Category 1 caesarean section [20]. Principles of this approach include using a 'no-touch' technique and using sterile gloves only, utilizing other staff members to perform i.v. cannulation, limiting the number of attempts to one and preparing the patient for general anaesthesia during attempted spinal insertion. The authors of this study reported successful reduction in the decision to delivery interval with this approach; however, concerns exist around minimizing the aseptic technique.

8.3.2 Epidural Analgesia

The role of epidural anaesthesia in emergency caesarean section is largely confined to when an existing labour epidural is extended to provide surgical anaesthesia. Epidural anaesthesia alone is generally not preferred for elective caesarean section as the quality of anaesthesia is less than that achieved by spinal anaesthesia. The ability to site an epidural when the woman is in labour and then utilize that epidural should caesarean section be required can avoid the need for general anaesthesia. The use of epidural analgesia in this context can be particularly useful in 'high-risk' women who may require intrapartum delivery.

Before extending a labour epidural block for caesarean section, it is vital to ensure that the epidural has been working well during labour. Other considerations when extending a labour epidural block for caesarean section include the choice of drug and where the top-up drug should be administered.

The choice of local anaesthetic agent to use in this situation has been widely but not extensively studied. Comparison of these studies is limited by a number of factors including differing end points and the use of different labour analgesia regimens. The ideal agent should have a fast onset but be associated with minimal side effects as a large bolus of local anaesthetic is being administered over a short time period. A meta-analysis on the subject looked at 11 randomized controlled trials, involving 779 parturients [21]. The local anaesthetic agents used in the various studies were classified into three groups: 0.5% bupivacaine or levobupivacaine; 2% lidocaine and 1: 200 000 epinephrine, with or without fentanyl; and 0.75% ropivacaine. The authors found that lidocaine and epinephrine, with or without fentanyl, resulted in a significantly faster onset of sensory. The bupivacaine or levobupivacaine group was associated with a significantly increased risk of intraoperative supplementation compared with the other groups. The addition of fentanyl to a local anaesthetic resulted in a significantly faster onset but did not affect the need for intraoperative supplementation. The authors concluded that if the speed of onset is important, then a lidocaine and epinephrine solution, with or without fentanyl, was preferable, but for quality of epidural block then 0.75% ropivacaine preferable. There were insufficient trials to assess the effect of adding sodium bicarbonate in this meta-analysis, although it was noted that the reduction in onset time appeared more pronounced when bicarbonate was added in two studies. However, the time required to prepare solutions of drugs could outweigh any reduction in onset times, and there are safety implications when mixing drugs in emergency situations [22].

The location where the epidural 'top-up' should be given is controversial and can be affected by a variety of factors including the urgency of delivery, local practice factors and the layout of an individual unit [23]. Initiating the 'top-up' in the labour ward can help to expedite the establishment of an adequate block height and minimize the decision to delivery interval. However, any large epidural top-up is associated with the risks of significant hypotension, high blockade and local anaesthetic toxicity. The anaesthetist's ability to effectively monitor for the development of these complications and manage them may be compromised by being in the delivery room. If the top-up is given only after the patient has arrived in the operating room there may not be sufficient time to allow an adequate block height to develop and general anaesthesia may be required [24]. A compromise would be to administer a small dose of local anaesthetic in the delivery room and then giving the rest of the top-up once the patient has arrived in theatre.

8.3.3 General Anaesthesia

The use of general anaesthesia for caesarean section has fallen dramatically in the past two decades particularly in the resourced world. It has been estimated that less than 5% of all elective caesarean deliveries in the United States and United Kingdom are performed under general anaesthesia. Recommendations from the United Kingdom are that less than 15% of emergency (Category 1, 2 and 3 caesarean sections) and 5% of elective (Category 4 CS) be performed with general anaesthesia [9].

Indications for general anaesthesia for caesarean section include:

- Contraindication to regional anaesthesia
- Maternal refusal
- Failure of regional anaesthesia
- Insufficient time to establish neuraxial anaesthesia for urgent delivery in the presence of severe maternal/foetal compromise

The safe delivery of general anaesthesia depends on rigorous planning and preparation. General anaesthesia is frequently performed in an urgent situation, and time for planning and preparation may be limited. Effective multidisciplinary team communication is essential so that high-risk women can be identified early before an emergency situation develops thus facilitating optimization, the administration of antacid prophylaxis, assessment of the haemoglobin and confirmation that a group and save sample has been sent for laboratory analysis.

The key elements of general anaesthesia include:

1. Pre-assessment is the cornerstone of maintaining safety, particularly in the emergency situation. This includes routine assessment for general co-morbidities and relevant pregnancy-related problems but most importantly a thorough appraisal of the airway. Airway assessment should not only evaluate possible difficulty with intubation but also with mask ventilation/supraglottic airway device insertion and front-of-neck access.
2. Prevention of pulmonary aspiration of gastric contents. Risk factors for aspiration include a prolonged gastric emptying time in labour, increased intra-abdominal pressure due to the gravid uterus and relaxation of the lower oesophageal sphincter due to hormonal changes. To reduce the risk, prophylaxis against acid aspiration should be given prior to anaesthesia.
3. The use of rapid sequence induction for induction and intubation.

The use of thiopental and succinylcholine for general anaesthesia for caesarean section has remained standard for many decades although propofol is also now widely used as the induction agent. The publication of a major investigation into accidental awareness during general anaesthesia has highlighted obstetric patients being at particular risk [25]. Factors associated with an increased risk of awareness include:

- Induction or emergence of anaesthesia
- Use of neuromuscular blockade
- Use of thiopentone
- Rapid sequence induction
- Obesity
- Difficult airway management
- Out-of-hours operating, emergencies.

Following general anaesthesia for a Category 1 caesarean section, surgery may commence very soon after induction. This is a period when rapid redistribution of the intravenous induction agent and slowly increasing partial pressure of the volatile anaesthetic may lead to a gap in effective anaesthetic depth and consequent awareness. Accidental awareness may lead to psychological morbidity, which can have a significant impact on the maternal experience and maternal-infant bonding. Anaesthetists should consider obstetric cases as having a high risk of awareness, and include the risk of awareness as part of the consent process. Recommended strategies to minimize the risk of awareness include an additional syringe of induction agent being available to maintain anaesthesia in case of airway difficulties at induction and intubation, strategies to ensure the rapid attainment of adequate end-tidal volatile levels after intravenous induction (additional uterotonics may be required to allow 'enough' volatile agent to be used) and the use of opioids at induction.

The advent of videolaryngoscopy, second-generation supraglottic devices and now transnasal humidified rapid-insufflation ventilatory exchange devices such as Optiflow™ is providing an increasingly safer environment for the emergency GA section. However, as there remains a relatively low rate of general anaesthesia for caesarean section, training remains challenging; it has been suggested that the use of emergency drills in the simulation environment can be helpful [26, 27].

8.4   Special Circumstances

8.4.1   The Bleeding Patient

Maternal haemorrhage is a leading cause of maternal mortality and morbidity, and if it occurs antenatally can cause foetal hypoxia and death. Antepartum haemorrhage has an incidence of 2–5% over 24 weeks gestation [28]. The major causes are abruption, uterine rupture and placenta previa. The anaesthetic management of these patients is key to ensuring a good outcome for mother and baby. Surgical intervention is lifesaving and must be accompanied by the safe provision of rapid anaesthesia. Particular features that complicate decision-making when choosing the best mode of anaesthesia relate to concerns about the presence of a coagulopathy and the administration of anaesthesia to a patient with cardiovascular compromise. Major obstetric haemorrhage may precipitate disseminated intra-vascular coagulopathy (DIC), which is incompatible with safe neuraxial blockade [29]. The most common cause of clinically significant consumptive coagulopathy in obstetrics is placental abruption accounting for approximately one third of cases of disseminated intra-vascular in the obstetric patient [30]. It is particularly likely to arise in the presence of antenatal foetal demise. It is more likely in a concealed abruption as the intrauterine pressure will increase and force more thromboplastin into the maternal venous system, leading to reduced fibrinogen levels with or without thrombocytopaenia [31].

A further concern when considering anaesthetic choice for a patient who has had an obstetric haemorrhage or has the potential to do so, for example a woman with placenta praevia, is an anxiety that the sympathetic blockade induced by neuraxial anaesthesia would make it difficult to manage blood pressure in the event of a haemorrhage.

In general, consensus advice appears to favour neuraxial blockade in situations in which the patient remains relatively haemodynamically stable and in which there are no clear contraindications [32]. The caveat remains that induction of any type of surgical anaesthesia will require appropriate fluid resuscitation and the use of vasopressors to avoid hypotension and cardiovascular collapse. A further consideration is that in a woman who has received neuraxial anaesthesia and suffered obstetric haemorrhage, significant reassurance or resuscitative management will require additional skilled anaesthetic assistance.

Other situations in which coagulation may be affected are in cases of massive transfusion, where there is altered haemostasis, dilution and consumption of clotting factors. This is particularly relevant when considering the timing of removal of an epidural catheter. The catheter should only be removed once the bleeding is controlled, the patient is stable and the coagulation can be assessed [29].

8.4.2 The Patient with Severe Pre-eclampsia

A hypertensive response to laryngoscopy and intubation in patients with pre-eclampsia requiring emergency operative delivery has been reported as a direct cause of mortality in UK Confidential Enquiry Reports [33]. In a woman with severe pre-eclampsia there is also an increased incidence of laryngeal oedema and therefore increased potential for difficult intubation. As a result, neuraxial blockade is considered the preferred choice in the absence of absolute contraindications [34, 35]; this includes circumstances following eclampsia seizures in which patients have regained a full level of consciousness [35].

Pre-eclampsia and particularly HELLP(Hemolysis, Elevated Liver enzymes and Low Platelet count) syndrome can be associated with thrombocytopenia, the extent of which may contraindicate neuraxial anaesthesia. There is no universally accepted optimum platelet count at which neuraxial anaesthesia procedures can be safely performed [29]. Obstetric neuraxial anaesthetic procedures are generally associated with a lower risk of the serious complications, including epidural haematoma [36]. Reports of epidural haematoma are often confounded by the presence of other risk factors including the use of anticoagulants or antiplatelet agents or in the case of pre-eclampsia with rapidly falling platelet counts. There are two important considerations in decision-making for the obstetric anaesthetist. Firstly, what the preferred mode of neuraxial anaesthesia is, spinal anaesthesia posing less risks than epidural anaesthesia; and secondly, the nature of the thrombocytopenia, a woman who has developed a physiological thrombocytopenia during pregnancy is at less risk of spinal haematoma than a woman who has severe pre-eclampsia with a falling platelet count.

In circumstances in which general anaesthesia cannot be avoided, care should be taken to reduce the hypertensive response to laryngoscopy using opiates, beta-blockers, magnesium or lidocaine and careful consideration to the likelihood of difficult intubation with appropriate provision made.

8.4.3 The Obese Patient

Obesity poses additional risks and difficulties for both general and neuraxial anaesthesia; an obese parturient presenting for emergency caesarean section may be particularly problematic [37]. Adequate multidisciplinary antenatal planning and early provision of epidural anaesthesia in labour are essential [38]. The safety of the mother is paramount and where possible general anaesthesia should be avoided.

Ultrasound may be a useful guide to establishing the midline when this proves difficult [39]; extra length spinal and epidural kits should be available when necessary, although it is generally considered that a standard set is suitable for most first attempts. Ultrasound may also be required for establishing intravenous access. Consideration should be made to the likelihood of increased surgical complexity and length of operation, which may make a combined spinal epidural approach the most suitable choice, as converting to general anaesthesia mid procedure would be less than ideal. Obstructive sleep apnoea is underdiagnosed in the obese pregnant population and confers additional risks peri-operatively, and is a further reason to avoid general anaesthesia [40].

Where general anaesthesia is unavoidable, comprehensive preparation even in the emergency is essential. This will include adequate monitoring which may mean establishing arterial access prior to attempting any anaesthetic procedure. Antacid treatment is essential and if the airway is assessed as difficult, awake fibreoptic intubation should be considered. Otherwise, a rapid sequence induction in the ramped position after thorough pre-oxygenation with the presence of an experienced anaesthetist and the availability of videolaryngoscope can assist with minimizing the otherwise inevitable desaturation following induction.

8.5   Planning for Failure

Despite all best efforts, occasionally the primary anaesthetic plan fails. Failure of neuraxial anaesthesia can mean the need to convert to general anaesthesia or conversion to a different form of anaesthesia [41–44]. In an audit of over 5000 caesarean sections, conducted over a 5-year period, the rate of general anaesthesia conversion of regional anaesthesia was 0.8% for elective and 4.9% for emergency caesarean sections, but for Category 1 caesarean sections the general anaesthesia conversion rate was 20% [45]. The rate of failure to achieve a pain-free operation was 6% with spinals, 24% with epidural top-up and 18% with combined spinal–epidural. A retrospective analysis of over 19,000 deliveries for failure rates for labour analgesia and caesarean section anaesthesia found that for caesarean section, 7.1% of pre-existing labour epidural catheters failed and 4.3% of patients required conversion to general anaesthesia. Spinal anaesthesia for caesarean section had a lower failure rate of 2.7%, with 1.2% of the patients requiring general anaesthesia [46].

When there is a problem in the emergency situation, rapid recognition and decision making is required to identify the next best course of action and an intrinsic part of anaesthetic training is the provision of a 'Plan B' in the case of failure. There is little evidence on which to make recommendations about the best mode of anaesthesia after failure of the primary technique. In addition, the options for an alternative mode of anaesthesia will be affected by the stage of the caesarean section; for example, if the regional block (spinal or epidural top-up) has not reached a sufficient height and maternal/foetal condition allows, there is the option to repeat the spinal anaesthetic. Some evidence suggest that performing a spinal anaesthetic after failure of an epidural top-up can be associated with the development of a high block

[47, 48]. If surgery has started, the options for alternative anaesthesia are more limited and conversion to general anaesthesia may be required. There is limited evidence to suggest superiority of a well-performed regional or general anaesthetic technique on neonatal outcome and the risk to mother for general anaesthesia varies in terms of the individual circumstances [49, 50].

Communication is also key, as decision for emergency caesarean section is a dynamic process, and the degree of urgency of a particular case may change. Decision-making should always be in the mother's best interests, and options should include seeking further assistance and advice as far as possible. There is increasing recognition of the impact of 'human factors' in these situations and how they can impact on a situation. In the 2014 UK Confidential Enquiry into Maternal Death, the MBRRACE Report (Mothers and Babies: Reducing Risk through Audits and Confidential Enquiries), fixation error was highlighted as an issue in anaesthetic-related maternal deaths [33]. A fixation error is said to occur when a practitioner concentrates solely upon a single aspect of a case to the detriment of other more relevant aspects; it can be associated with delayed diagnosis and a failure to change management plans appropriately. Training in non-technical skills is likely to become increasingly important in all areas of anaesthesia in the future.

References

1. http://www.oecd-ilibrary.org/sites/health_glance-2015-en/06/08/index.html?itemId=/content/chapter/health_glance-2015-37-en&mimeType=text/html. Accessed July 2016.
2. Morgan BM, Magni V, Goroszenuik T. Anaesthesia for emergency caesarean section. BJOG. 1990;97:420–4.
3. Classification of urgency of caesarean section—a continuum of risk, Good Practice No. 11. http://www.rcog.org.uk/classification-of-urgency-of-caesarean-section-good-practice-11.
4. Thomas J, Paranjothy S, James D. National cross sectional survey to determine whether the decision to delivery interval is critical in emergency caesarean section. BMJ. 2004;328:665–9.
5. Yentis SM. Whose distress is it anyway? 'Fetal distress' and the 30-minute rule. Anaesthesia. 2003;58:732–3.
6. James D. Caesarean section for fetal distress. BMJ. 2001;322:1316–7.
7. MacLennan A. For the international cerebral palsy task force. A template for defining a causal relation between acute intra-partum events and cerebral palsy: international consensus statement. BMJ. 1999;319:1054–9.
8. Bucklin BA, Hawkins JL, Anderson JR, Ullrich FA. Obstetric anesthesia workforce survey. Twenty year update. Anesthesiology. 2005;103:645–53.
9. Colvin JR. Raising the standard: a compendium of audit recipes. 3rd ed. London: RCOA; 2012.
10. http://www.oaa-anaes.ac.uk/assets/_managed/cms/files/NOAD%20REPORTS/National%20Obstetric%20Anaesthesia%20Data%20for%202012%20final.pdf. Accesses July 2016.
11. National Institute For Health And Care Excellence (Nice). Caesarean section. London: NICE; 2011.
12. Practice guidelines for obstetric anesthesia: an updated report by the American Society of Anesthesiologists Task Force on Obstetric Anesthesia and the Society for Obstetric Anesthesia and Perinatology. Anesthesiology. 2016;124:270–300.
13. Rout CC, Rocke DA, Levin J, Gouws E, Reddy D. A reevaluation of the role of crystalloid preload in the prevention of hypotension associated with spinal anesthesia for elective Cesarean section. Anesthesiology. 1993;79:262–9.

14. Ralston DH, Shnider SM, DeLorimier AA. Effects of equipotent ephedrine, metaraminol, mephentermine and methoxamine on uterine blood flow in the pregnant ewe. Anesthesiology. 1974;40:354–70.
15. Ngan Kee WD, Khaw KS, Lee BB, et al. A dose-response study of prophylactic intravenous ephedrine for the prevention of hypotension during spinal anaesthesia for cesarean delivery. Anesth Analg. 2000;90:1390–5.
16. Heesen M, Stewart A, Fernando R. Vasopressors for the treatment of maternal hypotension following spinal anaesthesia for elective caesarean section: past, present and future. Anaesthesia. 2015;70:252–7.
17. Heesen M, Klöhr S, Rossaint R, et al. Prophylactic phenylephrine for caesarean section under spinal anaesthesia: systematic review and meta-analysis. Anaesthesia. 2014;69:143–65.
18. Siddik-Sayyid SM, Taha SK, Kanazi GE, et al. A randomized controlled trial of variable rate phenylephrine infusion with rescue phenylephrine boluses versus rescue boluses alone on physician interventions during spinal anesthesia for elective cesarean delivery. Anesth Analg. 2014;118:611–8.
19. Kathirgamanathan A, Douglas MJ, Tyler J, Saran S, Gunka V, Preston R, Kliffer P. Speed of spinal vs. general anaesthesia for category-1 caesarean section: a simulation and clinical observation-based study. Anaesthesia. 2013;68:753–9.
20. Kinsella SM, Girgirah K, Scrutton MJL. Rapid sequence spinal anaesthesia for category-1 urgency caesarean section: a case series. Anaesthesia. 2010;65:664–9.
21. SG Hillyard, TE Bate, TB Corcoran, MJ Paech, G O'Sullivan; Extending epidural analgesia for emergency Caesarean section: a meta-analysis. Br J Anaesth 2011; 107: 668-678.
22. Lucas DN, Borra PJ, Yentis SM. Epidural top-up solutions for emergency caesarean section: a comparison of preparation times. Br J Anaesth. 2000;84:494–6.
23. Regan KJ, O'Sullivan G. The extension of epidural blockade for emergency Caesarean section: a survey of current UK practice. Anaesthesia. 2008;63:136–42.
24. Moore P, Russell IF. Epidural top-ups for category I/II emergency caesarian section should be given only in the operating theatre. IJOA. 2004;13:257–65.
25. Pandit JJ, Andrade J, Bogod DG, et al. The 5th National Audit Project (NAP5) on accidental awareness during general anaesthesia: summary of main findings and risk factors. Anaesthesia. 2014;69:1089–101.
26. Lipman S, Carvalho B, Brock-Utne J. The demise of general anesthesia in obstetrics revisited: prescription for a cure. IJOA. 2005;14:2–4.
27. Mushambi MC, Kinsella SM, Popat M, et al. Obstetric anaesthetists' association and difficult airway society guidelines for the management of difficult and failed tracheal intubation in obstetrics. Anaesthesia. 2015;70:1286–306.
28. Calleja-Aguus J, Custo R. Placental abruption and placenta previa. Eur J Clin Obstet Gynaecol. 2006;2:121–7.
29. Working Party. Regional anaesthesia and patients with abnormalities of coagulation: The Association of Anaesthetists of Great Britain & Ireland, the Obstetric Anaesthetists' Association, Regional Anaesthesia UK. Anaesthesia. 2013;68:966–72.
30. Rattray DD, O'Connell CM, Baskett TF. Acute disseminated intravascular coagulation in obstetrics: a tertiary centre population review (1980–2009). J Obstet Gynaecol Can. 2012;34:341–7.
31. Daflapurkar SB. High risk cases in obstetrics. 1st ed. London: JP Medical Ltd.; 2014. ISBN: 978-93-5152-218-8.
32. Walfish M, Neuman A, Wlody D. Maternal haemorrhage. Br J Anaesth. 2009;103:47–56.
33. Knight M, Kenyon S, Brocklehurst P, Neilson J, Shakespeare J, Kurinczuk JJ, editors., on behalf of MBRRACE-UK. Saving lives, improving mothers' care–lessons learned to inform future maternity care from the UK and Ireland Confidential Enquiries into Maternal Deaths and Morbidity 2009–12. Oxford: National Perinatal Epidemiology Unit, University of Oxford; 2014.
34. Dennis AT. Management of pre-eclampsia: issues for anaesthetists. Anaesthesia. 2012;67:1009–20.

35. Dyer RA, Piercy JL, Reed AR. The role of the anaesthetist in the pre-eclampsia patient. Curr Opin Anaesthesiol. 2007;20:168–74.
36. Cook TM, Counsell D, Wildsmith JAW. Major complications of central neuraxial block: report on the Third National Audit of the Royal College of Anaesthetists. Br J Anaesth. 2009;102:179–90.
37. Mace HS, Paech MJ, McDonnell NJ. Obesity and obstetric anaesthesia. Anaesth Intensive Care. 2011;39:559–70.
38. Members of the Working Party, Nightingale CE, Margarson MP, Shearer E, Redman JW, Lucas DN, Cousins JM, Fox WTA, Kennedy NJ, Venn PJ, Skues M, Gabbott D, Misra U, Pandit JJ, Popat MT, Griffiths R. Peri-operative management of the obese surgical patient 2015. Anaesthesia. 2015;70:859–76.
39. Sahin T, Balaban O, Sahin L, Solak M, Toker K. A randomized controlled trial of preinsertion ultrasound guidance for spinal anaesthesia in pregnancy: outcomes among obese and lean parturients: ultrasound for spinal anaesthesia in pregnancy. J Anesth. 2014;28:413–9.
40. Ankichetty SP, Angle P, Joselyn AS, Chinnappa V, Halpern S. Anesthetic considerations of parturients with obesity and obstructive sleep apnea. J Anaesthesiol Clin Pharmacol. 2012;28:436–43.
41. Shibli KU, Russell IF. A survey of anaesthetic techniques used for caesarean section in the UK in 1997. Int J Obstet Anesth. 2000;9:160–7.
42. Jenkins JG, Khan MM. Anaesthesia for caesarean section: a survey in a UK region from 1992 to 2002. Anaesthesia. 2003;58:1114–8.
43. Riley ET, Papasin J. Epidural catheter function during labor predicts anesthetic efficacy for subsequent cesarean delivery. Int J Obstet Anesth. 2002;11:81–4.
44. Garry M, Davies S. Failure of regional blockade for caesarean section. Int J Obstet Anesth. 2002;11:9–12.
45. Kinsella SM. A prospective audit of regional anaesthesia failure in 5080 Caesarean sections. Anaesthesia. 2008;63:822–32.
46. Pan PH, Bogard TD, Owen MD. Incidence and characteristics of failures in obstetric neuraxial analgesia and anesthesia: a retrospective analysis of 19,259 deliveries. Int J Obstet Anesth. 2004;13:227–33.
47. Dresner M, Brennan A, Freeman J. Six year audit of high regional blocks in obstetric anaesthesia. Int J Obstet Anesth. 2003;12:S10.
48. D'Angelo R, Smiley RM, Riley ET, Segal S. Serious complications related to obstetric anesthesia: the serious complication repository project of the society for obstetric anesthesia and perinatology. Anesthesiology. 2014;120:1505–12.
49. Afolabi BB, Lesi FEA, Merah NA. Regional versus general anaesthesia for caesarean section. Cochrane Database Syst Rev. 2006,(4):CD004350. doi: 10.1002/14651858.CD004350.pub2.
50. Dyer RA, Els I, Farbas J, et al. Prospective, randomised trial comparing general with spinal anaesthesia for Caesarian delivery in preeclamptic patients with a non reassuring fetal heart trace. Anaesthesiology. 2003;99:561–9.

Surgical Difficulties and Complications

9

Vincenzo Scotto di Palumbo

9.1   History

We cannot be sure when the term cesarean was derived. In past centuries the procedure was known as cesarean operation. In 1598, Jacques Guillemeau in his book on midwifery introduced the term section and this replaced the term operation.

The purpose of this procedure was essentially to retrieve the infant from a dead or dying mother.

In Western societies, women for the most part were not allowed to perform cesarean sections until the late nineteenth century because they were largely denied admission to medical schools. The first recorded successful cesarean in the British Empire, however, was conducted by a woman, James Miranda Stuart Barry, who in 1815 performed the operation while masquerading as a man and serving as a physician to the British army in South Africa.

In 1879, for example, one British traveller, R.W. Felkin, witnessed cesarean section performed by Ugandans. The healer used banana wine to semi-intoxicate the woman and to cleanse his hands and her abdomen prior to surgery. He used a midline incision and applied cautery to minimize hemorrhaging. He massaged the uterus to make it contract but did not suture it; the abdominal wound was pinned with iron needles and dressed with a paste prepared from roots. The patient recovered well, and Felkin concluded that this technique was well-developed and had clearly been employed for a long time.

In the mid-1860s, Joseph Lister, a British surgeon, introduced an antiseptic method using carbolic acid, and many operators adopted some part of his antisepsis.

Using those techniques, the procedure continued to produce many complications and deaths. According to one estimate, not a single woman survived cesarean

V.S. di Palumbo
UOC Ostetricia e Ginecologia, Ospedale S Spirito, Rome, Italy
e-mail: vscottodipalumbo@gmail.com

© Springer International Publishing Switzerland 2017
G. Capogna (ed.), *Anesthesia for Cesarean Section*,
DOI 10.1007/978-3-319-42053-0_9

section in Paris between 1787 and 1876. Surgeons were afraid to suture the uterine incision because they thought internal stitches, which could not be removed, might produce infections and cause uterine rupture in subsequent pregnancies. So some women died of hemorrhage or infection.

In 1876, an Italian doctor Eduardo Porro suggested performing an hysterectomy at the time of the cesarean section to control uterine hemorrhage and prevent systemic infection. This enabled him to reduce the incidence of postoperative sepsis. But his mutilating elaboration on cesarean section was soon obviated by the employment of uterine sutures.

Between 1880 and 1925, obstetricians experimented with transverse incisions in the lower segment of the uterus. This refinement reduced the risk of infection and of subsequent uterine rupture in pregnancy.

After the discovery of penicillin by Alexander Fleming in 1928 and its purification as a drug in 1940, the procedure became safer and maternal mortality decreased dramatically.

While the operation was historically performed largely to protect the health of the mother, more recently the health of the fetus has played a larger role.

An operation that virtually always resulted in a dead woman and dead fetus now almost always results in a living mother and baby.

In this chapter the complications and the difficulties that can occur performing a cesarean delivery (CD) will be examined.

9.2 Delivering the Fetal Head in Advanced Labor

Sometimes, when the CD is performed in the second stage, with the head strongly engaged in the pelvis, the removal of the head can be very difficult, and severe head trauma can occur, especially nowadays when forceps and vacuum delivery are not so common as before.

In this condition, the head is deeply engaged in the pelvis. Open the lower segment of the uterus and insert the hand; wait until the contraction disappears, avoid fighting against the contraction, because it can produce head trauma. Then when your hand does not feel the pressure, gently with flection or rotation, easily disengage the head of the baby. Never use the forceps to pull up the head. In some cases, when this maneuver is unsuccessful ask the anesthetist to administer terbutaline or glyceryltrinitrate 250 mcg i.v.to relax the uterus. The effect is quite immediate and of short duration.

When accessing the uterus in advanced labor remember that the lower segment is stretched and the incision must be made 3–4 cm higher than usual to avoid entering straight into the vagina.

Accessing a uterus which has fibroids is sometimes very difficult. In this case it is very useful to have a perfect knowledge of the position of the fibroids especially in the anterior part of the uterus and the thickness of the lower segment; this can be obtained by performing an ultrasound immediately before the procedure. Sometimes a large fibroid can rotate the uterus and in this case great attention must be made in choosing where to cut the uterus to effect the delivery in order to avoid cutting the uterine vessels.

Some difficulties in accessing the baby can occur when the position is unstable or abnormal because of uterine anomalies or amniotic bands. In this case it is better to try to understand the reason prior to surgery and to be helped by an experienced obstetrician.

9.3   Anterior Placenta

In the case of anterior placenta, it is better, before beginning the procedure, to check the placental position by ultrasound in order to cut the uterus below the placenta and so avoid going through it. In some cases, however, this is not possible and the obstetrician must pay attention when cutting the placenta to avoid the cord and must immediately clamp the cord itself to minimize any fetal blood loss. If it occurs advise the neonatologist in case the baby shows signs of acute hemorrhage.

9.4   Breech

In the CD for a breech presentation make a large incision of the skin and the uterus. If the incision of the uterus does not seem large enough, continue with a J-shaped incision avoiding the uterine vessels. Remember not to pull the baby, but invite your assistant to apply pressure from above; do not lift the baby until the nape is visible; if the head is trapped, ask the anesthetist to relax the uterus or apply a small forceps avoiding the hyperextension of the neck during application and traction must flex the neck.

9.5   Uterine Vessel Injury

If the incision injures the blood vessel a severe hemorrhage occurs and it expands into the broad ligament. The suggestion in this case is to exteriorize the uterus and pull it up in order to identify the bleeding vessel and contemporarily to move the bladder and the ureter away.

Always remember to stop the bleeding first, avoiding catching the ureter in the suture; when the bleeding has stopped, however, you can open the peritoneum and identify the ureter following it until the suture. If you are not able, call for the help of an expert gynecologist or urologist.

9.6   Shoulder Presentation

When the fetal arm is prolapsed through the vagina, perform a large incison of the skin and the uterus, if necessary also J-shaped and palpate the fetal leg and try to deliver the breech with Patwardhan's maneuver [1]. This maneuver can also be used when the head is deeply engaged in the pelvis in advanced labor.

9.7 Placenta Accreta

It occurs when the placenta becomes abnormally adherent to the myometrium rather than the uterine decidua. After delivery of the baby the placenta does not separate from the uterus leading to severe hemorrhaging. If the placenta invades the myometrium it is *increta*, if it invades the uterine serosa and/or adjacent organs it is termed *percreta.*

Placenta accreta is associated with severe maternal morbidity, including large volume blood transfusion, hysterectomy, intensive care unit (ICU) admission, and prolonged hospitalization. Severe hemorrhage can produce disseminated intravascular coagulation (DIC) and multiorgan failure (MOF). Fetal risks are similar to those for placenta previa and consist of complications related to preterm birth. Rates of placenta accreta are increased especially in relation to the increased rate of CD. The incidence was 1:30,000 in the 1960s to 1:500 in 2002 and also more in recent years.

Usually the trophoblast invades the decidua until a certain level, called Nitabuch's layer, and then stops.

In some conditions, after cesarean section or myomectomy there could be a relative hypoxia at the site of the scar, resulting in the cytotrophoblast invading the myometrium to an abnormal degree and sometimes the serosa and also adjacent organs like the bladder. It is therefore evident that the major risk factor for placenta accrete is multiple prior cesarean deliveries. The combination of placenta previa and prior cesarean delivery increases the risk of placenta accreta because the placenta lies on the uterine scar. Obviously, the risk increases with the number of CD, from 11% for the second CD to 61% for the fifth CD [2, 3].

Prior curettage and hysteroscopic surgery are considered risk factors for placenta accreta; also patients who develop Asherman syndrome, or any injury of the normal architecture of the endometrium, are at high risk of placenta accreta.

9.7.1 Screening and Diagnosis for Placenta Previa and Accreta

The gold standard for diagnosis of placenta accreta is histology that is possible only if an hysterectomy is performed. The suspicion, however, of adherent placenta must be present in any woman who has had previous cesarean or uterine surgery. In those cases, an ultrasound assessment of the placental site must be done at 32 weeks and prior to surgery.

9.7.2 Clinical Diagnosis

Clinical suspicion should be raised in all women with vaginal bleeding after 20 weeks of gestation. A high presenting part, an abnormal lie, and painless or provoked bleeding, irrespective of previous imaging results, are more suggestive of a low-lying placenta but may not be present, and definitive diagnosis usually relies on ultrasound imaging [4].

9.7.3   Which Kind of Screening Can Be Done?

Routine ultrasound at 20 weeks of gestation should include placental localization [4] (evidence level 4).

Sonographic features that suggest accreta are the following: (from NICE Green-top Guideline no. 27)

9.7.3.1 With Gray Scale
The sonographic features that suggest placenta accreta are:

Loss of retroplacental sonolucent zone
Irregular retroplacental sonolucent zone
Thinning or disruption of the hyperechoic serosa–bladder interface
Presence of focal exophytic masses invading the urinary bladder
Abnormal placental lacunae

9.7.3.2 With Color Doppler
Diffuse or focal lacunar flow
Vascular lakes with turbulent flow (peak systolic velocity over 15 cm/s)
Hypervascularity of serosa–bladder interface
Markedly dilated vessel over peripheral subplacental zone

9.7.3.3 With Three-Dimensional Power Doppler
Numerous coherent vessels involving the whole uterine serosa–bladder junction
    (basal view)
Hypervascularity (lateral view)
Inseparable cotyledonal and intervillous circulation, chaotic branching, detour vessels (lateral view)

The sensitivity of the three-dimensional power Doppler is 100%, the specificity 85%, and the positive predictive value 88% [5], higher in comparison with gray scale and color doppler.

MRI is indicated when the ultrasound scan is inconclusive or percreta is suspected.

9.7.4   Complications

The primary risk of placenta accreta is hemorrhage and the associated complications such as DIC and MOF. Bladder and ureter injury occurs in 10–15% of cases; 30–40% of patients require ICU admission for complications such as thromboembolism and pyelonephritis and pneumonia. Maternal death is reported in 5–7% of cases. Outcome is related to the severity of the case and the expertise of the center treating the patient. Vesicovaginal fistula is a late complication of cesarean hysterectomy as a result of placenta accreta.

9.7.5 Management

The milestone for the management of placenta accreta is prenatal diagnosis. This allows for the best obstetric management and a significant reduction of morbidity. The suspicion arises from prior multiple cesarean sections, placenta previa, and Asherman syndrome.

There are no randomized trials, but the following recommendations are based on retrospective studies and expert opinions and recommendations of the recent NICE guideline cited above.

9.7.6 Antepartum for Suspected Accreta

Ultrasound to assess the probability as written above

Bed rest or hospitalization in the case of antepartum bleeding

Corticosteroid administration in the case of antepartum bleeding or at the time of hospitalization

Consultation with the patient and her parents about delivery and risks, including also the chance of hysterectomy, leaving the placenta in situ, cell salvage, and interventional radiology; make a note on the chart of all of these.

Prepare a multidisciplinary team at the operating theater

The time of delivery should be between 34 and 36 weeks balancing the risk of maternal hemorrhage and prematurity of the baby

Heavy bleeding requires immediate delivery

9.7.7 Surgery for Suspected Accreta

Present in the main operating theater:

Consultant obstetrician

Consultant anesthesiologist

Blood and blood products on site

Interventional radiologist to decide if preoperative placement of introducer or balloon is required

Neonatal team especially if surgery is far away from the delivery room

Availability of ICU bed

A vertical skin incision should be made, regardless of a prior abdominal or pelvic scar.

The choice of anesthetic technique (loco, regional, or general) for cesarean section for placenta previa or suspected accreta must be made by the anesthetist conducting the procedure; there is insufficient evidence to support one technique over another [6, 7].

It could be prudent to insert a bilateral ureteral stent preoperatively.

In the case of strongly suspected accreta, a planned cesarean hysterectomy should be accomplished. A classical hysterotomy that does not disturb the placenta should be done to deliver the baby [8]. Do not attempt to remove the placenta! The hysterotomy has to be sutured to achieve hemostasis, followed by an hysterectomy [9].

Consideration may be given to leaving the placenta in situ and planning a delayed hysterectomy 6 weeks later [10]. This technique has been advocated in the case of percreta to avoid bladder resection.

9.7.8 Conservative Management

Some women with placenta accreta desire to preserve fertility. Many strategies have been suggested to avoid hysterectomy, such as leaving the placenta in situ after delivery, uterine devascularization made during surgery, embolization of uterine vessels or intraoperative aorta balloon occlusion [11], oversewing the placental vascular bed or the use of methotrexate to inhibit trophoblast growth, and induce postpartum involution of the placenta. The cited techniques, however, may result in increased morbidity. We do not know what the risk of obstetric complication and recurrent accrete could be in a future pregnancy. Conservative management can be done in selective cases such as posterior or fundal placenta (Timmerman).

9.7.9 Prevention

The only prevention is to reduce or avoid multiple cesarean deliveries and of course the primary cesarean. Also the technical modality of suture can be considered as closing the hysterotomy at cesarean; a two layer suture versus one layer could facilitate the endometrial integrity and vascularization.

9.8 Cesarean Myomectomy

The management of myomas during a cesarean delivery is a controversial topic.

In some patients cesarean myomectomy can be associated with increased morbidity, but it can be useful if the myoma compromises the fetal extraction or hysterotomic suture and in all cases with pedunculated and subserous myomas of the anterior wall to avoid multiple hysterotomies for deep intramural nodules, fundal, and cornual associated with severe surgical complications [12].

9.9 Infections

The most important risk factor for postpartum maternal infection is cesarean section. Although all guidelines endorse the use of prophylactic antibiotics for women undergoing cesarean section, there is not a uniform interpretation of this recommendation.

The Cochrane review (2014) identified 95 studies enrolling 15,000 women and stated that the use of a prophylactic antibiotic in women undergoing cesarean section reduced the incidence of wound infection (RR 0.40, C.I. 0.35–0.46), endometritis (RR 0.38, C.I. 0.34–0.42), and maternal serious infection complications (RR 0.31, C.I. 0.20–0.49). For women undergoing elective cesarean section, the protective effect of a prophylactic antibiotic is slightly inferior: for wound infection (RR 0.62, C.I. 0.47–0.82) and for endometritis (RR 0.38, C.I. 0.24–0.61). There was no difference if the prophylactic antibiotics were administered before or after the cord was clamped. No study reported the incidence of oral candidiasis as being a possible effect of the antibiotic in the babies nor if they could effect the baby's immune system. The authors conclude that prophylactic antibiotics should be administered to all women undergoing cesarean section to prevent infections [13].

9.10 How to Control Major Hemorrhage During Cesarean Section

Major causes of obstetric hemorrhage are:

Uterine atony
Placenta previa
Retained placenta or placental fragments
Broad ligament hematoma
Uterine rupture
Uterine anatomical anomalies and myomas

All the procedures to control hemorrhage are well recommended in the Green-top Guideline 52 of the Royal College of Obstetrician and Gynaecologist "Prevention and Management of Postpartum Haemorrhage" [14]. In this paragraph, we will examine the advanced techniques adopted when the pharmacological options fail to control the hemorrhage.

9.10.1 Intrauterine Tamponade with Balloon

The intrauterine tamponade with balloon is suggested in the case of uterine atony and placenta previa. At the beginning, a Rusch balloon or a condom catheter was used, but now the Bakri® balloon by Cook Medical is widely used. This balloon has a drainage lumen that allows blood loss monitoring. It can be inserted after a spontaneous delivery or cesarean section, filled with saline until the bleeding is controlled, maintained in situ for 12–24 h, and removed by vaginal route under uterotonic drugs (syntocinon infusion) and antibiotic regimen [15–17].

In terms of mechanism of action, the intrauterine balloon is believed to act by exerting inward to outward pressure against the uterine wall, resulting in a reduction in persistent capillary and venous bleeding from the endometrium and the myometrium.

The Bakri balloon is used for temporary control or reduction of postpartum hemorrhage when conservative management of uterine bleeding is warranted, after bleeding from genital tract lacerations, and retained product of conception has been excluded.

When uterotonics fail to cause sustained uterine contractions and satisfactory control of hemorrhage after vaginal delivery, tamponade of the uterus can be effective in decreasing hemorrhage secondary to uterine atony.

Although the use of an intrauterine balloon catheter is often successful and serves as a definite therapy, it can also be used as a temporary measure to decrease hemorrhage while waiting and preparing for other definite treatments (i.e., uterine artery ligation, uterine compression suture, hysterectomy) or while the patient is being transferred to another unit with more experience and resources.

The use of the balloon is contraindicated in heavy arterial bleeding requiring surgical exploration or angiographic embolization, congenital uterine anomaly, uterine distorting pathology (leiomyoma), suspected uterine rupture, purulent infection of the vagina, cervix, or uterus, and allergy to balloon material (silicone).

9.10.2 Hemostatic Brace Sutures

The B-Lynch brace suture [18] was devised to control atony after cesarean section in order to avoid hysterectomy; it is a procedure to keep the uterus contracted when bimanual pressure has stopped.

With the uterus exteriorized a rapidly absorbable stitch (chromic catgut in the paper by B-Lynch) with a needle 70 mm diameter is passed 3 cm from the right lower edge of the uterine incision and 3 cm from the right lateral border.

The stitch is threaded through the uterine cavity to emerge at the upper incision margin 3 cm above and approximately 4 cm from the lateral border.

The stitch, now visible, is passed over to compress the uterine fundus approximately 3–4 cm from the right cornual border.

The stitch is fed posteriorly and vertically to enter the posterior wall of the uterine cavity at the same level as the upper anterior entry point.

The stitch is pulled under moderate tension assisted by manual compression exerted by the first assistant.

The length of the stitch is passed back posteriorly through the same surface marking as for the right side, the suture lying horizontally.

The stitch is fed through posteriorly and vertically over the fundus to lie anteriorly and vertically compressing the fundus on the left side, as occurred on the right. The needle is passed in the same fashion on the left side through the uterine cavity and out approximately 3 cm anteriorly and below the lower incision margin on the left side.

The two lengths of stitch are pulled taught assisted by bimanual compression to minimize trauma and to achieve or aid compression. During such compression, the vagina is checked so that the bleeding is controlled.

As good hemostasis is secured and while the uterus is compressed by an experienced assistant the principal surgeon throws a knot (double throw) followed by two or three further throws to secure tension.

The lower transverse uterine incision is now closed in the normal way, in two layers, with or without closure of the lower uterine segment peritoneum.

It is not clear at the moment if fertility can be saved after the procedure. Cases of Asherman syndrome [19] and successful pregnancy have been reported [20].

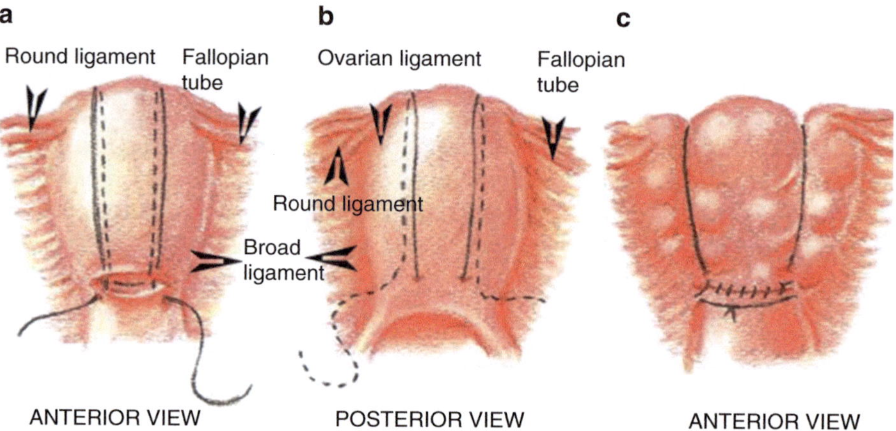

Figure (a) and (b) demonstrate the anterior and posterior views of the uterus showing the application of the B-Lynch Brace suture. Figure (c) shows the anatomical appearance after competent application.

9.10.3 Stepwise Uterine Artery Ligation and Bilateral or Unilateral Internal Lliac Artery Ligation

This procedure is rarely indicated because it has to be performed by a very experienced gynecologist and may make the subsequent interventional radiology very difficult.

References

1. Patwardhan BD, Motashaw ND. Cesarian section. J Obstet Gynaecol India. 1957;8:1–15.
2. Rosen T. Placenta accreta and caesarean scar pregnancy: overlooked cost of rising caesarean section rate. Clin Perinatol. 2008;35:519–29.
3. Gilliam M, Rosenberg D, Davis E. The likeliwood of placenta praevia with greater number of, caesarean deliveries and higher parity. Obstet Gynecol. 2002;99:976–80.
4. RCOG. Greentop Guideline N° 27. Placenta praevia, placenta praeviaaccreta and vasapraevia; diagnosis and management. London: RCOG; 2011.

5. Shih JC, Palacios JM, Su YN, Shyu MK, et al. Role of three-dimensional power Doppler in the antenatal diagnosis of placenta accrete: comparison with gray scale and color Doppler tecniques. Ultrasound Obstet Gynecol. 2009;33:193–203.
6. Bonner SM, Haynes SR, Ryall D. The anesthetic management of caesarean section for placenta praevia: a questionary survey. Anaesthesia. 1995;50:992–4.
7. Parekh N, Husaini SW, Russell IF. Caesarean section for placenta praevia: a retrospective study of anaesthetic management. Br J Anaesth. 2000;84:725–30.
8. Wong HS, Hutton J, Zucollo J, Tait J, Pringle KC. The maternal outcome in placenta accrete: the significance of antenatal diagnosis and non separation of placenta delivery. NZ Med J. 2008;121:30–8.
9. Eller AG, Porter TF, Soisson P, Silver RM. Optimal management strategies for placenta accreta. BJOG. 2009;116:648–54.
10. Timmermans S, van Hof AC, Duvekot JJ. Conservative management of abnormally invasive placentation. Obstet Gynecol Surv. 2007;62:52939.
11. Panici PB, Anceschi M, Borgia ML, et al. Intraoperative aorta balloon occlusion: fertility preservation in patients with placenta praeviaaccreta/increta. J Matern Fetal Neonatal Med. 2012;25:2512–6.
12. Sparić R, Malvasi A, Kadija S, et al. Caesarean myomectomy trends and controversies: an appraisal. J Matern Fetal Neonatal Med. 2016;21:1–38.
13. Smaill FM, Grivell RM. Antibiotic prohylaxis versus no prophylaxis for preventing infection after caesarean section. Cochrane Database Syst Rev. 2014.
14. Royal College of Obstetrician and Gynecologist. Greentop Guideline 52 Prevention and Management of Postpartum Haemorrhage. London: RCOG; 2011.
15. Bakri YN, Amri A, Abdul JF. Tamponade-balloon for obstetrical bleeding. Int J Gynaecol Obstet. 2001;74(2):139–42.
16. Georgiou C. Balloon tamponade in the management of postpartum haemorrhage: a review. BJOG. 2009;116(6):748–57.
17. Lo A, St Marie P, Yadav P, Belisle E, Markenson G. The impact of bakri balloon tamponade on the rate of postpartum hysterectomy for uterine atony. J Matern Fetal Neonatal Med. 2016;30:1–15.
18. B-Lynch C, Coker A, Lawal AH, Abu J, Cowen MJ. The B-Lynch surgical technique for the control of massive postpartum haemorrhage: an alternative to hysterectomy? Five cases reported. BJOG. 1997;104:372–5.
19. Goojha CA, Case A, Pierson R. Development of Asherman syndrome after conservative surgical management of intractable postpartum haemorrhage. Fertil Steril. 2010;94(3):1098.
20. Sentilhes L, Gomez A, Trichot C, et al. Fertility after B-Lynvh suture and stepwise uterine devascularization. Fertil Steril. 2009;91:934–9.

Complications Due to Regional and General Anaesthesia

P.Y. Dewandre and J.F. Brichant

10.1 Introduction

Caesarean delivery is the most frequently performed inpatient surgical procedure [1]. Compared with vaginal delivery, caesarean delivery is associated with a significantly increased risk of anaesthesia-related adverse events (ARAEs) [2–5]. These obstetric ARAEs are usually preventable because most of them are caused by substandard care [3, 5, 6].The risk of ARAEs increases when caesarean delivery is performed under general anaesthesia (GA) [2, 7]. Hence, unless existing contraindication, neuraxial anaesthesia techniques are recommended for caesarean delivery [8, 9]. The actual incidence of serious complications related to obstetric anaesthesia remains largely unknown but is considered as very rare. Changes in the obstetric anaesthesia practice in recent decades have improved patient safety, and the increased use of neuraxial anaesthesia techniques for caesarean deliveries has contributed to this safety improvement [10].

The Serious Complications Repository project (SCORE project) of the Society for Obstetric Anesthesia and Perinatology (SOAP), collecting data from 2004 to 2009 on 257,000 parturients in the USA, concluded to an overall incidence of serious complications related to obstetric anaesthesia of 1 in 3000 patients [11]. The serious complications tracked in this database were maternal death, cardiac arrest, epidural abscess, meningitis, epidural hematoma, serious neurologic injury, aspiration, failed intubation, high neuraxial block, anaphylaxis and respiratory arrest. Caesarean deliveries represented 31.3% of all the deliveries, neuraxial anaesthesia was used in 94.4% of the cases and GA was used in 5.6%. Another recent study collecting data from 785,864 caesarean deliveries in the state of New York between 2003 and 2012 reported a global incidence of ARAEs of 0.7%. This incidence increased to 7% in the subgroup of caesarean deliveries under GA. Minor ARAEs

P.Y. Dewandre • J.F. Brichant (✉)
Centre Hospitaliere Universitaire de Liège, Liège, Belgium
e-mail: anesrea@ulg.ac.be

© Springer International Publishing Switzerland 2017
G. Capogna (ed.), *Anesthesia for Cesarean Section*,
DOI 10.1007/978-3-319-42053-0_10

represented 94% of all ARAEs and major ARAEs accounted for 6% of the total. In this cohort, no maternal death was related to anaesthesia [12].

10.2 Complications Due to Neuraxial Anaesthesia

10.2.1 Hypotension

Hypotension is a common complication of neuraxial anaesthesia for caesarean delivery.

Its incidence may be as high as 80% after spinal anaesthesia.

The most widely accepted definition for maternal hypotension is a systolic blood pressure (SBP) lower than 100 mmHg or a decrease in SBP of more than 20% to 30% from baseline values [13]. Spinal anaesthesia-induced hypotension is principally related to a decrease in systemic vascular resistances rather than a decrease in cardiac output which is commonly increased [14]. In case of severe hypotension, the uteroplacental perfusion may be impaired, resulting in fetal hypoxia, acidosis and neonatal depression. In the parturient, hypotension may result in nausea and vomiting, altered consciousness, aspiration, apnoea and cardiac arrest. The severity of hypotension is related to the rate and extent of the sympathetic blockade [13]. Therefore, hypotension is less common with epidural anaesthesia than with spinal anaesthesia because of the slower onset of sympathetic blockade and the earlier recognition and treatment [15]. Although some physical methods (leg wrapping, thromboembolic stockings) and prevention of aorto-caval compression by left displacement of the uterus are useful, main prevention relies on two pharmacological methods, vasopressor therapy and intravascular fluid loading generally in combination [16]. Phenylephrine is now the vasopressor of choice since it has been demonstrated that as compared to ephedrine, phenylephrine decreases the risk of fetal acidosis [17]. Crystalloid preloading is ineffective and should be abandoned. Crystalloid coloading is more effective. Preloading or coloading with hydroxyethyl starch is equally effective. Combining phenylephrine infusion with hydroxyethyl starch preloading or with crystalloids coloading is the method of choice to prevent and reduce the severity of spinal hypotension during caesarean delivery [16].

10.2.2 Failure of Neuraxial Blockade

It is not uncommon that a neuraxial blockade does not provide adequate anaesthesia to initiate or to complete a caesarean delivery. This can occur in up to 4% of the cases following spinal anaesthesia and 13% of the cases following epidural anaesthesia [18, 19].

In the UK, pain is the most common cause of litigation related to regional anaesthesia in obstetrics [20]. In the recent SCORE project of the SOAP, the incidence of failed neuraxial anaesthesia that required an alternate technique for caesarean delivery was 1.7% [11]. Initiation of surgery should be delayed until adequate level of thoracic and sacral sensory blockade has been achieved. Management of breakthrough pain begins with acknowledgement of patient's discomfort and consideration of fetal, surgical and anaesthetic implications. In case of partial block in an elective procedure, a second neuraxial technique may be performed with caution. A second epidural after a failed epidural caries the risk of local anaesthetics toxicity. A second spinal after a partial but failed spinal or a spinal after a failed epidural is controversial because the intrathecal administration of a standard dose of bupivacaine in those settings may result in a high spinal block. Combined spinal-epidural anaesthesia (CSE) is recommended by many practitioners to allow a cautious titration of the rescue neuraxial anaesthesia [13]. If discomfort arises after the start of surgery and if an epidural catheter is in place, an additional dose of local anaesthetic with an opioid should be administered. Inhalation of nitrous oxide or intravenous administration of an opioid or ketamine in 5–10 mg increments, combined with small doses of midazolam, may be helpful. Care must be taken to avoid deep sedation and loss of consciousness given the risk of aspiration [13]. Finally, conversion to general anaesthesia may be necessary and should be offered to the patient in case of persisting pain or discomfort.

10.2.3 High Neuraxial Blockade

High neuraxial blockade can result from an excessive spread of spinal or epidural drugs or an accidental intrathecal or subdural administration of an "epidural dose".

When a T2 sensory level is achieved, patient may complain of dyspnoea or the inability to cough. Impaired phonation, impaired ventilation, unconsciousness, bradycardia and hypotension are potential sequelae of high neuraxial blockade. Tracheal intubation and circulatory support are required in this setting [13].

In the SCORE project of the SOAP, high neuraxial block has been reported with an incidence of 1 in 4336 anaesthesia. Forty percent of the cases followed a spinal anaesthesia, 36% an epidural and 24% an unrecognized spinal catheter. Obesity and spinal technique after failed epidural were the most common associated risk factors.

No maternal death was reported as the consequence of high neuraxial block [11].

Similarly, in the last MBBRACE-UK report, no maternal death was related to a high neuraxial block [4]. It is recommended that anaesthetists remain vigilant for a potentially misplaced catheter. Aspiration of an epidural catheter for CSF or blood has a high sensitivity and specificity [21]. The routine use of a test dose in an epidural catheter to detect an inadvertent intrathecal placement is controversial and does not guarantee proper placement as the majority of epidural anaesthesia associated with high neuraxial block and maternal death can occur after an uneventful test dose [6].

10.2.4 Local Anaesthetic Toxicity

Local anaesthetic toxicity (LAST) after epidural anaesthesia is a rare but potentially catastrophic complication with an incidence of 4 in 10,000 epidural procedures [22–24]. Clinical signs of LAST range from prodromal signs such as auditory change, metallic taste, and agitation to seizures, CNS depression and cardiovascular collapse. The incidence of LAST has decreased during the last decades due to the implementation of routine safety procedures such as catheter aspiration, test dose administration and slow injection of divided doses of local anaesthetics [22–24]. No maternal death related to LAST was reported in the SCORE project of the SOAP or in the last MBBRACE-UK report [4, 11]. The American Society of Regional Anesthesia and Pain Medicine (ASRA) and the Association of Aaesthesiologists of Great Britain and Ireland (AAGBI) have released recommendations for the treatment of LAST. They include prompt and effective airway management in order to prevent hypoxia and acidosis; treatment of seizures with benzodiazepine, propofol or thiopental; consideration of lipid emulsion administration at the first signs of LAST and modified ACLS (Advanced Cardiac Life Support) in the setting of cardiac arrest. The suggested modifications to ACLS include avoidance of high-dose epinephrine, vasopressin, calcium-channel and beta-adrenergic blockers and treatment of ventricular dysrhythmias with amiodarone instead of lidocaine. The currently recommended regimen for intravenous 20% lipid emulsion administration for LAST is an initial bolus of 1.5 mL/kg followed by an infusion of 0.25 mL/kg/min with a maximal dose of 10 mL/kg [25, 26].

10.2.5 Neurologic Complications of Neuraxial Anaesthesia

Most of neurologic injuries after childbirth are related to obstetric rather than anaesthetic causes. However, in such circumstances, neuraxial anaesthesia is often wrongly considered as the cause of the neurologic deficit. In the SCORE project of the SOAP, the incidence of serious neurologic injury following obstetric anaesthesia was 1 for 35,923 [11].

When neurologic symptoms arise after childbirth, an accurate and prompt diagnosis is essential. History, clinical examination and other diagnostic tools such as radiology, electromyography and nerve conduction studies are paramount. They allow to localize the lesion and differentiate mononeuropathy or plexus lesions which are more likely obstetrical complications from radiculopathy or cord lesions, which are more likely related to neuraxial anaesthesia. The reported incidence of peripheral nerve palsy which has an obstetric cause ranges between 0.6 and 92/10,000. The most commonly reported lesions are: (a) compression of the lumbosacral trunks, (b) obturator nerve palsy, (c) femoral nerve palsy, (d) meralgia paresthetica, (e) sciatic nerve palsy, (f) peroneal nerve palsy. The complete description of these obstetric palsies are out of the scope of this chapter, but anaesthesiologists should have an adequate knowledge of segmental and peripheral sensory nerve distributions useful in the diagnosis of central and peripheral nerve lesions [27, 28].

10.2.5.1 Trauma to Nerve Roots and Spinal Cord
Paraesthesia may occur during insertion of a spinal needle or an epidural catheter. An epidural catheter with a flexible tip is unlikely to produce persisting damage to a nerve root. However, an epidural catheter may ensnare a nerve root if an excessive

length is inserted in the epidural space. In case of tethered cord or of undetected spina bifida, attempts to identify the epidural space may result in spinal cord injury.

Insertion of a spinal needle below the conus medullaris may elicit paraesthesia in a dermatome that may persist, suggesting nerve root injury. Symptoms in more than one dermatome suggest a spinal cord lesion. Conus medullaris injuries have been reported after spinal and after CSE blockade [29]. In these cases, the supposed vertebral interspace is L2–L3 and the parturient complains of pain during the spinal needle insertion before any injection. Subsequently, a normal CSF flow and an easy local anaesthetic injection lead to a normal neural blockade. After recovery, numbness is followed by pain; paresthesia in the L5–S1 distribution is observed. Foot drop and urinary symptoms can be observed. MRI may exhibit small syrinx or hematoma within the conus medularis. Sensory symptoms may last for months or years.

Anaesthesia providers must keep in mind that identification of lumbar interspace with anatomical landmarks is far from being accurate. The use of Tuffier's line, joining the iliac crest, is supposed to identify the L4 spinous process. However, this landmark can lie anywhere between the L3–L4 and L5–S1 interspace. Moreover, this method is particularly inaccurate in obese and pregnant patients. Frequently, the selected interspace is higher by one or two levels. In adults, the spinal cord typically ends at the level of the lower body of L1 or at the L1–L2 interspace. At the L1–L2 interspace, the spinal needle can reach the conus medularis in 27% of men and 43% of women [29].

For all these reasons, the spinal needle should not be inserted above the L3 spinous process.

10.2.5.2 Epidural Hematoma after Neuraxial Blockade

Epidural hematoma after neuraxial blockade is a very rare complication, making the quantification of its probability very difficult. From an analysis of 850,000 epidural blocks and 650,000 spinal blocks, its incidence has been quoted as 1:150,000 after epidural block and 1:220,000 after spinal block [30]. A review of 61 published cases of spinal hematoma between 1906 and 1994 and involving central nervous blocks identified five cases in pregnant women. Among these five cases, three had associated risk factors: pre-eclampsia, thrombocytopenia and epidural ependymoma [31]. A 10-year review (1990–1999) in Sweden collecting 1,260,000 spinal anaesthesia and 450,000 epidural blocks (200,000 during labour) identified 33 spinal hematoma and only two cases in obstetrics. Both cases were associated with a Hellp syndrome and apparent signs of coagulopathy, one case after a spinal anaesthesia and one case after removal of an epidural catheter. The calculated incidence of epidural hematoma following an epidural block in obstetrics was 1:200,000 [32]. More recently, an extensive review of the complications associated with spinal and epidural anaesthesia in Finland between 2000 and 2009, and collecting 1,400,000 neuraxial blocks, identified 13 epidural hematomas of which none was in obstetrics [33]. In the SCORE project of the SOAP, one epidural hematoma has been described among 251,463 parturients [11]. The most common risk factors for this complication are multiple attempts, bloody tap, the use of LMWH (Low Molecular Weight Heparin) and other haemostasis abnormalities more specifically in the context of severe pre-eclampsia.

Even if rare, this complication must be promptly recognized. Signs and symptoms of spinal/epidural hematoma include acute onset of back and radicular lower limbs pain, weakness and numbness of legs and bladder and bowel dysfunction. These complaints should generate prompt neurological evaluation and MRI to allow a surgical decompression within 6 h of the onset of symptoms.

10.2.5.3 Epidural Abscess and Meningitis

Epidural abscess and meningitis are rare but potentially devastating complications of neuraxial blocks. They can lead to permanent disability or even to death.

These complications seem to occur less frequently in obstetric patients than in general surgery patients. In a 10-year retrospective study in Sweden (1990–1999) on severe neurological complications after neuraxial block, 29 meningitis cases were identified among 1,260,000 patients receiving spinal anaesthesia. None of the cases was described among the 55,000 patients receiving spinal anaesthesia for caesarean section. Similarly, 12 epidural abscess cases were identified among 460,000 patients who received an epidural in general surgery versus 1 in 200,000 patients who received an epidural for labour analgesia [32].

In a 10-year retrospective study in Finland (2000–2009) on complications associated with 1,400,0000 neuraxial procedures, 4 epidural abscess cases were identified in general surgery and in chronic pain but 0 in obstetric anaesthesia. In the same study, none of the 8 observed meningitis cases was a complication of spinal anaesthesia in obstetrics [33].

A recent review dedicated to neurological infections after neuraxial anaesthesia in obstetrics calculated a risk of meningitis of 1/39,000 spinals and the risk of epidural abscess of 1/303,000 epidurals [34]. Of note, only 16 epidural abscess cases have been reported in the literature until 2005 as a complication of neuraxial blocks in obstetrics.

In the SCORE project of the SOAP, infectious complications (epidural abscess and meningitis) occurred with a frequency of 1 for 62,866 procedures [11].

Most of the time, meningitis is a complication of a dural puncture and an uneventful spinal anaesthesia. The most frequently identified pathogen is a *Streptococcus viridans* or *Streptococcus α-hemolyticus* and the source of the pathogen is either the upper airway of the operator or the vagina. This complication is less frequent when a spinal anaesthesia is performed in an operating room and for an elective caesarean section than during labour. The use of an antibiotic prophylaxis, the absence of Streptococcus bacteraemia during elective C-section and a better aseptic technique in an operating room as compared to a delivery room might contribute to the reduced incidence of meningitis in this situation [34–36].

The classical clinical picture of meningitis is of headache, fever, altered consciousness, emesis and meningism. Symptoms appear a few hours or days after anaesthesia. Diagnosis is confirmed by lumbar puncture and CSF analysis. CSF is cloudy and exhibits hyperleucocytosis, decreased glucose (<30 mg/dl) and increased proteins (>150 mg/dl). One third of cultures yield no growth. The initial antibiotic therapy relies on vancomycin and a third-generation cephalosporin pending further information [28]. Delay of a few hours worsens neurologic outcome [34]. The outcome of meningitis ranges from complete recovery to cerebral oedema, coma or death.

Epidural abscess is almost exclusively a complication of an epidural catheter and almost never a complication of single-shot spinal. This complication increases with the prolonged duration of the catheter and patient's comorbidities. This may explain why epidural abscess is so rare in obstetric anaesthesia. The most commonly identified pathogen is a *Staphylococcus aureus*, the source being the patient's skin.

Symptoms appear a few days or even weeks after anaesthesia. The clinical picture of an epidural abscess is of backache, local tenderness, local inflammation and fluid leak at the insertion point, fever, hyperleucocytosis, increased CRP, radiating root pain, weakness of legs, bladder disturbance and cauda equina syndrome. MRI is the most sensitive diagnostic tool. Blood culture may identify the microorganism. Lumbar puncture is contraindicated.

The treatment relies on antibiotic therapy and surgical treatment. Outcome varies according to early diagnosis and treatment and neurologic symptoms at the time of diagnosis. Here again, a delay of a few hours worsens the neurologic outcome [34–36].

Adequate aseptic technique is paramount to prevent infectious complications.

Chlorhexidine in alcohol is preferred for skin disinfection. It is recommended that anaesthesia providers wear cap, mask, gown and sterile gloves [37, 38]. The use of sterile drape is also recommended. Handwashing, removal of watch and jewelry and appropriate catheter dressing are also important components of sterile technique.

10.2.5.4 Ischemic Injury to the Spinal Cord

The blood supply of the spinal cord depends on a single anterior spinal artery and bilateral posterior spinal arteries. Posterior spinal arteries receive reinforcement by radicular arteries but the single anterior artery, which supplies the anterior two third of the spinal cord, receives only sporadic reinforcement mainly from the Adamkiewicz artery. Anterior spinal artery syndrome is characterized by a predominant motor deficit with or without pain and temperature-sensitive loss but with sparing of proprioception.

Ischemic injury of the spinal cord following neuraxial anaesthesia is extremely rare in the obstetric population. Hypotension and epinephrine-containing solutions are associated risk factors [29].

10.2.5.5 Transient Neurologic Syndrome

Transient neurologic syndrome (TNS) is characterized by pain in the lower back, buttocks and thighs without any detectable neurologic deficit. It occurs approximately 12 h after an uncomplicated spinal anaesthesia and resolves typically in a few days. No permanent sequelae have been reported. The aetiology of this syndrome is unclear; however, the distribution of pain mirrors the distribution of nerve damage in cauda equina syndrome, supporting the theory of neurotoxicity or nerve irritation by the intrathecal injection. TNS is much more frequent with spinal lidocaine than with bupivacaine and is also more common with lidocaine in surgical (10–30%) than in obstetric patients (0–10%) [39–41].

10.2.5.6 Chemical Injury

Chemical injury of the neuraxis may lead to cauda equina syndrome or arachnoiditis.

The epidural space is remarkably tolerant of potentially neurotoxic substances because of two protective factors. Vascular uptake removes a large proportion of solutions injected in the epidural space and nerve roots in the epidural space are protected by a cuff of dura, arachnoid and pia mater. There are many case reports of accidental injections of substances in the epidural space, including antibiotics, thiopental and potassium chloride without permanent sequelae.

In the subarachnoid space, nerve roots are only covered by the pia mater and the sacral roots are poorly myelinated. Therefore, there is a high risk for adverse outcome after accidental injection of toxic substances. Many substances are neurotoxic, including drug preservatives and high doses of local anaesthetics [28, 29].

10.2.6 Postdural Puncture Headache

Postdural puncture headache (PDPH) is the most common serious complication resulting from epidural or spinal anaesthesia. The overall incidence of PDPH following spinal, epidural or CSE is approximately 1%. The estimated incidence of headache after planned spinal anaesthesia with small pencil-point needles is 0.5–2%. In the recent SCORE project of the SOAP, the percentage of patients who developed PDPH after receiving a neuraxial anaesthesia was 0.7%, of which 55.7% required one epidural blood patch (EBP) and 10.7% required a second EBP [11]. With 16–18G epidural needles, wet tap occurs 0.5–4% of the time with a resulting incidence of PDPH of 45–80% [42]. The rate of PDPH following dural puncture is extremely variable (ranging from 1 to 75%) due to the large number of factors influencing its incidence. Young adults are at high risk and pregnant women constitute the highest risk group [43]. Large defects in the meninges cause a higher incidence of PDPH. Size and type of spinal needle are therefore two of the most important factors for decreasing the risk for PDPH [44, 45]. Concerning the technique used to identify the epidural space during epidural placement, the continuous loss of resistance to saline technique, whether midline or paramedian, theoretically offers the practitioner a decreased risk of accidental dural puncture [46]. However, no robust data support a difference in outcome with different techniques. Similarly, there are no definitive conclusions regarding a reduction of risk when using standard epidural as compared to combined spinal epidural (CSE). According to the ASA closed claims project, headache is the third most common cause of lawsuits against anaesthesiologists in obstetrics [6].

Even if the exact pathophysiology of PDPH remains controversial, it certainly involves the leakage of CSF out of the intrathecal space. The decreased CSF volume and pressure result in a caudad excursion of the brain and cerebral vasodilation. Headaches probably result from traction on pain-sensitive structures of the meninges and from a mechanism similar to vascular headaches [47].

PDPH occurs within 72 h after meningeal puncture in 90% of patients and is evident by a headache typically worsening within 20 s of standing and resolving within 20 s of recumbency [47], although the international headache society (IHS) defines it as occurring within 15 min of standing and resolving within 30 min of recumbency [48]. Headache occurs probably earlier and is more severe after puncture with larger needles. If the postural component is not present, the diagnosis should be questioned. The IHS defines PDPH as self-limited and resolving within 14 days (usually within 1 week) even if prolonged symptomatology is reported in patients who may require treatment years later, probably more frequently following larger punctures but reported with all sizes of needles [49].

Headache is usually frontal but may be occipital with or without neck irradiation. Associated symptoms are present in 50% of the patients, including nausea, tinnitus, vertigo and photophobia. CSF hypotension may cause caudad brain displacement with cranial nerve traction, resulting in auditory, ocular or vestibular symptoms.

These headaches can be severe and debilitating. They limit the interaction between mother and baby, prolong hospitalization and increase health care cost.

Long-term consequences and permanent disability have been reported, including cranial nerve palsy, chronic headache, subdural hematoma, intracerebral bleeding, cerebral venous thrombosis and aneurysm rupture [50, 51].

The diagnosis of PDPH is clinical, but radiologic imaging can be useful to rule out another pathology or to confirm the diagnosis of PDPH in case of unclear presentation.

In case of CSF hypotension, MRI findings consist of enhancement of the pachymeninges, decreased size of subarachnoidal cisterns and cerebral ventricles, downward displacement of the brain and subdural collection [52].

There is no accepted algorithms for the treatment of PDPH. Even if supine position alleviates symptoms, there is no evidence supporting bed rest or fluid administration to prevent PDPH or to hasten recovery [53]. Medical therapies are overall disappointing.

Caffeine neither provides sustained improvement nor reduction of the rate of EBP and may be associated with side effects [48]. Sumatriptans and other "triptans" are ineffective [53, 54]. Gabapentin and pregabalin might confer some benefits [55, 56] but are contraindicated in nursing mothers. Finally, ACTH 1.5 units/kg IV and cosyntropin have been associated with conflicting results [57–59].

First described in 1960, epidural blood patch (EBP) is the most effective treatment to date. The injection of 20–30 mL of autologous blood in the epidural space provides up to 95% immediate short-term relief with up to 70% headache-free several days later. Up to 30% of patients will require a second EBP due to return of symptoms. Some practitioners recommend waiting at least 48–72 h after known meningeal puncture prior to EBP considerations. This recommendation relies on results of non-randomized studies demonstrating a higher success rate when EBP is delayed as compared to an earlier EBP performed within the first 24–48 h. This practice is controversial, and other authors recommend performing the EBP earlier, particularly in cases of dural puncture with a large bore needle and in patients with severe headache or cranial nerve symptoms.

Prophylactic epidural blood patch performed through the epidural catheter after delivery and intrathecal catheter left in situ for at least 24 h are two controversial strategies to reduce the incidence of PDPH and the need for a therapeutic epidural blood patch [42, 60].

10.3 Complications of General Anaesthesia

10.3.1 Aspiration

Aspiration pneumonitis (Mendelson's syndrome) is an alveolar chemical injury caused by the inhalation of gastric acid content. Clinical signs consist of dyspnoea, tachypnoea, bronchospasm and hypoxemia. Radiographic signs of alveolar infiltrates are seen in up to 90% of patients with aspiration. In severe cases, aspiration pneumonitis may progress to ARDS [61].

Maternal mortality from pulmonary aspiration of gastric contents has dramatically decreased over the last decades. According to the data from six reports covering the period from 1994 to 2012, only three cases of maternal death from aspiration had occurred in the UK. The exact total number of procedures performed under GA during this period is unknown, but aspiration was the cause of maternal death in less than 1 in 4.5 million deliveries [4]. In the United States, prior to 1990, aspiration was the most common cause of anaesthesia-related maternal death, and the relative risk (RR) of maternal mortality following GA compared to RA was 17. This ratio decreased to 1.7/1 in 2002 [7]. In the recent SCORE project of the SOAP, no case of pulmonary aspiration was identified in 257,000 procedures, including 5000 GA on the 5-year period 2004–2009 [11]. This finding is consistent with other recent reports and suggests that the frequency of this complication has decreased [62].

Several factors have contributed to the decline of this complication. They include the increased use of neuraxial anaesthesia for CS, the routine use of antacids and anti-H2 or proton-pump inhibitors before administering GA for CS, the use of rapid-sequence induction of GA and a better training of anaesthesia providers.

10.3.2 Difficult Airway and Failed Intubation

Difficult airway is defined as difficult facemask ventilation, difficult tracheal intubation or a combination of both. In the obstetric population, the incidence of failed intubation has long been estimated to be 1 in 250–300. This is 8–10 times higher than in the general population. This increased difficulty is mainly related to physiologic and anatomic changes during pregnancy. This higher incidence of difficult airway in obstetric patients has been the main reason for the long-lasting high incidence of general anaesthesia-related maternal death. In case of failed intubation, maternal death results from hypoxemia, aspiration or oesophageal intubation [63–65]. The recent Score project of the SOAP has reported an incidence of failed intubation of 1 in 533 [11]. A recently published literature review calculated an incidence of failed intubation of 1 in 390 for obstetric general anaesthesia and of 1 in 443 for caesarean section under general anaesthesia [66]. The last MBBRACE-UK survey reported no maternal death related to failed intubation [4]. Risk factors for failed intubation in obstetrics are maternal age, BMI and Mallampati score.

Approved guidelines for the management of difficult or failed intubation must be followed to further decrease the incidence of morbidity and mortality associated with this condition. Patient awakening, use of supraglottic airway devices, use of video-laryngoscopes, cricothyrotomy and tracheotomy must be considered [67]. Decreasing further maternal morbidity and mortality related to failed intubation might be difficult as maternal obesity and age are increasing whereas the anaesthesiologists' experience with general anaesthesia for Caesarean section decreases. In addition, many emergent deliveries under general anaesthesia are performed during off hours.

10.3.3 Awareness and Recall

Caesarean delivery is considered as a high-risk procedure for accidental awareness during general anaesthesia (AAGA). Risk factors for AAGA include female sex, younger adults, obesity, use of neuromuscular blocking agents and emergency procedure [68]. All these risk factors are frequently present during GA for CS.

Historically, when GA for CS relied on thiopental and nitrous oxide until delivery of the baby, AAGA has been reported with an incidence up to 26% [69].

The introduction of 0.5% halothane with 50% nitrous oxide reduced this incidence to 1% [70]. The use of higher concentrations of volatile halogenated agents further decreased the incidence of AAGA to 0.26% [71]. In the UK, the last national audit project (NAP5) on accidental awareness during GA reported an incidence of AAGA of 0.15% during caesarean delivery. This incidence is 28 times higher than in the general surgery population [68]. AAGA is also the first cause of litigations in obstetrics general anaesthesia [72].

Concerns about neonatal depression and uterine atony have been the main reasons for the use of low concentrations of volatile halogenated agents. However, although pregnancy reduces the MAC (Minimum Alveolar Concentration) of volatile halogenated agents by 25–45% [73, 74], administration of 0.5 MAC of a volatile halogenated agent does not consistently prevent AAGA. The MAC is defined by the absence of motor response to a noxious stimulus and is related to a spinal mechanism. Unconsciousness and absence of recallare related to a cerebral mechanism. A recent BIS (bispectral index) study has demonstrated that pregnancy does not enhance the hypnotic effect of volatile anaesthetics [75]. This is consistent with the results of another study demonstrating that 0.75 MAC of a volatile halogenated agent with 50% nitrous oxide is required to maintain a BIS value <60 and to prevent AAGA during caesarean section [76].

References

1. Centers for Disease Control and Prevention: impatients surgery 2010. http://www.cdc.go/nchs/fastats/inpatient-surgery.htm.
2. Cheesman K, Brady JE, Flood P, et al. Epidemiology of anesthesia-related complications in labor and delivery, New York State, 2002–2005. Anesth Analg. 2009;109:1174–81.
3. Cantwell R, Clutton-Brock T, Cooper G, et al. Saving mother's lives: reviewing maternal deaths to make motherhood safer: 2006–2008. The eighth report of the confidential enquieries into maternal deaths in the United Kingdom. BJOG. 2011;118(suppl. 1):1–203.
4. Freedman RL, Lucas DN. MBRRACE-UK: saving lives, improving mother's care: implications for anaesthetists. Int J Obstet Anesth. 2015;24:161–73.
5. Saucedo M, Deneux-Tharaux C, Bouvier-Colle MH. French National Experts Committee on Maternal Mortality: ten years of confidential inquieries into maternal deaths in France: 1998–2007. Obstet Gynecol. 2013;122:752–60.
6. Davies JM, Posner KL, Lee LA, et al. Liability associated with obstetric anesthesia: a closed claims analysis. Anesthesiology. 2009;110:131–9.
7. Hawkins JL, Chang J, Palmer SK, et al. Anesthesia-related maternal mortality in the United States: 1979–2002. Obstet Gynecol. 2011;117:69–74.
8. American Society of Anesthesiologists Task Force on Obstetric Anesthesia. Parctice guidelines for obstetric anesthesia: An updated report by the American Society of Anesthesiologists Task Force on Obstetric Anesthesia. Anesthesiology. 2007;106:843–63.
9. Van de velde M, Vercauteren M, Stockman W, et al. On behalf of the Obstetric Anesthesia Working Group. Recommendations and Guidelines for Obstetric Anesthesia in Belgium. Acta Anaesth Belg. 2013;64:97–104.
10. Bucklin BA, Hawlins JL, Anderson JR, et al. Obstetric anesthesia workforce Survey: twenty-year update. Anesthesiology. 2005;103:645–53.
11. D'Angelo R, Smiley R, Riley ET, Segal S. Serious complications related to obstetric anesthesia. The serious complications repository project of the Society for Obstetric Anesthesia and Perinatology. Anesthesiology. 2014;120:1505–12.
12. Guglielminotti J, Wong CA, Landau R, et al. Temporal trends in anesthesia-related adverse évents in cesarean deliveries: New York State, 2003–2012. Anesthesiology. 2015;123:1013–23.
13. Tsen LC. Anesthesia for cesarean delivery. In: Chestnut DH, Wong CA, Tsen LC, Ngan Kee W, Beilin Y, Mhyre JM, editors. Obstetric anesthesia principles and practice. 5th ed. Philadelphia: Elsevier Saunders; 2014. p. 545–603.
14. Langesaeter E, Rosseland LA, Stubhaug A. Continuous invasive blood pressure and cardiac output monitoring during cesarean delivery. A randomized, double blind comparison of low dose versus high dose spinal anesthesia with intravenous phenylephrine or placebo infusion. Anesthesiology. 2008;109:856–63.
15. Ng K, Parsons J, Cyna AM, et al. Spinal versus epidural anaesthesia for caesarean section. Cochrane Database Syst Rev. 2004;2:CD003765.
16. Mercier FJ, Auge M, Hoffmann C, et al. Maternal hypotension during spinal anesthesia for cesarean delivery. Minerva Anesthesiol. 2013;79:62–73.
17. Veeser M, Hofmann T, Roth R, et al. Vasopressors for the management of hypotension after spianl anesthesia for elective caesarean section. Systematic review and cumulative Mataanalysis. Acta Anesthesiol Scand. 2012;56:810–6.
18. Pan PH, Bogard TD, Owen MD. Incidence and characteristics of failures in obstetrics neuraxial analgesia and anesthesia: a rétrospective analysis of 19259 deliveries. Int J Obstet Anesth. 2004;13:227–33.
19. Bauer ME, Koutanis JA, Tsen LC, et al. Risk factors for failed conversion of labor epidural analgésia to caesarean delivery anesthesia: a systematic review and méta-analysis of observational trials. Int J Obstet Anesth. 2012;21:294–309.
20. Szypula K, Ashpole KJ, Bogod D, et al. Litigation related to régional anaesthesia: an analysis of claims against the NHS in England 1995–2007. Anaesthesia. 2010;65:443–52.

21. Norris MC, Fogel ST, Dalman H, et al. Labor epidural analgesia without an intravenous "test dose". Anesthesiology. 1998;88:1495–501.
22. Toledo P. What's new on onstetric anesthesia: the 2011 Gerad W Ostheimer Lecture. Int J Obstet Anesth. 2012;21:68–74.
23. Toledo P, Nixon HC, Mhyre JM, et al. Availability of lipid emulsion in United States obstetric Units. Anesth Analg. 2013;116:406–8.
24. Mulroy MF. Systemic toxicity and cardiotoxicity from local anesthetics: incidence and préventive measures. Reg Anesth Pain Med. 2002;27:556–61.
25. Neal JM, Bernards CM, Butterworth JFT, et al. ASRA practice advisory on local anesthetic sytemic toxicity. Reg Anesth Pain Med. 2010;35:152–61.
26. The association of Anaesthetist of Great Britain and Ireland. AAGBI safety guidelines: Management of severe local anaesthetic toxicity 2010.
27. Wong CA, Scavone BM, Dugan S, et al. Incidence of postpartum lumbosacral spine and lower extremity nerve injuries. Obstet Gynecol. 2003;101:279–88.
28. Wong CA. Nerve injuries after neuraxial anaesthesia and their medicolegal implications. Best Pract Res Clin Obstet Gynaecol. 2010;24:367–81.
29. Reynolds F. Neurologic complication of pregnancy and neuraxial anesthesia. In: Chestnut DH, Wong CA, Tsen LC, Ngan Kee W, Beilin Y, Mhyre JM, editors. Obstetric anesthesia principles and practice. 5th ed. Philadelphia: Elsevier Saunders; 2014. p. 739–63.
30. Tryba M. Epidural régional anesthesia and low molecular weight heparin: pro (German). Anästh Intensimed Notfallmed Schmerzther. 1993;28:179–81.
31. Vandermeulen EP, Van Aken H, Vermylen J. Anticoagulants and spinal-epidural anesthesia. Anesth Analg. 1994;79:1165–77.
32. Moen V, Dahlgren N, Irestedt L. Severe neurological complications after central neuraxial blockades in Sweden 1990–1999. Anesthesiology. 2004;101:950–9.
33. Pitkänen MT, Aromaa U, Cozanitis DA, et al. Serious complications associated with spinal and epidural anaesthesia in Finland from 2000 to 2009. Acta Anaesthesiol Scand. 2013;57:553–64.
34. Reynolds F. Neurological infections after neuraxial anaesthesia. Anesthesiol Clin. 2008;26:23–52.
35. Hebl JR. The importance and implication of aseptic techniques during régional anesthesia. Reg Anesth Pain Med. 2006;31:311–23.
36. Infection control in anaesthesia. Anaesthesia 2008;63:1027–36.
37. Horlocker T, Wedel D. Infectious complications of regional anesthesia. Best Pract Res Clin Anesthesiol. 2008;22(3):451–75.
38. Hebl JR, Niesen AD. Infectious complications of régional anesthesia. Cur Opin Anesthiol. 2011;24:273–80.
39. Pollock JE. Transient neurologic syndrome: etiology, risk factors and management. Reg Anaesth Pain Med. 2002;27:581–6.
40. Aouad MT, Siddik SS, Jalbout MI, et al. Does pregnancy protect against intrathecal lidocaine-induced transient neurologic symptoms? Anesth Analg. 2001;92:401–4.
41. Philip J, Sharma SK, Gottumukkala VN, et al. Transient neurologic symptoms after spinal lidocaine in obstetric patients. Anesth Analg. 2001;92:405–9.
42. Van de Velde M, Schepers R, Berends N, et al. Ten years of expérience with accidental dural puncture and post-dural puncture headache in a tertiary obstetric anesthesia department. Int J Obstet Anesth. 2008;17:329–35.
43. De Almeida SM, Shumaker SD, Leblanc SK, et al. Incidence of post-dural puncture headache in research volunteers. Headache. 2011;51:1503–10.
44. Halpern S, Preston R. Postdural puncture headache and spinal needle design. Metaanalyses Anesthesiology. 1994;81:1376–83.
45. Vallejo MC, Mandell GL, Sabo DP, et al. Postdural puncture headache: a randomized comparison of five spinal needles in obstetric patients. Anesth Analg. 2000;91:916–20.
46. Shenouda PE, Cunningham BJ. Assessing the superioruty of saline versus air for use in the epidural loss of resistance technique: a littérature review. Reg Anesth Pain Med. 2003;28:48–53.

47. Sachs A, Smiley R. Post-dural puncture headache: the worst common complication in obstetric anesthesia. Semin Perinat. 2014;38:386–94.
48. Headache Classification Subcommittee of the International Headache Society. The international classification of headache disorders: 2nd édition. Cephalalgia. 2004;24(suppl. 1):9–160.
49. Ahmed SV, Jayawarna C, Jude E. Post lumbar puncture headache, diagnosis and management. Postgrad Med J. 2006;82:713–6.
50. Paech MJ, Doherty DA, Christmas T, et al. Epidural blood patch trial group. The volume of blood for epidural blood patch in obstetrics: a randomized, blinded clinical trial. Anesth Analg. 2011;113:126–33.
51. Paech MJ, Whybrow T. The prévention and treatment of post dural puncture headache. ASEAN J Anesthesiol. 2007;8:86–96.
52. Algin O, Taskapiliogliu O, Zan E, et al. Detection of CSF leaks with magnetic résonance imaging in intracranial hypotension syndrome. J Neuroradiol. 2011;38:175–7.
53. Arevalo-Rodriguez I, Ciapponi A, Munoz L, et al. Posture and fluids for preventing post-dural puncture headache. Cochrane Database Syst Rev. 2013;7:CD009199.
54. Bussone G, Tullo V, d'Onoffrio F, et al. Frovatriptan for the prévention of postdural puncture headache. Cephalalgia. 2007;22:809–13.
55. Erol DD. The analgesic and antiemetic efficacy of gabapentin or egotamine/caffeine for the treatment of post-dural puncture headache. Adv Med Sci. 2011;56:25–9.
56. Zencirci B. Postdural puncture headache and pregabalin. J Pain Res. 2010;3:11–4.
57. Basurto Ona X, Uriona Tuma SM, Martinez Garcia L, et al. Drug therapy to prevent post-dural puncture headache. Cochrane Database Syst Rev. 2013;2:CD001792.
58. Gupta S, Agrawal A. Postdural puncture headache and ACTH. J Clin Anesth. 1997;9:258.
59. Hakim SM. Cosyntropin for prophylaxis against postdural puncture headache aftyer accidental dural puncture. Anesthesiology. 2010;113:413–20.
60. Scavone BM, Wong CA, Sullivan JT, et al. Efficacy of prophylactic epidural blood patch in preventing postdural puncture headache in parturients after inadvertent dural puncture. Anesthesiology. 2004;101:1422–7.
61. O'Sullivan G. Aspiration: risk, prophylaxis and treatment. In: Chestnut DH, Wong CA, Tsen LC, Ngan Kee W, Beilin Y, Mhyre JM, editors. Obstetric anesthesia principles and practice. 5th ed. Philadelphia: Elsevier Saunders; 2014. p. 665–83.
62. Mhyre JM, Riesner MN, Poley LS, et al. A series of anesthesia-related maternal death in Michigan, 1985–2003. Anesthesiology. 2007;106:1096–104.
63. Quinn AC, Milne D, Columb M, et al. Failed trachéal intubation in obstetric anaesthesia: 2 year national case-control study in the UK. Br J Anaesth. 2013;110:74–80.
64. Mc Donnel NJ, PAech MJ, Clavisi OM, Scott KL, ANZCA Trials Group. Difficult and failed intubation in obstetric anaesthesia: an observational study of airway management and complications associated with general anaesthesiafor caesarean section. Int J Obstet Anesth. 2008;7:292–7.
65. Tsen LC, Pitner R, Camann WR. General anesthesia for cesarean section at a tertiary care hospital 1990–1995: indications and implications. Int J Obstet Gynecol. 1998;7:147–52.
66. Kinsella SM, Winton AL, Mushambi MC, et al. Failed tracheal intubation during obstetric general anaesthesia: a literature review. Int J Obstet Anaesth. 2015;24:356–74.
67. Mushambi MC, Kinsella SM, Popat M, et al. Obstetric Anaesthetists Association and Difficult Airway Society guidelines for the management of difficult and failed tracheal intubation in obstetrics. Anaesthesia. 2015;70:1286–306.
68. Pandit JJ, Andrade J, Bogod DG, et al. 5th National Audit Project (NAP5) on accidental awareness during general anaesthesia: summary of main findings and risk factors. Br J Anaesth. 2014;113:549–59.
69. Crawford JS. Awareness during opérative obstetrics under general anaesthesia. Br J Anaesth. 1971;43:179–82.
70. Moir DD. Anaesthesia for caesarean section: an evaluation of a method using low concentrations of halothane and 50% of oxygen. Br J Anaesth. 1970;42:136–42.

71. Robins K, Lyons G. Intraoperative awareness during general anesthesia for cesarean delivery. Anesth Analg. 2009;109:886–90.
72. Ashpole KJ, Cook TM. Litigation in obstetric general anaesthesia: an analysis of claims against the NHS in England 1995–2007. Anaesthesia. 2010;65:529–30.
73. Palahniuk RJ, Schnider SM, Eger 2nd EI. Pregnancy decreases the requirement for inhaled anesthetic agents. Anesthesiology 1974;41:82–3.
74. Gin T, Chan MT. Decreased minimum alveolar concentration of isoflurane in pregnat humans. Anesthesiology. 1994;81:829–32.
75. Ueyama H, Hagihira S, Takashina M, et al. Anesthesiology 2010;113:577–84.
76. Chin KJ, Yeo SW. A BIS-guided study on sevoflurane requirements for adequate depth of anaesthesia in caesarean section. Anaesthesia. 2004;59:1064–8.

Postoperative Analgesia

11

Michela Camorcia

11.1 Introduction

Cesarean section (CS) is a unique surgery, accompanied by significant hormonal and emotional pregnancy modifications, the arrival of the newborn with consequent care responsibilities, the expectation to recover rapidly, and sleep deprivation resulting from maternal neonatal interactions. Indeed the period after cesarean surgery is not only a postoperative but also a postpartum period (puerperium).

Cesarean section can be classified as a major surgery and commonly causes moderate to severe pain for the first 48 h after surgery [1].

An adequate control of postoperative pain after cesarean section is actually of paramount importance for many reasons: a pain-free mother is able to care for her newborn baby in the immediate postpartum period helping an early interaction between mother and infant to be created and breastfeeding carried out effectively, thereby significantly increasing maternal satisfaction.

However, despite recent improvements in postoperative pain management, many parturients still suffer from moderate to severe postoperative pain after CS. This results in distress for the parturients with an increase in maternal morbidity such as an increased risk of thromboembolic disease and therefore prolonged hospitalization and delayed return to normal activities [2–4].

In addition, the failure to provide good acute pain control after cesarean birth may cause important and detrimental psychological consequences such as a significant increase in the incidence of postpartum depression [5] and failure of breastfeeding [6].

M. Camorcia
Department of Anesthesiology, Città di Roma Hospital,
Via Maidalchini 20, Rome 00152, Italy
e-mail: michelaca.mc@gmail.com

© Springer International Publishing Switzerland 2017

153

G. Capogna (ed.), *Anesthesia for Cesarean Section*,
DOI 10.1007/978-3-319-42053-0_11

Furthermore, inadequately controlled pain in the postoperative period is primary as, if not adequately treated, it can lead to the development of chronic pain. In fact, it has been observed that the severity of acute pain after delivery is associated with the risk of experiencing persistent postpartum pain and that, in turn, the development of chronic pain is associated with the risk of maternal postpartum depression with significant negative effects on daily activities [7–9].

11.2 Pain Pathways

Pain after cesarean section is due to the skin, the anterior abdominal wall and the uterine incisions. Surgical techniques, such as type of incision (Joel-Cohen compared to the Pfannenstiel) [10], skin closure method [11], and exteriorization of the uterus for repair of the uterine incision [12], may affect the intensity of postoperative pain.

This intensity can also be affected by the way pain is assessed [13].

Pain after cesarean section is characterized by both somatic and visceral components.

Somatic pain is due to the incision of the skin and the anterior abdominal wall and is conducted by the ileoinguinal and ileohypogastric nerves that are located in the lateral portion of the abdominal wall, between the transversus abdominis and the internal oblique muscle layers, and enter the spinal cord via the T10-L1 dermatomes.

Visceral pain that is due to peritoneal trauma and uterine breech is transmitted via the inferior hypogastric nerve and then enters the spinal cord via the T10-L1 dermatomes.

The analgesic management of postoperative pain therefore has to focus on both the visceral pain and the somatic pain.

11.3 Postoperative Analgesia Practice

An ideal method of pain relief after cesarean section should be cost-effective, safe for the mother, require minimal monitoring, and use drugs that are not secreted into breast milk.

Moreover, the mother should not be sedated or impeded by equipment that prevents her from moving freely and caring for the newborn. Minor side effects, acceptable in the general population, like nausea and vomiting, pruritus, and shivering may restrict the care of the new born, leading to less maternal satisfaction.

There are several analgesic agents that can be used to treat post-cesarean pain. These can be used alone or as part of a therapy (multimodal approach) and the route of administration can be systemic, neuraxial, oral, or local.

To date, there is not a "gold standard" for the management of post-cesarean pain. There are many options and the choice of the analgesic management depends on the type of anesthesia performed, drug availability, anesthesiologist preference, institutional protocols, and also costs.

11.4 Opioids

Opioids represent the most commonly administered analgesic agents for the treatment of postoperative pain in both surgical and obstetric populations. These can be administered systemically or neuraxially, alone or in combination with other drugs, such as the NSAIDs as part of a multimodal approach.

Analgesia from neuraxial opioid administration is primarily mediated by binding pre- and postsynaptic mu-opioid receptors sited in the dorsal horn of the spinal cord.

The onset of action, duration, and efficacy depends primarily on their lipid solubility and also on the route of administration.

With regard to the occurrence of side effects, at clinical doses, no respiratory depression is usually observed with any of the routes of administration while the administration of intrathecal morphine was associated with a significant incidence of pruritus plus nausea and vomiting [14]. The presence of these side effects must not be underestimated as it is associated with a negative impact on maternal satisfaction [15].

11.4.1 Morphine: Neuraxial Administration

Neuraxial administration of morphine includes the epidural or the intrathecal route depending mainly on the type of anesthesia performed (spinal or epidural). There seems to be a better clinical profile for epidural morphine as opposed to its intrathecal administration but there is no clear evidence to recommend one technique over the other. However, the dose under investigation chosen by all studies that have compared the two different routes of administration was based on the doses commonly used in clinical practice rather than the exact potency ratio of intrathecal versus epidural morphine as this remains undetermined. The results therefore, might not be completely reliable.

After epidural administration, variable quantities (depending on which opioid is used) will diffuse across the dura and arachnoid mater into the subarachnoid space to bind opioid receptors in the dorsal horn of the spinal cord. Lipid solubility is the most important factor affecting the rate of diffusion and the subsequent onset and duration of analgesia. Lipophilic opioids such as fentanyl and sufentanil diffuse rapidly across the dura into the CSF compared to hydrophilic opioids such as morphine. Lipophilic opioids produce rapid onset of analgesia which is of short overall duration. After epidural delivery, CSF opioid levels peak at 6 min for sufentanil, 20 min for fentanyl, and 1–4 h for morphine. The epidural space is extremely vascular and there is extensive absorption of opioids via the epidural venous plexus into the systemic circulation. Systemic opioids reach the CNS and bind receptors in areas of the brain that modulate pain perception and response.

11.4.2 Epidural Morphine

Morphine is currently the "gold-standard" neuraxial opioid for post-cesarean analgesia primarily due to its long-acting effect that can last for many hours after a single administration [16].

Morphine is a hydrophilic agent that is not easily absorbed by the blood vessels and fat and therefore it has high central nervous system availability and a very long duration of action.

Epidural morphine is generally administered as a single bolus rather than with a continuous infusion technique.

The administration of epidural morphine follows a precise dose–response relationship: as the dose of epidural morphine is increased, the quality and duration of analgesia increases accordingly until a sailing effect is reached, at 3.75 mg, where the quality of analgesia does not increase [17].

Many studies have been performed in order to find the best balance between drug efficacy and reduced side effects for epidural morphine. The administration of 2–4 mg of epidural morphine is suggested as it can provide optimal analgesia for the first postoperative day, minimizing at the same time the risk of side effects such as nausea, vomiting, and respiratory depression [17–20].

Side effects after epidural morphine administered as a single 2–4 mg bolus are characterized by mild pruritus that can occur in approximately 50% of patients, nausea and vomiting in approximately 30–40% of patients, and dizziness in 10%.

Respiratory depression after epidural morphine may occur early after its administration, approximately in the first hour thanks to its vascular absorption or it can be observed later, after approximately 6–18 h due to its slow cephalad spread in the cerebrospinal fluid and consequent penetration into the brainstem [21, 22]. The incidence of respiratory depression after clinical doses of epidural morphine is unlikely to occur. However, if the doses are increased above 5 mg, even young and healthy parturients can develop clinically detectable respiratory depression. In such cases, clinical respiratory monitoring might be indicated.

11.4.3 Epidural Fentanyl and Sufentanil

Both fentanyl and sufentanil are highly lipophilic opioids that act with different affinity for the mu receptor [23]. They are both characterized by a fast onset of analgesia and shorter duration when compared to morphine due to their high lipid solubility. Epidural fentanyl 50–100 µg or sufentanil 10–20 µg represent the dose currently used in clinical practice and usually provide effective analgesia that lasts for approximately 4–5 h. The increase in the dose of these opioids is not associated with an increase in the efficacy or the duration of action.

When used epidurally, sufentanil is 5.9 times more potent than fentanyl [24] although no differences were observed in both the onset and the duration of analgesia between the two opioids [25].

Neuraxially administered fentanyl and sufentanil can be effectively used to improve intraoperative analgesia and provide early postoperative analgesia [26] while their short duration make them unsuitable agents for the treatment of post-cesarean analgesia.

The side effects associated with these two short-acting opioids are comparable to that observed with the administration of morphine but with an earlier onset.

Both these two opioids can cause early onset respiratory depression in less than 1 h after their administration due to vascular absorption and rostral spread in cerebrospinal fluid [27].

11.4.4 Intrathecal Opioids

Spinal anesthesia is the most commonly used technique for cesarean delivery; therefore, the addition of opioids to the spinal solution in order to enhance and prolong intraoperative and postoperative analgesia has become the standard practice worldwide.

Intrathecal opioids exert their action primarily by directly binding pre- and post-synaptic mu-opioid receptors in the substantia gelatinosa of the dorsal horn of the spinal cord and they are also transported supra-spinally by CSF flow where they modulate descending inhibitory pain pathways.

A large variety of opioids have been investigated as suitable options for postoperative analgesia such as morphine [28–30], fentanyl [30, 31], and sufentanil [32].

11.4.5 Intrathecal Morphine

Morphine is the most commonly used intrathecal opioid as it can provide excellent analgesia with a long duration of action. Analgesia provided by morphine is generally characterized by a slow onset and a long duration of action, generally up to 24 h [33].

Unlike epidural morphine, its intrathecal administration does not follow a precise dose–response relationship for analgesia. Dose–response studies have in fact found that the analgesic efficacy of intrathecal morphine increases until the dose of 50–150 µg [28]. The incidence of side effects such as nausea and vomiting did not appear to follow a dose-related effect while the incidence of pruritus increases in a dose-dependent fashion and can be observed in up to 90% of the cases [28, 33].

The optimal intrathecal dose for morphine was investigated by several studies and meta-analyses which examined doses ranging from 0.1 to 0.5 mg and found that doses from 0.1 to 0.2 mg are associated with optimal analgesia lasting up to 27 h (from 11 to 29 h) and reduced side effects while doses above 0.2 mg do not provide an improvement in the quality of analgesia [20]. However, the use of 0.2 mg intrathecal morphine instead of 0.1 mg is associated with only a little improvement in the analgesic efficacy, but with a twofold increase of side effects such as nausea, vomiting, use of antiemetics, and pruritus. The use of 0.1 mg, therefore, might represent the preferable choice for nursing parturients although in most cases it is still associated with nausea and pruritus [34].

One other potential complication that can be observed with intrathecal morphine is the rostral spread in the cerebrospinal fluid and consequent penetration in the brainstem due to its extremely low lipid solubility that can possibly lead to late respiratory depression. This however, is much more frequent when administered intravenously, and with the intrathecal doses commonly used in clinical practice it is very unlikely to observe this harmful complication.

Nevertheless, it is important to take into account that the sole administration of morphine either intrathecally or epidurally is often accompanied by the request for additional pain medications (multimodal approach).

A randomized controlled trial examined the dose–response relationship of intrathecal morphine comparing 0.05, 0.1, or 0.15 mg combined with 30 mg intravenous ketorolac in patients undergoing elective cesarean section with 12 mg of hyperbaric bupivacaine and fentanyl 15 µg. The results of the study indicate that 0.05 mg of intrathecal morphine produces similar analgesia as 0.1 or 0.15 mg when used as part of a multimodal therapy. The only difference observed was the incidence of pruritus, greater in the 0.1 and 0.15 mg, while the incidence of nausea and vomiting was comparable in the three groups [35].

11.4.6 Intrathecal Fentanyl and Sufentanil

Intrathecal fentanyl and sufentanil can be used to provide optimal intraoperative analgesia as they are highly lipid soluble so characterized by a fast onset of action. In fact, when added to intrathecal bupivacaine they allow for a reduction in antiemetic medications and provide early postoperative analgesia. However, they also have a brief duration of action and are therefore not suitable as postoperative agents [32].

The use of intrathecal fentanyl and sufentanyl were found to provide some early postoperative analgesia [30] and contributed to an increase in the quality of intraoperative analgesia in a small percentage of parturients [20, 32].

11.4.7 Diamorphine

Diamorphine is a lipophilic opioid that rapidly diffuses in the cerebrospinal fluid after its administration [36] and can be used either epidurally or intrathecally. It is available only in the UK.

In comparison to morphine, diamorphine is more lipid soluble so its onset of action is shorter while its duration is comparable to that obtained with morphine into which it is rapidly metabolized once it reaches the CSF. In terms of safety, diamorphine is unlikely to produce late respiratory depression as there is little drug that gains access to the spinal cord and brainstem from the cerebrospinal fluid due to its rapid clearance.

Its efficacy after being administered epidurally and intrathecally has been investigated in several trials.

Dose–response studies have found that increasing the dose of intrathecal diamorphine is associated with an increase in analgesia efficacy without a ceiling effect and with a concurrent increase in the incidence of side effects [37, 38].

One study which investigated the ED95 of intrathecal diamorphine suggested the use of 0.4 mg in clinical practice that was able to provide effective analgesia with a mean duration of action of approximately 10 h [39]. However, this was obtained at the expense of a significant increase in the incidence of side effects such as nausea and vomiting and pruritus observed in more than 50% of parturients. For this reason, many authors have suggested reducing the dose of this analgesia medication to 0.3 mg [39, 40].

Epidural diamorphine has a fast onset and a long duration of action and it is clinically used in doses ranging from 2.5 to 5 mg with good analgesic efficacy and a duration of approximately 14 h [41, 42]. The increase in the dose of the drug is associated with an increase in the duration of analgesia at the expense of an increase in the incidence and severity of side effects. For this reason, the suggested dose for epidural diamorphine is about 3 mg [43].

The epidural administration of diamorphine was found to be as equally effective as its intrathecal administration with regard to both prolonged duration and good quality of analgesia [42], although the epidural administration is associated with an increased incidence of side effects such as nausea and vomiting. The authors of the study in fact suggest the use of intrathecal diamorphine due to its favorable side effect profile as part of a spinal or a combined spinal epidural technique.

11.4.8 Extended-Release Epidural Morphine (Depodur)

Recently extended-release epidural morphine (EREM) formulations have been investigated in comparison to the conventional neuraxial morphine that can provide good post-cesarean analgesia but for only 1 day after surgery.

Extended-release epidural morphine was found to significantly improve pain scores after cesarean section and prolong post-cesarean analgesia when compared with conventional epidural morphine, with no significant increase in the incidence and severity of side effects [43, 44].

11.4.9 Opioid: Systemic Administration

The administration of systemic morphine is commonly used for postoperative analgesia when cesarean section is performed under general anesthesia and consists of the intravenous, intramuscular, and subcutaneous routes.

The intramuscular and subcutaneous routes are less commonly used when compared with the intravenous route as the use of repeated injections is uncomfortable for the parturients, and because there is a large interindividual variability in opioid requirement, onset of action, duration, and pharmacokinetics [14], although they are associated with fewer side effects. These latter factors can contribute to intermittent and suboptimal levels of analgesia obtained with intramuscular or subcutaneous administrations.

Morphine is often administered intravenously as part of a patient-controlled intravenous anesthesia technique (PCIA). Its advantages are represented by more stable levels of analgesia due to the low fluctuations in plasma opioid levels and great analgesic efficacy when compared with the intramuscular administration that leads to higher maternal satisfaction [45]. In addition, the feeling of control that women can have with using PCIA administration contributes to providing good overall parturient satisfaction.

On the other hand, major disadvantages of the PCIA technique are that women must be correctly instructed on the proper use of the device and also that new mothers are often concerned about the potential entry of the drug into their milk leading to a reduction in the demand doses.

Some authors suggest the use of the PCIA technique associated with a background infusion of the solution. However, the efficacy of this technique is controversial [46], more side effects can be seen, and also there is concern on its safety.

11.5 Multimodal Approach

The multimodal analgesia technique consists of the use of different pharmacological agents that act via different mechanisms of action providing synergistic or additive analgesia, thereby enhancing the quality of analgesia but minimizing the incidence and severity of side effects. This approach was extensively studied and clinically used in obstetric as well as in nonobstetric patients [47].

The multimodal approach involves the use of coanalgesic or adjuvant drugs or the use of nerve block or wound infiltration.

11.6 NSAIDs

The anti-inflammatory and antipyretic properties of nonsteroidal anti-inflammatory drugs (NSAIDs) may reduce visceral pain originating from the uterus, complementing the somatic wound pain relief from the opioid. The addition of NSAIDs has been shown to potentiate opioid effect, decrease opioid consumption, and reduce side effects when systemic or neuraxial opioids are administered for post-cesarean delivery analgesia [48, 49].

However, even if they are effective in blunting the inflammatory component of the surgical site, their use alone is associated with poor postoperative analgesia [49]. On the other hand, NSAIDs can be used to effectively treat post-cesarean pain as part of a multimodal approach.

The use of NSAIDs, in fact, can enhance the analgesic effect provided by opioids allowing the reduction in the consumption of opioids and, in turn, minimizing their side effects.

NSAIDs drugs exert a significant opioid-sparing effect.

The use of an NSAID such as intramuscular diclofenac 75 mg significantly enhances the efficacy of analgesia of IT morphine allowing doses as low as 0.025 mg morphine to produce effective postoperative pain relief for up to 24 h [50, 51].

However, these agents have potential gastrointestinal side effects and platelet dysfunction that can limit their use. The use of COX 2 inhibitors that do not interfere with gastrointestinal or platelet function is not recommended as they are secreted into the breast milk, and there is no evidence regarding their safe used in breastfeeding mothers.

The use of NSAIDs can be performed as an on-demand or a fixed schedule.

11.7 Epidural vs. Systemic Administration

The administration of opioids neuraxially rather than systemically is far more effective, as has been shown in a number of studies performed in obstetrics [14, 52], the latter usually being chosen when general anesthesia is performed.

The administration of neuraxial opioids is in fact associated with lower pain scores when compared with intravenous patient-controlled analgesia (PCIA) in the first 24 h.

When an epidural technique is used for cesarean section, the epidural catheter can be effectively used for postoperative analgesia.

In the nonobstetric setting, it has been demonstrated that the use of epidural postoperative analgesia can decrease perioperative complications, thereby improving postoperative outcomes [53, 54].

Several studies have concluded that the use of postoperative epidural analgesia is associated with greater analgesic efficacy when compared with systemic analgesia [55, 56] in the surgical population.

This better postoperative analgesia was consistent at all the tested intervals and for up to 4 days after surgery. The quality of analgesia was higher at rest and on movement with every combination of local anesthetics with or without an opioid when compared with systemic analgesia [57].

Postoperative epidural analgesia is generally administered using a patient-controlled epidural analgesia (PCEA) technique or a continuous infusion (CEI) technique.

A meta-analysis performed on obstetric patients reported the significant superiority of the patient-controlled epidural analgesia (PCEA) and the continuous epidural infusion (CEI) over the PCIA technique. In fact, the visual analogue pain scale (VAPS) values, at rest and on movement, obtained with the PCEA or the CEI technique were significantly lower than the PCIA in all the intervals tested and for 3 days after cesarean section [58].

The use of PCEA with fentanyl and bupivacaine was found to provide greater analgesia than CEI [59, 60].

In addition, the PCEA technique is associated with a decreased dose of local anesthetic solution with less need for physician-administered additional rescue boluses and therefore with a greater sense of control by parturients and thus an increase in maternal satisfaction [61].

However, some evidence has shown that this technique might be poorly tolerated by mothers as their mobility may be reduced by the use of infusion systems which in turn reduces their ability to nurse their babies [62, 63].

Preliminary observations reported that the programmed epidural intermittent bolus (PIEB) technique has the potential to decrease motor block maintaining adequate analgesia when compared to CEI for post-cesarean analgesia even for a prolonged period of time [64].

In my institution, almost all cesarean sections have been performed under combined spinal epidural anesthesia. For this reason, we use the epidural catheter to provide postoperative analgesia. By using a very diluted local anesthetic solution (such a levobupivacaine 0.0625%) plus an opioid (such as sufentanil) given by PIEB (programmed intermittent epidural bolus) pumps, we have usually been able to provide satisfactory analgesia avoiding the concurrent administration of NSAIDs and allowing for early maternal ambulation and breastfeeding. An additional PCEA (patient-controlled epidural analgesia) rescue bolus is also part of our post-cesarean section analgesia program.

In all cases, it must be remembered that when using the epidural catheter for postoperative analgesia, given the widespread use of postpartum low molecular weight heparin (LMWH), there is concern about the correct timing of catheter removal and the risks due to its inadvertent dislocation and therefore proper training of personnel and adequate guidelines are needed.

11.8 Transversus Abdominis Plane Block (TAP Block)

The TAP block is a regional technique that consists of blocking of the neural afferents deriving from the abdominal wall. This is obtained by administering local anesthetics in the neurofascial plane that is located between the internal oblique and the transversus abdominis muscles [65]. This technique, therefore, is able to partially reduce the severity of cesarean section as it acts only on its somatic component.

TAP block was found to provide effective post-cesarean analgesia in particular when the technique is performed under ultrasound imaging [66].

A Cochrane systematic review examining three trials suggested that local anesthetic wound infiltration and TAP block might improve the quality of postoperative analgesia after cesarean section as demonstrated by a reduction in the dose of opioid consumption when compared to a placebo [67]. However, the studies examined suffered from some methodological flaws and the sample examined was in all cases small.

More recent studies that investigated TAP block as a part of multimodal analgesia gave conflicting results with regard to its efficacy when compared with intrathecal morphine [68, 69].

A recent meta-analysis on the efficacy of TAP block found that this technique provides more effective post-cesarean analgesia, reduces the need for postoperative opioid medications and the time for first request for further analgesia, and reduces the incidence of opioid-related side effects [70].

TAP block technique may be used as a part of a multimodal analgesic regimen and can be recommended when it is not possible to provide other types of analgesia such as in the case of general anesthesia.

11.9 Analgesic Drugs and Breastfeeding

It is well recognized that breastfeeding is essential to improve neonatal and maternal well-being [71, 72].

However, one of the major concerns with post-cesarean analgesia is the potential passage of the analgesic medication into the milk that might expose the newborn to the analgesic drugs administered to the mother. For this reason, mothers sometimes choose to abandon breastfeeding in order to be able to get the medications or choose to avoid the use of analgesic drugs to continue breastfeeding.

It is, therefore, essential to identify the drugs that can be safely used in early postpartum to allow for a pain-free postpartum period but with no negative interference on breastfeeding.

Multiple factors should be considered, such as the potential effects of the drug on milk production, the amount of the drug excreted into human milk, the extent of oral absorption by the breastfeeding infant, and the potential adverse effects on the breastfeeding infant.

Generally, nonopioid medications such as NSAIDs or acetaminophen are considered to be safer than the opioid medications as they do not cause sedation either to the neonate or to the mother. Acetaminophen and paracetamol can be safely used in nursing mothers although being used alone is associated with poor analgesic efficacy.

NSAIDs are generally considered to be compatible with breastfeeding for short-term therapies with the exception of aspirin.

The use of ketorolac and ibuprofen are, in fact, clinically well accepted and considered to be safe for the infant due to their extremely low transfer into the milk [73, 74]. However, ketorolac received a "black box" warning on its use in both laboring and nursing mothers [75].

Although some studies found that the passage of COX 2 inhibitors in the milk is very low, their use is still not recommended as there is insufficient evidence to suggest their safe use during lactation.

However, when considering the use of drugs during breastfeeding, it should be taken into account that the effective concentration of the drug detected on the neonates' blood is extremely low and is unlikely to have any clinical effect.

The concern arising from the use of opioids derives from the potential negative effect on neonatal and maternal alertness with the consequent negative effect on the neonatal suckling reflex that is likely to delay the initiation of breastfeeding or is associated with its failure.

The administration of morphine is considered the gold standard during lactation as its passage into the milk is very low and its bioavailability in the newborn is poor [76, 77].

The use of meperidine (pethidine) is contraindicated in breastfeeding mothers as its metabolite causes significant and long-lasting neonatal sedation and inhibition of the suckling reflex [76].

Given these data, it is reasonable to encourage mothers to effectively treat their pain after cesarean section with morphine or/and NSAIDs considering that these drugs are practically not excreted into the milk, the bioavailability is very low, and when used in clinical doses they do not appear to affect neonatal behavior and the quality of breastfeeding. Drug delivery via patient-controlled anesthesia or administration by the epidural route may also minimize infant exposure. In addition, it is very important to note that maternal pain itself is associated with the failure of breastfeeding and is associated with postpartum depression and negatively affects the bonding between the mother and her child.

References

1. Bonnet MP, Mignon A, Mazoit JX, Ozier Y, Marret E. Analgesic effect and adverse effects of epidural morphine compared to parenteral opioids after elective caesarean section: a systematic review. Eur J Pain. 2010;14:894–9.
2. Wu CL, Naqibuddin M, Rowlingson AJ, Lietman SA, Jermyn RM, Fleisher LA. The effect of pain on health-related quality of life in the immediate postoperative period. Anesth Analg. 2003;97:1078–85.
3. Ismail S, Shahzad K, Shafiq F. Observational study to assess the effectiveness of postoperative pain of patients undergoing elective cesarean section. J Anaesthesiol Clin Pharmacol. 2012;28:36–40.
4. Leung A. Postoperative pain management in obstetric—new challenges and solutions. J Clin Anesth. 2004;16:57–65.
5. Cooper PJ, Murray L. Post natal depression. BMJ. 1988;316:1884–6.
6. Annika Karlström A, Engström-Olofsson R, Norbergh KG, Sjöling M, Hildingsson I. Postoperative pain after cesarean birth affects breastfeeding and infant care. J Obstet Gynecol Neonatal Nurs. 2007;36:430–40.
7. Eisenach JC, Pan PH, Smiley R, et al. Severity of acute pain after childbirth, but not type of delivery, predicts pain and post partum depression. Pain. 2008;15:87–94.
8. Kehlet H, Jensen TS, Woolf CJ. Persistent postsurgical pain: risk factors and prevention. Lancet. 2006;367:1618–25.
9. Perkins FM, Kehlet H. Chronic pain as an outcome of surgery—a review of predictive factors. Anesthesiology. 2000;93:1123–33.
10. Mathai M, Hofmeyr GJ, Mathai NE. Abdominal surgical incisions for caesarean section. Cochrane Database Syst Rev. 2013;5:CD004453.
11. Rousseau JA, Girard K, Turcot-Lemay L, Thomas N. A randomized study comparing skin closure in cesarean sections: staples vs. subcuticular sutures. Am J Obstet Gynecol. 2009;200:265.e1–4.
12. Nafisi S. Influence of uterine exteriorization versus in situ repair on post-cesarean maternal pain: a randomized trial. Int J Obstet Anesth. 2007;16:135–8.
13. Chooi CLS, White AM, Tan SGM, Dowling K, Cyna AM. Pain vs. comfort scores after caesarean section: a randomized trial. Br J Anaesth. 2013;110:780–7.
14. Lim Y, Jha S, Sia AT, et al. Morphine for post cesarean section analgesia: intrathecal, epidural or intravenous? Singapore Med J. 2005;46:392–6.
15. Cade L, Ashley J. Towards optimal analgesia after caesarean section: comparison of epidural and intravenous patient-controlled opioid analgesia. Anaesth Intensive Care. 1993;21:696–9.

16. Vercauteren M, Vereecken K, La Malfa M, et al. Cost-effectiveness of analgesia after caesarean section. A comparison of intrathecal morphine and epidural PCA. Acta Anaesthesiol Scand. 2002;46:85–9.
17. Palmer CM, Nogami WM, Van Maren G, et al. Post cesarean epidural morphine: a dose-response study. Anesth Analg. 1990;90:887–91.
18. Ready LB. Acute postoperative pain. In: Miller RD, editor. Anaesthesia, vol. 2. New York: Churchill Livingstone; 1994. p. 2327–44.
19. Fuller JG, McMorland GH, et al. Epidural morphine for analgesia after caesarean section: a report of 4880 patients. Can J Anaesth. 1990;37:636–40.
20. Dahl JB, Jeppesen IS, Jorgesen H, et al. Intraoperative and postoperative analgesic efficacy and adverse effects of intrathecal opioids in patients undergoing cesarean section with spinal anesthesia: a qualitative and quantitative systematic review of randomized controlled trials. Anesthesiology. 1999;91:1919–27.
21. Cousins MJ, Mather LE. Intrathecal and epidural administration of opioids. Anesthesiology. 1984;61:276–310.
22. Bromage PR, Camporesi EM, Durant PA, Nielsen CH. Rostral spread of epidural morphine. Anesthesiology. 1982;56:431–6.
23. Leysen JE, Commereu W, Niemegeers CJE. Sufentanil, a superior ligand for μ-opiate receptors: binding properties and regional distribution in rat brain and spinal cord. Eur J Pharmacol. 1983;87:209–25.
24. Camorcia M, Capogna G, Columb MO. Minimum analgesic doses of fentanyl and sufentanil for epidural analgesia in the first stage of labor. Anesth Analg. 2003;96:1178–82.
25. Grass JA, Sakima NT, Schmidt R, Michtisch R, Zuckerman RL, Harris AP. A randomized, double-blind, dose-response comparison of epidural fentanyl versus sufentanil analgesia after cesarean section. Anesth Analg. 1997;85:365–71.
26. Palmer CM, Voulgaropoulos D, Alves D. Subarachnoid fentanyl augments lidocaine spinal anesthesia for cesarean delivery. Reg Anesth. 1995;20:389–94.
27. Bernards CM. Recent insights into the pharmacokinetics of spinal opioids and the relevance to opioid selection. Curr Opin Anaesthesiol. 2004;17:441–7.
28. Palmer CM, Emerson S, Volgoropolous D, et al. Dose response relationship of intrathecal morphine for post cesarean analgesia. Anesthesiology. 1999;90:437–44.
29. Sarvela J, Halonen P, Soikkeli A, et al. A double blinded randomized comparison of intrathecal and epidural morphine for elective cesarean delivery. Anesth Analg. 2002;95:436–40.
30. Sibilla C, Albertazzi P, Zatelli R, et al. Perioperative analgesia for caesarean section: comparison of intrathecal morphine and fentanyl alone or in combination. Int J Obstet Anaesth. 1997;6:43–8.
31. SM S-S, Aouad MT, Jalbout MI, et al. Intrathecal versus intravenous fentanyl for supplementation of subarachnoid block during cesarean delivery. Anesth Analg. 2002;95:209–13.
32. Dahlgren G, Hulstrand C, Jakobsson J, et al. Intrathecal sufentanil, fentanyl, or placebo added to bupivacaine for cesarean section. Anesth Analg. 1997;85:1288–93.
33. Milner AR, Bogod DG, Harwood RJ. Intrathecal administration of morphine for elective caesarean section. Anaesthesia. 1996;51:871–3.
34. Wong JY, Carvalho B, Riley ET. Intrathecal morphine 100 and 200 µg for post-cesarean delivery analgesia: a trade-off between analgesic efficacy and side effects. Int J Obstet Anaesth. 2013;22:36–41.
35. Berger JS, Gonzalez A, Hopkins A, et al. Dose-response of intrathecal morphine when administered with intravenous ketorolac for post-cesarean analgesia: a two-center, prospective, randomized, blinded trial. Int J Obstet Anesth. 2016;28:3–11.
36. Moore A, Bullingham R, McQuay H, et al. Spinal fluid kinetics of morphine and heroin. Clin Pharmacol Ther. 1984;35:40–5.
37. Skilton RW, Kinsella SM, Smith A, et al. Dose response study of subarachnoid diamorphine for analgesia after elective caesarean section. Int J Obstet Anaesth. 1999;8:231–5.
38. Kelly MC, Carabine UA, Mirakhur RK. Intrathecal diamorphine for analgesia after caesarean section. A dose finding study and assessment of side-effects. Anaesthesia. 1998;53:231–7.

39. Saravan S, Robinson APC, Qayoum D, et al. Minimum dose if intrathecal diamorphine required to prevent intraoperative supplementation of spinal anaesthesia for caesarean section. Br J Anaesth. 2003;91:368–72.
40. Lyons G. Dose of intrathecal diamorphine for caesarean section and position for spinal insertion. Br J Anaesth. 2004;92:448–9.
41. Roulson CJ, Bennett J, Shaw M, et al. Effect of extradural diamorphine on analgesia after cesarean section under subarachnoid block. Br J Anaesth. 1993;71:810–3.
42. Hallworth SP, Fernando R, Bell R, et al. Comparison of intrathecal and epidural diamorphine for elective caesarean section using a combined spinal epidural technique. Br J Anaesth. 1999;82:228–32.
43. Bloor GK, Thompson M, Chung N. A randomized, double blind comparison of subarachnoid and epidural diamorphine for elective caesarean section using a combined spinal epidural technique. Int J Obstet Anesth. 2000;9:233–7.
44. Carvalho B, Roland LM, Chu LF, et al. Single-dose, extended-release epidural morphine (DepoDur) compared to conventional epidural morphine for post-cesarean pain. Anesth Analg. 2007;105:176–83.
45. Eisenach JC, Grice SC, Dewan DM. Patient controlled analgesia following cesarean section: a comparison with epidural and intramuscular narcotics. Anesthesiology. 1988;68:444–8.
46. Parker RK, Holtman B, White PF. Patient controlled analgesia: does a concurrent opioid infusion improve pain management after surgery? JAMA. 1991;266:1947–52.
47. Jenkins JG, Khan MM. Anaesthesia for caesarean section: a survey in the UK region from 1992 to 2001. Anaesthsia. 2003;58:1114–8.
48. Wilder-Smith CH, Hill L, Dyer RA, Torr G, Coetzee E. Postoperative sensitization and pain after cesarean delivery and the effects of single IM doses of tramadol and diclofenac alone and in combination. Anesth Analg. 2003;97:526–33.
49. Lowder JL, Shackelford DP, Holbert D, Beste TM. A randomized, controlled trial to compare ketorolac tromethamine versus placebo after cesarean section to reduce pain and narcotic usage. Am J Obstet Gynecol. 2003;189:1559–62.
50. Cardoso M, Carvalho J, Amaro A, et al. Small doses of intrathecal morphine combined with systemic diclofenac for postoperative pain control after cesarean delivery. Anesth Analg. 1998;86:82–6.
51. Hodsman NBA, Burns J, Blyth A. The morphine sparing effects of diclofenac sodium following abdominal surgery. Anaesthesia. 1987;42:1005–8.
52. Cohen SE, Subak LL, Brose WG, Halpern J. Analgesia after cesarean delivery: patient evaluations and costs of five opioid technique. Reg Anesth. 1991;16:141–9.
53. Guay J. The benefits of adding epidural analgesia to general anesthesia: a metaanalysis. J Anesth. 2006;20:335–40.
54. Richman JM, Wu CL. Epidural analgesia for postoperative pain. Anesthesiol Clin North Am. 2005;23:125–40.
55. Cooper DW, Ryall DM, Desira WR. Extradural fentanyl for postoperative analgesia: predominant spinal or systemic action? Br J Anaesth. 1995;74:184–7.
56. Correll DJ, Viscusi ER, Grunwald Z, et al. Epidural analgesia compared with intravenous morphine patient controlled analgesia: postoperative outcome measures after mastectomy with immediate TRAM flap breast reconstruction. Reg Anesth Pain Med. 2001;26:444–9.
57. Block BM, Liu SS, Rowlingson AJ. Efficacy of postoperative epidural analgesia. A meta analysis. JAMA. 2003;290:2455–63.
58. Wu CL, Cohen SR, Richman JM, et al. Efficacy of postoperative patient controlled and continuous infusion epidural analgesia versus intravenous patient controlled analgesia with opioids. Anesthesiology. 2005;103:1079–88.
59. Lubenow TR, Tanck EN, Hopkins EM, et al. Comparison of patient—assisted epidural analgesia with continuous-infusion epidural analgesia for postoperative patients. Reg Anesth. 1994;19:206–11.
60. Nightingale JJ, Knight MV, Higgins B, et al. Randomized, double-blind comparison of patient-controlled epidural infusion vs. nurse administered epidural infusion for postoperative analgesia in patients undergoing colonic resection. Br J Anaesth. 2007;98:380–4.

61. Liu SS, Allen HW, Olsson GL. Patient-controlled epidural analgesia with bupivacaine and fentanyl on hospital wards: prospective experience with 1,030 surgical patients. Anesthesiology. 1998;88:688–95.
62. Ellis DJ, Millar WL, Reisner LS. A randomized double blind comparison of epidural versus intravenous fentanyl infusion for analgesia after cesarean section. Anesthesiology. 1990;72:981–6.
63. Cohen S, Pantuck CB, Amar D, et al. The primary action of epidural fentanyl after cesarean delivery is via a spinal mechanism. Anesth Analg. 2002;94:674–9.
64. Stirparo S, Laudani A, Haiberger E, et al. Postoperative analgesia after cesarean section: a comparison between programmed intermittent epidural bolus (PIEB) versus continuous epidural infusion (CEI). Reg Anesth Pain Med. 2011;36:E1–E27.
65. Mc Donnell JG, Curley G, Carney J, et al. The analgesic efficacy of transversus abdominis plane block after cesarean section. Anesth Analg. 2008;106:186–91.
66. Barrington MJ, Ivanusic JJ, Rozen WM, Hebbard P. Spread of injectate after ultrasound-guided subcostal transversus abdominis plane block: a cadaveric study. Anaesthesia. 2009;64:745–50.
67. Bamigboye AA, Hofmeyr GJ. Local anesthetic wound infiltration and abdominal nerves block during cesarean section for postoperative pain relief. Cochrane Database Syst Rev. 2009;3:CD006954.
68. McMorriw RC, Mhuircheartaigh RJ, Ahmed KA, et al. Comparison of transversus abdominis plane blocks vs. spinal morphine for pain relief after caesarean section. Br J Anaesth. 2011;106:706–12.
69. Belavy D, Cowlishaw PJ, Howes M, et al. Ultrasound guided transverse abdominis plane block for analgesia after caesarean delivery. Br J Anaesth. 2009;103:726–30.
70. Siddiqui MR, Sajid MS, Uncles DR, Baig MK. A meta-analysis on the clinical effectiveness of transverse abdominis plane block. J Clin Anesth. 2011;23:7–14.
71. Kramer MS. "Breast is best": the evidence. Early Hum Dev. 2010;86:729–32.
72. Section B, et al. Breastfeeding and the use of human milk. Pediatrics. 2012;129:e827–41.
73. Bennett PN. Drugs and human lactation. 2nd ed. Amsterdam: Elsevier; 1996.
74. Bar-Oz B, Bulkowstein M, et al. Use of antibiotic and analgesic drugs during lactation. Drug Saf. 2003;26:925–35.
75. Drugs and lactation database (LactMed). U.S. National Library of Medicine, TOXNET Toxicology Data Network.
76. Wittels C, Scott DT, Sinatra RS. Exogenous opioids in human breast milk and acute neonatal neurobehaviour: a preliminary study. Anesthesiology. 1990;73:864–9.
77. Feilberg VL, Rosemborg D, Broen CC, et al. Excretion of morphine in human breast milk. Acta Anaesthesiol Scand. 1989;33:426–8.

Long-Term Problems and Chronic Pain After Caesarean Section

12

Patricia Lavand'homme

12.1 Introduction

Caesarean section is one of, if not, the most common surgical procedure performed over the world as estimated number was 22.9 million in 2012 [1]. In developing countries, surgical volume is growing with caesarean deliveries accounting for nearly a third (29.6%) of all the procedures. In high-resource developed countries, the rate of caesarean sections has strongly rised reflecting changes in obstetric practice toward increasing medical interventions in relation with older age of the mothers, obstetrician's fear of litigation, repeated caesarean deliveries, and also maternal preference [1]. Regarding women's health after caesarean delivery, most of the reports have focused on maternal mortality and short-term morbidity, e.g., infections, adhesions, need for resection, increased risk for abnormal placentation [2]. In contrast, longer term consequences on the mother's quality of life have received little interest probably because after delivery, the attention of both the caregivers and the mothers themselves has shifted to the neonate.

This chapter will focus on the long-term potential consequences of a previous caesarean delivery for the upcoming life of a woman (Fig. 12.1). Further, as a consequence to the rise in caesarean section rate, two questions stand as important issues. Do the long-term problems directly related to childbirth differ between caesarean delivery and vaginal delivery? Did the incidence of the long-term problems related to caesarean section change over the last decade?

P. Lavand'homme
Department of Anaesthesiology, St Luc Hospital University Catholic of Louvain,
Av Hippocrate 10-UCL 1821, 1200 Brussels, Belgium
e-mail: patricia.lavandhomme@uclouvain.be

© Springer International Publishing Switzerland 2017
G. Capogna (ed.), *Anesthesia for Cesarean Section*,
DOI 10.1007/978-3-319-42053-0_12

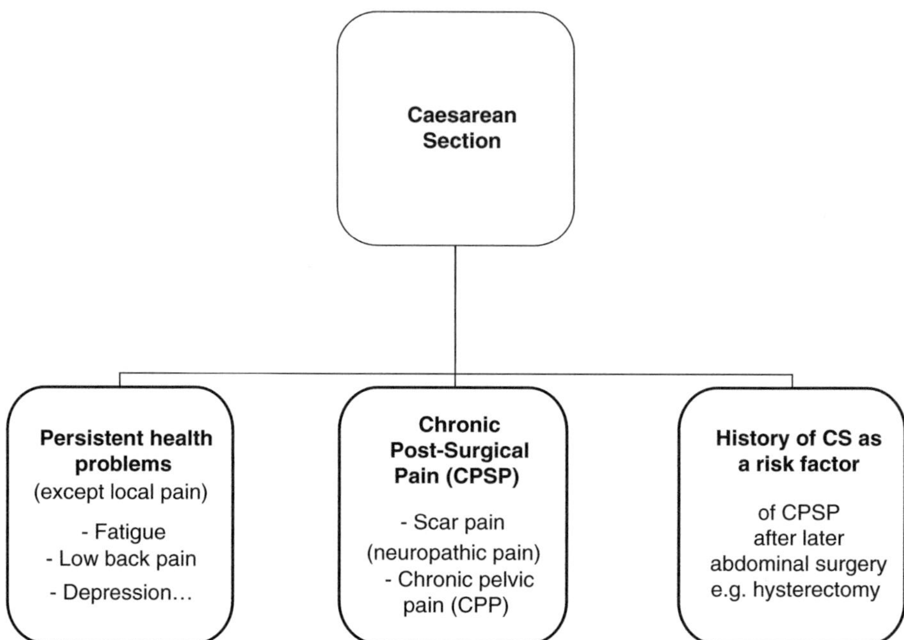

Fig. 12.1 Long-term potential consequences of a caesarean section for the upcoming life of a woman

12.2 Long-Term Health Problems: Except Local Pain—After Caesarean Section

Childbirth is a major event in life, associated with both physical and psychological changes which may affect the woman's quality of life. The awareness on long-term maternal, physical, and emotional health problems after childbirth is increasing, with some recent study including a 5-year follow-up [3]. The global perception of her health status as well as the overall perceived health-related quality of life by the women herself is interesting. Childbirth is generally an expression of good health and thereby, self-rated health in women after childbirth is higher than in a population sample of women of same age [4]. Nevertheless, the mode of delivery seems to affect the health-related quality of life up to 5 years after birth of the first child because women who have undergone an emergency caesarean section or a caesarean section due to medical indication are more likely to report health concerns than women who had vaginal delivery, instrumental vaginal delivery, or caesarean section on request [3].

The most common problems at 8 weeks and later after childbirth are reported in Table 12.1. Two large prospective cohort studies published in 2002 [5] and 2012 [6] confirm the high prevalence of health problems which persist or recur after childbirth by either vaginal route or caesarean section. Tiredness is by far the most common physical symptom after childbirth [4]. However, women who had a

Table 12.1. Prevalence of the most common health problems (except local pain) reported as significant problems after childbirth

	2 months (%)	6 months (%)	12–24 months (%)
Physical exhaustion	50–66	45–50	58–60
Low back pain	51–53	43–47	42–44
Urinary incontinence	21–27	11–12	20–23
Bowel problems	35–37	17–21	9–11
Painful intercourse	36–56	–	8–9
Breast problems	14–18	6–9	4–6
Headaches, migraine	18–22	16–19	23–25
Depressive symptoms	10–13	7–10	10–12
Others: colds, illnesses…	19–23	16–19	36–39

From Thompson et al. [5], Woolhouse et al. [6], Hannah et al. [10], and Declercq et al. [23]

caesarean section are more likely to report major fatigue (adjusted OR: 1.4; 95% CI: 1.06–1.83) and to suffer back pain at 6 and 12 months postpartum than women who had a vaginal delivery. Fatigue is often associated with sleeping problems which are very frequent in the early postpartum period but may persist [4, 5]. Furthermore, the presence of pain also interferes with sleep as sleep disturbances are frequently reported in questionnaires assessing the quality of life in patients with chronic pain. Between 10 and 25% of women with chronic pain at 6 months and later after childbirth mention associated sleeping problems [4, 5, 7–9], unrelated to the mode of delivery.

Besides, whether caesarean section causes less urinary incontinence, it seems to induce more bowel problems, i.e., constipation [5, 10]. The risk of intra-abdominal adhesions and hence intestinal obstruction is higher in women with a history of caesarean section (OR 2.1; 95% CI: 1.8–2.4) by comparison with women who had vaginal birth [11]. Having a caesarean section is often thought to avoid trauma to the genital tract and to protect postpartum sexual function. However, over 6 weeks after childbirth, sexual function does not seem to be affected by the mode of delivery [12].

Postpartum depression is a specific mental disorder, with 13–15% of women experiencing a major depressive episode during the first postpartum year [13]. Accordingly, the prevalence of self-reported postpartum depressive symptoms range from 12 to 20% and mood lability is common after childbirth. Suicide in mothers with postpartum depression accounts for 17% of late-pregnancy-related death [14]. Beyond the distress of the mother, postpartum depression and maternal mental health in general affect the child's health outcomes in terms of cognitive, behavioral problems and risk of subsequent depression at adolescence [15]. Regarding depressive symptoms, assessed by a questionnaire used in the general population, a prospective Chinese study found a higher prevalence at 3 months (46% vs. 38%) but not later after caesarean delivery [12]. In contrast, a few prospective studies using the same specific questionnaire and scoring, i.e., the Edinburgh Postnatal Depression Scale (EPDS) [7, 10], report an incidence of 10.5% postpartum depression at either 2 months and 2 years after delivery, whatever the mode of delivery [7, 10, 16]. Both studies confirm the previous results of a large prospective population cohort study ($N = 14{,}663$) which already found no different risk among elective caesarean section, emergency caesarean section, and spontaneous vaginal delivery [13]. Finally, several studies on the quality of life after delivery also mention mood alterations caused by the presence of persistent pain (prevalence of 10–25% in women who underwent a caesarean section) [7, 9, 17].

At 2 years postpartum, maternal outcomes (i.e., fatigue, back pain, incontinence, sexual problem, menstrual problem, depression) after planned caesarean section are similar to planned vaginal birth as found in a prospective study on breech presentation at term [10]. For other physical health problems, the pattern of morbidity does not differ between caesarean section and spontaneous vaginal birth. Breast problems are very common, such as sore nipples and mastitis, but resolve with time. Interestingly, breast problems are also experienced by women who did not breastfeed at all [6]. In contrast to breast problems which decrease with time, the frequency of colds and coughs increases with time and they are more frequent in multiparas [4, 6].

12.3 Chronic Postsurgical Pain After Caesarean Section

Chronic pain is recognized as pain that persists past normal healing time and hence lacks the acute warning function of physiological nociception. Moderate to severe pain that persists at least 3 months (by definition, *Chronic Post-Surgical Pain*, CPSP) is frequent after surgery and may concern up to 6–10% of the patients [18, 19]. Depending the type of surgery, CPSP often involves a neuropathic component (average 30% of the cases, range 6–54%). In this case, pain is usually more severe and affects the quality of life more adversely. CPSP has become a health priority and will be included in the new version of the *International Classification of Diseases* (ICD-11) [18] because adequate pain treatment is a human right and also because CPSP represents a complex biopsychosocial problem. Further, the prevention of CPSP is currently a challenge for the clinicians as an indicator of the quality of healthcare [20]. Chronic pain related to caesarean section has received little attention until the first study was published in 2004 [21]. According to the definition of CPSP, chronic pain after caesarean section should persist at least 3 months after delivery and should not be present before or during pregnancy (Table 12.2).

The first studies on the topic were retrospective ones with inherent bias and have reported on global CPSP without distinction between parietal scar pain and deeper abdominal or pelvic pain. According to these studies ($N = 220$–1573), the prevalence of CPSP at 6 months and later was 12–18%. The prevalence of disabling pain with a negative impact on the mother's quality of life and on the mother-child relationship was consistently 4–7% [8, 21–24]. Reported incidence of CPSP after caesarean section did not really change over time from 2004 [21] until 2016 [22]. In contrast, the relative risk of developing chronic pain after caesarean delivery compared with spontaneous vaginal delivery differed from one study to another [8, 22], probably because most of the retrospective studies did not characterize chronic pain, i.e., parietal abdominal pain versus deep intra-abdominal pain versus pelvic pain.

Table 12.2. Type and incidence (*) of chronic postsurgical pain after caesarean section compared with hysterectomy for a benign condition

Caesarean section	
Scar pain	
With predominant neuropathic pain	4–5% (2% severe pain)
	50–60% at 6 months; 26% at 12 months
Visceral pain	
Deep intra-abdominal pain	5.4–7.6%
Chronic pelvic pain	2.9% at 6 months; 1.3% at 18 months
Hysterectomy	
Scar pain	
With predominant neuropathic pain	16–25% at 4 months; 8–10% at 1 year and later
	33% at 6 months and later
Visceral pain	
Deep intra-abdominal pain	15.3%
Chronic pelvic pain	16.7%

(*) from prospective studies

Because of the increasing interest on the topic, prospective studies emerged, focusing on new pain related to the procedure and excluding preexisting pain. In these studies, the incidence of CPSP at 6 months and later ranges from less than 1% [7, 17] to 4–9% [25, 26] (mainly pain of moderate intensity with only 2.1% of women complaining of severe pain [26]). Two studies have reported a very low incidence of CPSP after caesarean section, 1.8–3% at 6 months and 0.3–0.6% at 1 year [7, 17] but possible bias may exist. One study [7] only followed up at 6 months and later patients who reported pain at 2 months while it is now evident that CPSP may develop later after surgery [19]. The other study mostly included Brazilian women who underwent planned caesarean section at their own request [17]. By comparison, the incidence of CPSP after gynecologic surgery (i.e., hysterectomy for benign causes) decreases from 16–25% at 4 months post-surgery [27] to 8–10% at 1 year [26, 28] and to 7% at 2 years post-surgery [29]. The majority of theses studies report 4–6% moderate pain and only 1–2% severe pain [26, 28, 29].

12.3.1 Scar Pain and Neuropathic Pain Component in Chronic Pain After Caesarean Section

As scar pain predominates, being the major complaint in more than 83% of the women with CPSP after caesarean section [7, 17], some studies have focused on scar pain and/or have distinguisched scar pain from deep intra-abdominal and pelvic pain. The prevalence of scar pain remains constant over years and ranges from 4 to 5% with less than 2% severe pain [6, 10, 25]. Recent arguments are in favor of a predominant neuropathic origin as the presence of CPSP and the presence of sensory abnormalities in the area of surgery are commonly associated despite wide ranges for normal variability in sensory function [30]. A Pfannenstiel incision is commonly used for caesarean delivery; its advantages include a low incidence of incisional hernia and an aesthetic scar. However, the risk of ilio-inguinal and ilio-hypogastric nerve entrapment related to the technique is real. Among the 32% of women who had undergone obstetric or gynecologic procedures with a Pfannenstiel incision and suffered CPSP at incision site at 2 years after surgery (including 7% with severe pain), neuropathic descriptors were used by 50% of them, and pain was located at lateral ends of the incisional scar in 70% of the patients [29]. Few studies have used adequate screening tools to characterize scar pain after caesarean section. In one study, when pain quality was assessed using the Short-Form McGill Pain Questionnaire Revised (SF-MPQ2), chronic pain was qualified as predominantly neuropathic, respectively, in 56%, 50%, and 26% of the patients at 3, 6, and 12 months after surgery [17, 31]. In another study, the prospective epidemiologic French study "EDONIS" aimed to assess the prevalence and possible neuropathic character of postsurgical pain using the Douleur Neuropathic 4 (DN4) questionnaire, the 6-months cumulative incidence of CPSP after caesarean section was approximately 20% with an established neuropathic origin in 61% of the cases [32]. It is interesting to note that the reported pain intensity was generally low (pain score > 3/10 in only 2% of the patients). The low intensity of neuropathic pain diagnosed after caesarean delivery is intriguing. According to the EDONIS results [32] and findings from other studies [26], neuropathic characteristics are generally associated with severe CPSP (average pain score of 5–6 on a scale from 0 to 10) and functional impairement. By comparison, the prevalence of neuropathic characteristics in chronic pain after abdominal hysterectomy is less, around 33% [33, 34]. The variability in the incidence of the neuropathic origin of CPSP relates not only on the different modalities of assessment but also on the fact that chronic pain intensity and characteristics fluctuate considerably over time [30, 32].

12.3.2 Visceral Pain Component in Chronic Pain After Caesarean Section

Studies on sex-gender differences demonstrate that females have a higher incidence of severe pain, which is more anatomically diffuse and longer lasting pain than males [35] with the prevalence of visceral pain being more frequent. The abdomen (47%) and the perineal region (38%) are often mentioned as locations for CPSP by patients attending pain clinics [36]. In the classification of chronic pain for ICD-11, *chronic visceral pain* represents persistent or recurrent pain that originates from the internal organs including abdominal and pelvic cavities [18]. Pain is perceived in the somatic tissues of the body wall (skin, muscles), in the areas that receive the same sensory innervation as the internal organ at the origin of the symptom (referred to as visceral pain). By consequence, visceral pain related to caesarean section should be perceived as diffuse abdominal wall pain, not localized at the surgical scar, and in some cases felt as a deep intra-abdominal pain. Few studies about CPSP after delivery have assessed deep abdominal pain. Three prospective studies however report a very low incidence at 6 months and later because the incidence of CPSP itself was already very low [7, 10, 17]. Also, because of the low incidence of CPSP and thereby abdominal pain, it is difficult to determine if caesarean section carries a higher risk than vaginal delivery but it does not seem to be the case [10]. At 2 years after a planned caesarean section for breech delivery, intra-abdominal pain was mentioned by 5.4% of the women versus 4.3% of the women who had planned vaginal birth. By comparison, 15.3% of the women undergoing gynecological surgery for a non-painful condition will develop chronic intra-abdominal pain (prevalence around 3.6% in general female population) [37].

Among the various "chronic visceral pain conditions," *chronic pelvic pain* (CPP) is a common problem in women of reproductive age with a prevalence rate of 15–25% [38]. The definition proposed by the American College of Obstetricians and Gynecologists includes noncyclic pelvic pain of at least 6 months duration that localizes to anatomical pelvis, anterior abdominal wall at or below umbilicus, lumbosacral back, or buttocks, sufficient to cause functional disability or to lead to medical care [39]. CPP is a multifactorial disease, difficult to treat. A retrospective case-control study including patients (mean age of 34 years; range 19–52 years) who underwent a laparoscopy for CPP found a significantly higher incidence of caesarean section history (67% of the cases) [40]. The risk factor associated with previous caesarean section was almost 4 times greater (OR 3.7; 95% CI: 1.7–7.7). Possible causes for CPP after caesarean section include adhesions, inflammation, and abnormal healing of bladder, round ligaments, and adjacent structures. Myofascial pain and neuroma may also be involved. While a relationship between caesarean section and CPP is easy to understand, CPP prevalence has been rarely assessed in most of the studies about CPSP after delivery. Furthermore, most of these studies did not exclude women with preexisting pelvic pain; hence, the true incidence of CPP, i.e., new onset of pelvic pain secondary to caesarean section was not evaluated. Two retrospective studies mention an incidence of 9% new onset CPP at 1 year after delivery [41, 42]. Both studies report an important impact on the daily quality of life, upon a wide range of sexual and nonsexual activities. The median duration of CPP was 24 months (IQR 6–51 months). A few prospective studies looking into physical health problems and pain after delivery mention an incidence of 5–7.6% CPP between 6 months and 2 years after delivery, with no difference regarding the mode of delivery [6, 10]. A recent longitudinal population study dedicated to assess the new onset of pelvic pain after delivery ($N = 20,248$) found a global incidence of 4.5% at 6 months and 1.7% at 18 months [43]. Both planned and emergency caesarean section was associated with a reduced risk of CPP (2.9% at 6 months and 1.3% at 18 months) by comparison with vaginal delivery. In patients with CPP, mean pelvic pain score was low, did not change over time and did not differ according to the mode of delivery. No information about the duration of pain was available. These results may support those of a recent retrospective study ($N = 495$) which also found a protective effect of caesarean section over spontaneous vaginal delivery regarding chronic pain at 2 years (odd ratio 0.13; 95% CI: 0.01–0.63) [22].

12.4 Caesarean Section as a Risk for Chronic Pain After Later Obstetric or Gynecologic Surgery

Although a history of caesarean delivery does not preclude further vaginal delivery, it is often a cause of resection. The initial publication related to CPSP after caesarean section [21] did not report previous caesarean section or previous abdominal surgery as a cause of CPSP, a finding supported by later publications, either retrospective ones [8] and prospective ones [25]. Nevertheless, the report from Loos [29] about the Pfannenstiel incision as a source of chronic pain ($N = 866$, including >90% caesarean sections) mentioned repeated surgeries as an independent risk factor (OR 2.92; 95% CI: 1.44–5.93) whereas the length of the scar was not. In this study, around 50% of the patients presented with characteristics of neuropathic pain in their chronic pain description and the presence of numbness also significantly predicted CPSP (OR 3.01; 95% CI: 2.05–4.4). Modifications of skin sensitivity surrounding the scar of a previous caesarean section was also reported by others [44] who found the presence of scar hyperalgesia in 41% of women scheduled for a repeat procedure at 55 ± 33 months after their first caesarean section. The presence of scar hyperalgesia was correlated with higher acute postoperative pain and with the presence of increased central sensitization processing assessed by mechanical temporal summation [44]. Thereby, it is not excluded that nerve lesion during repeat section might lead to CPSP in some patients with a predisposed background as demonstrated by Martinez and colleagues in a different surgical model [45].

Finally, as aforementioned, a history of caesarean section was common is women who underwent a laparoscopy for chronic pelvic pain (CPP) [40]. Both preoperative pelvic pain and previous caesarean section actually represent significant risk factors (respective odds ratio of 3.25 [2.40–4.41] and 1.54 [1.06–2.26]) for the development of CPSP after hysterectomy for a benign indication [46].

12.5 Risk Factors of Chronic Pain After Caesarean Section

As any other chronic conditions, CPSP is a complex phenomenon involving peripheral and central processes as well as psychological components. Predictive factors for CPSP may be surgery specific, i.e., in relation to the tissue trauma, or patient specific [47]. The later factors seem to be prominent because all the patients are not equally at risk of severe acute pain and/or persistent pain after either surgery or trauma [48]. The knowledge of the risk factors associated with the development of persistent pain after a specific surgical procedure is mandatory to implement preventive strategies.

12.5.1 Surgery and Tissue Damage-Specific Risk Factors

Elective versus unplanned caesarean delivery. As the risk of abdominal wall nerve injury may be higher during emergency procedures, emergency caesarean section may carry a higher risk of chronic neuropathic pain by comparison with an elective procedure [29]. Interestingly, labor and trial of vaginal birth have not been associated with an increased risk of developing persistent pain after caesarean delivery [8, 10, 23].

Extent of tissue damage during caesarean delivery. The type of abdominal wall incision, i.e., vertical or transverse incision only has an impact on acute pain and does not affect persistent pain [7]. Today, most of the procedures are performed via a transverse incision, i.e., the Pfannenstiel incision or the modified Joel-Cohen (Misgav-Ladach) incision. As previously mentioned, the Pfannenstiel incision carries a risk of injury of the lower abdominal wall nerves leading to a risk of developing chronic neuropathic pain [29]. In comparison, the Misgav-Ladach technique seems associated with better outcomes up to 5 years post-surgery in term of improved quality of life, reduced incidence of chronic pain, neuropathic pain, and decreased pain intensity [49, 50]. Besides the type of abdominal incision, some variations of operative techniques have also been investigated. Closure versus nonclosure of the visceral and/or parietal peritoneum to reduce pelvic adhesions is still debated. A systematic review on the topic however reported reduced chronic abdominal pain and pelvic discomfort after nonclosure of the peritoneum [51].

12.5.2 Patient-Specific Risk Factors

Some individuals may be predisposed to the development of persistent pain. To support this, the recent literature on CPSP, specifically the research on the transition from acute to chronic postsurgical pain, has moved from general risk factors, such as gender, age, and obesity, to more individualized risk factors reported in a risk index for the prediction of CPSP [52]. Among the predictors, pain itself is the strongest one what indicates that individual changes in the processing of pain are involved in the development of CPSP [20]. Both preoperative pain in the body part to be operated on, preoperative pain distant from the operative site and severe acute postoperative pain are part of the risk index and have been mentioned in different studies concerning caesarean section. Preoperative pain is found in more than 50% of patients undergoing surgery [26]. Both the presence of a chronic pain condition and the potential regular intake of analgesics may sensitize the central nervous system and so may favor pain chronicity after tissue injury [20]. All the retrospective studies on chronic pain after childbirth mention the presence of pain elsewhere as major risk factor for the development of persistent pain after delivery [8, 21] with an odds ratio even superior to that related to the recall of intense acute post-delivery pain (2.5 vs. 1.3) [9]. Further, clinical observations show that patients reporting pelvic pain often suffer from more than one pain what raises the question of potential alterations of endogenous pain modulatory mechanisms rather than only local organ-based mechanisms [48]. Similarly, a previous history of a peripheral neuropathic event predicted the occurrence of chronic neuropathic pain after caesarean section, supporting the role of an endogenous nerve fragility [53].

In the retrospective studies, patients with CPSP often recall severe acute postpartum pain [9, 21] although that point should be taken with caution because the memory of pain may be influenced by the meaning and the affective value of the pain experience. In example, patients who have given birth by caesarean section are more accurate at recalling acute postoperative pain than patients who have had vaginal delivery or patients who have undergone gynecological surgery [54].

The clinical reality shows severe acute postpartum pain in 17% of women within the first 36 h of caesarean section, caesarean delivery being associated with a 32.5% increase in acute pain scores by comparison with vaginal delivery [16]. Acute pain severity, independent of the type of delivery, may predict an 2.5-fold increase in the risk of persistent pain at 2 months but not later after childbirth [7, 16], a fact that argues for the major role played by individual factors in CPSP beyond the initial degree of tissue injury which is more involved in acute pain severity. Similar findings have been found for hysterectomy [27, 33].

Psychosocial vulnerability represents an important individual risk factor. Mental health has an impact on the patient's willingness to recover. Psychological mechanisms of pain processing (emotion and when pain is perceived as a threat) already known to play a role in chronic pain conditions have recently attracted interest in perioperative conditions [20]. Obviously, there is a vulnerable population who presents with a reduced ability to cope with pain, to anticipate pain, and to control pain when confronted with it. In the context of childbirth, the influence of preoperative psychological factors on the development of CPSP seems quite mild [53] in contrast with the weight of the same factors in the context of other surgical procedures including hysterectomy [55] what supports the hypothesis of a context effect in the development of CPSP [53].

12.5.3 Genetic Predisposition as an Individual Risk Factor

Over the last few years, major developments in genomic research have shown how genetic variability may affect not only the response to medications including analgesics but also may account for the side effects of the medication. An actual challenge would be to find "pain genes" allowing to identify individuals with an increased vulnerability to pain and genes which confer an increased risk of developing intense acute pain and chronic pain after tissue injury [56]. To date, the value of clinical factors remains superior to that of genetic factors for predicting CPSP. In example, clinical factors (surgery, age, physical and mental health, preoperative pain) predicted 73% of CPSP that developed after various procedures including hysterectomy while no specific genetic marker did it [28].

12.6 Management of Long-Term Health Problems After Caesarean Delivery

The majority of women may expect a certain amount of physical symptoms as a consequence of pregnancy and childbirth. They consider those problems as natural and of temporary nature. However, for some of them, the problems may persist what can seriously impact the quality of life and interfere with the mother–child bonding.

Several studies pointed out that a majority of women do not consult a health professional even if they feel that they need advice [4, 41, 42]. Pain complaints localized to areas that are related to sexual function and urination are still often considered taboo and are complicated by psychological issues [39]. However, among the women reporting chronic pain localized to abdominal scar after caesarean delivery, only 4–8% mentioned to have visited a physician [21, 29] and less than 25% were taking pain medications. There is still a lack of education regarding pain relief in the postpartum period. A previous report from 2002 [5] already underlined mothers'needs for help and advice. When questioned at 2 and 6 months after delivery, 40% of them reported they had missed emotional support and medical advices. Other authors have pointed out that postnatal checkup at 6 weeks is likely to provide only a limited protection for some health problems that may persist after delivery [3]. Physicians should continue to ask mothers about any pain related to delivery, beyond the first year postpartum, to make appropriate referrals for pain management [41]. It is important to note that the use of systemic analgesics is restricted in breastfeeding women due to the concerns about the excretion of drugs in the breast milk and hence the potential toxicity for the infant. Therefore, if indicated, local analgesic treatments will be preferable, e.g., scar infiltration of the abdominal wall [57], intravaginal injection [58], or pudendal block [59], using a combination of corticosteroids and local anaesthetics. Beyond their diagnostic value, these nerve blocks may provide long-term pain relief in some patients. In case of intractable persistent pain caused by a nerve entrapment, the surgical neurectomy may represent an effective solution [57, 60].

Conclusion

Giving birth is a major event in the life of a woman. The majority of women may expect a certain amount of physical symptoms as a consequence of pregnancy and childbirth. They consider those problems as natural and of temporary nature. However, for some of them, the problems may persist what can seriously impact the quality of life and interfere with the mother–child relationship. The mode of delivery, thereby the degree of tissue trauma has only a short-term impact, long-lasting problems and specifically chronic pain are more related to individual factors. No change in the incidence of health problems related to delivery occurred during the last decade despite an increased recognition of their reality. Women's health after childbirth whatever the mode of delivery should be a shared responsibility between the caregivers and the mothers. Finally, it is important to notice that long-lasting health problems after childbirth certainly occur in low-income countries which have a high rate of CS but very few data are available and the problems remain hidden with a limited access to healthcare for a majority of these patients.

References

1. Molina G, Weiser TG, Lipsitz SR, Esquivel MM, Uribe-Leitz T, Azad T, Shah N, Semrau K, Berry WR, Gawande AA. Relationship between cesarean delivery rate and maternal and neonatal mortality. JAMA. 2015;314(21):2263–70.

2. Clark EA, Silver RM. Long-term maternal morbidity associated with repeat cesarean delivery. Am J Obstet Gynecol. 2011;205(6 Suppl):S2–10.

3. Carlander AK, Andolf E, Edman G, Wiklund I. Health-related quality of life five years after birth of the first child. Sex Reprod Healthc. 2015;6(2):101–7.

4. Schytt E, Lindmark G, Waldenstrom U. Physical symptoms after childbirth: prevalence and associations with self-rated health. BJOG. 2005;112(2):210–7.

5. Thompson JF, Roberts CL, Currie M, Ellwood DA. Prevalence and persistence of health problems after childbirth: associations with parity and method of birth. Birth. 2002;29(2):83–94.

6. Woolhouse H, Perlen S, Gartland D, Brown SJ. Physical health and recovery in the first 18 months postpartum: does cesarean section reduce long-term morbidity? Birth. 2012;39(3):221–9.

7. Eisenach JC, Pan P, Smiley RM, Lavand'homme P, Landau R, Houle TT. Resolution of pain after childbirth. Anesthesiology. 2013;118(1):143–51.

8. Kainu JP, Sarvela J, Tiippana E, Halmesmaki E, Korttila KT. Persistent pain after caesarean section and vaginal birth: a cohort study. Int J Obstet Anesth. 2010;19(1):4–9.

9. Sng BL, Sia AT, Quek K, Woo D, Lim Y. Incidence and risk factors for chronic pain after caesarean section under spinal anaesthesia. Anaesth Intensive Care. 2009;37(5):748–52.

10. Hannah ME, Whyte H, Hannah WJ, Hewson S, Amankwah K, Cheng M, Gafni A, Guselle P, Helewa M, Hodnett ED, et al. Maternal outcomes at 2 years after planned cesarean section versus planned vaginal birth for breech presentation at term: the international randomized term breech trial. Am J Obstet Gynecol. 2004;191(3):917–27.

11. Andolf E, Thorsell M, Kallen K. Cesarean delivery and risk for postoperative adhesions and intestinal obstruction: a nested case-control study of the Swedish Medical Birth Registry. Am J Obstet Gynecol. 2010;203(4):406 e401–6.

12. Chang SR, Chen KH, Ho HN, Lai YH, Lin MI, Lee CN, Lin WA. Depressive symptoms, pain, and sexual dysfunction over the first year following vaginal or cesarean delivery: a prospective longitudinal study. Int J Nurs Stud. 2015;52(9):1433–44.

13. Patel RR, Murphy DJ, Peters TJ. Operative delivery and postnatal depression: a cohort study. BMJ. 2005;330(7496):879.

14. Gissler M, Deneux-Tharaux C, Alexander S, Berg CJ, Bouvier-Colle MH, Harper M, Nannini A, Breart G, Buekens P. Pregnancy-related deaths in four regions of Europe and the United States in 1999–2000: characterisation of unreported deaths. Eur J Obstet Gynecol Reprod Biol. 2007;133(2):179–85.

15. Pearson RM, Evans J, Kounali D, Lewis G, Heron J, Ramchandani PG, O'Connor TG, Stein A. Maternal depression during pregnancy and the postnatal period: risks and possible mechanisms for offspring depression at age 18 years. JAMA Psychiat. 2013;70(12):1312–9.

16. Eisenach JC, Pan PH, Smiley R, Lavand'homme P, Landau R, Houle TT. Severity of acute pain after childbirth, but not type of delivery, predicts persistent pain and postpartum depression. Pain. 2008;140(1):87–94.

17. Ortner CM, Turk DC, Theodore BR, Siaulys MM, Bollag LA, Landau R. The short-form McGill pain questionnaire-revised to evaluate persistent pain and surgery-related symptoms in healthy women undergoing a planned cesarean delivery. Reg Anesth Pain Med. 2014;39(6):478–86.

18. Treede RD, Rief W, Barke A, Aziz Q, Bennett MI, Benoliel R, Cohen M, Evers S, Finnerup NB, First MB, et al. A classification of chronic pain for ICD-11. Pain. 2015;156(6):1003–7.

19. Werner MU, Kongsgaard UE. I. Defining persistent post-surgical pain: is an update required? Br J Anaesth. 2014;113(1):1–4.

20. Lavand'homme P. The progression from acute to chronic pain. Curr Opin Anaesthesiol. 2011;24(5):545–50.

21. Nikolajsen L, Sorensen HC, Jensen TS, Kehlet H. Chronic pain following caesarean section. Acta Anaesthesiol Scand. 2004;48(1):111–6.

22. Bijl RC, Freeman LM, Weijenborg PT, Middeldorp JM, Dahan A, van Dorp EL. A retrospective study on persistent pain after childbirth in the Netherlands. J Pain Res. 2016;9:1–8.

23. Declercq E, Cunningham DK, Johnson C, Sakala C. Mothers' reports of postpartum pain associated with vaginal and cesarean deliveries: results of a national survey. Birth. 2008;35(1):16–24.
24. Nardi N, Campillo-Gimenez B, Pong S, Branchu P, Ecoffey C, Wodey E. Chronic pain after cesarean: impact and risk factors associated. Ann Fr Anesth Reanim. 2013;32(11):772–8.
25. Liu TT, Raju A, Boesel T, Cyna AM, Tan SG. Chronic pain after caesarean delivery: an Australian cohort. Anaesth Intensive Care. 2013;41(4):496–500.
26. Fletcher D, Stamer UM, Pogatzki-Zahn E, Zaslansky R, Tanase NV, Perruchoud C, Kranke P, Komann M, Lehman T, Meissner W, et al. Chronic postsurgical pain in Europe: an observational study. Eur J Anaesthesiol. 2015;32(10):725–34.
27. Brandsborg B, Dueholm M, Nikolajsen L, Kehlet H, Jensen TS. A prospective study of risk factors for pain persisting 4 months after hysterectomy. Clin J Pain. 2009;25(4):263–8.
28. Montes A, Roca G, Sabate S, Lao JI, Navarro A, Cantillo J, Canet J, Group GS. Genetic and clinical factors associated with chronic postsurgical pain after hernia repair, hysterectomy, and thoracotomy: a two-year multicenter cohort study. Anesthesiology. 2015;122(5):1123–41.
29. Loos MJ, Scheltinga MR, Mulders LG, Roumen RM. The Pfannenstiel incision as a source of chronic pain. Obstet Gynecol. 2008;111(4):839–46.
30. Johansen A, Schirmer H, Nielsen CS, Stubhaug A. Persistent post-surgical pain and signs of nerve injury: the Tromso Study. Acta Anaesthesiol Scand. 2016;60(3):380–92.
31. Bollag L, Richebe P, Siaulys M, Ortner CM, Gofeld M, Landau R. Effect of transversus abdominis plane block with and without clonidine on post-cesarean delivery wound hyperalgesia and pain. Reg Anesth Pain Med. 2012;37(5):508–14.
32. Duale C, Ouchchane L, Schoeffler P, Group EI, Dubray C. Neuropathic aspects of persistent postsurgical pain: a French multicenter survey with a 6-month prospective follow-up. J Pain. 2014;15(1):24 e21–0.
33. Brandsborg B, Dueholm M, Kehlet H, Jensen TS, Nikolajsen L. Mechanosensitivity before and after hysterectomy: a prospective study on the prediction of acute and chronic postoperative pain. Br J Anaesth. 2011;107(6):940–7.
34. Haroutiunian S, Nikolajsen L, Finnerup NB, Jensen TS. The neuropathic component in persistent postsurgical pain: a systematic literature review. Pain. 2013;154(1):95–102.
35. Hurley RW, Adams MC. Sex, gender, and pain: an overview of a complex field. Anesth Analg. 2008;107(1):309–17.
36. Crombie IK, Davies HT, Macrae WA. Cut and thrust: antecedent surgery and trauma among patients attending a chronic pain clinic. Pain. 1998;76(1–2):167–71.
37. Sperber AD, Morris CB, Greemberg L, Bangdiwala SI, Goldstein D, Sheiner E, Rusabrov Y, Hu Y, Katz M, Freud T, et al. Development of abdominal pain and IBS following gynecological surgery: a prospective, controlled study. Gastroenterology. 2008;134(1):75–84.
38. Weijenborg PT, Greeven A, Dekker FW, Peters AA, Ter Kuile MM. Clinical course of chronic pelvic pain in women. Pain. 2007;132(Suppl 1):S117–23.
39. Wesselmann U. Chronic pelvic and urogenital pain syndromes. Pain Clinical Updates (IASP). 2008;XVI(6):1–4.
40. Almeida EC, Nogueira AA, Candido dos Reis FJ, Rosa e Silva JC. Cesarean section as a cause of chronic pelvic pain. Int J Gynaecol Obstet. 2002;79(2):101–4.
41. Paterson LQ, Davis SN, Khalife S, Amsel R, Binik YM. Persistent genital and pelvic pain after childbirth. J Sex Med. 2009;6(1):215–21.
42. Li WY, Liabsuetrakul T, Stray-Pedersen B, Li YJ, Guo LJ, Qin WZ. The effects of mode of delivery and time since birth on chronic pelvic pain and health-related quality of life. Int J Gynaecol Obstet. 2014;124(2):139–42.
43. Bjelland EK, Owe KM, Pingel R, Kristiansson P, Vangen S, Eberhard-Gran M. Pelvic pain after childbirth: a longitudinal population study. Pain. 2016;157(3):710–6.
44. Ortner CM, Granot M, Richebe P, Cardoso M, Bollag L, Landau R. Preoperative scar hyperalgesia is associated with post-operative pain in women undergoing a repeat caesarean delivery. Eur J Pain. 2013;17(1):111–23.

45. Martinez V, Ben Ammar S, Judet T, Bouhassira D, Chauvin M, Fletcher D. Risk factors predictive of chronic postsurgical neuropathic pain: the value of the iliac crest bone harvest model. Pain. 2012;153(7):1478–83.
46. Brandsborg B, Nikolajsen L, Hansen CT, Kehlet H, Jensen TS. Risk factors for chronic pain after hysterectomy: a nationwide questionnaire and database study. Anesthesiology. 2007;106(5):1003–12.
47. Lavand'homme P. Chronic pain after childbirth. Curr Opin Anaesthesiol. 2013;26(3):273–7.
48. Edwards RR. Individual differences in endogenous pain modulation as a risk factor for chronic pain. Neurology. 2005;65(3):437–43.
49. Belci D, Di Renzo GC, Stark M, Duric J, Zoricic D, Belci M, Peteh LL. Morbidity and chronic pain following different techniques of caesarean section: a comparative study. J Obstet Gynaecol. 2015;35(5):442–6.
50. Gizzo S, Andrisani A, Noventa M, Di Gangi S, Quaranta M, Cosmi E, D'Antona D, Nardelli GB, Ambrosini G. Caesarean section: could different transverse abdominal incision techniques influence postpartum pain and subsequent quality of life? A systematic review. PLoS One. 2015;10(2):e0114190.
51. Bamigboye AA, Hofmeyr GJ. Closure versus non-closure of the peritoneum at caesarean section: short- and long-term outcomes. Cochrane Database Syst Rev. 2014;8:CD000163.
52. Althaus A, Hinrichs-Rocker A, Chapman R, Arranz Becker O, Lefering R, Simanski C, Weber F, Moser KH, Joppich R, Trojan S, et al. Development of a risk index for the prediction of chronic post-surgical pain. Eur J Pain. 2012;16(6):901–10.
53. Richez B, Ouchchane L, Guttmann A, Mirault F, Bonnin M, Noudem Y, Cognet V, Dalmas AF, Brisebrat L, Andant N, et al. The role of psychological factors in persistent pain after cesarean delivery. J Pain. 2015;16(11):1136–46.
54. Babel P, Pieniazek L, Zarotynski D. The effect of the type of pain on the accuracy of memory of pain and affect. Eur J Pain. 2015;19(3):358–68.
55. Pinto PR, McIntyre T, Almeida A, Araujo-Soares V. The mediating role of pain catastrophizing in the relationship between presurgical anxiety and acute postsurgical pain after hysterectomy. Pain. 2012;153(1):218–26.
56. Clarke H, Katz J, Flor H, Rietschel M, Diehl SR, Seltzer Z. Genetics of chronic post-surgical pain: a crucial step toward personal pain medicine. Can J Anaesth. 2015;62(3):294–303.
57. Loos MJ, Scheltinga MR, Roumen RM. Surgical management of inguinal neuralgia after a low transverse Pfannenstiel incision. Ann Surg. 2008;248(5):880–5.
58. Doumouchtsis SK, Boama V, Gorti M, Tosson S, Fynes MM. Prospective evaluation of combined local bupivacaine and steroid injections for the management of chronic vaginal and perineal pain. Arch Gynecol Obstet. 2011;284(3):681–5.
59. Vancaillie T, Eggermont J, Armstrong G, Jarvis S, Liu J, Beg N. Response to pudendal nerve block in women with pudendal neuralgia. Pain Med. 2012;13(4):596–603.
60. Ducic I, Moxley M, Al-Attar A. Algorithm for treatment of postoperative incisional groin pain after cesarean delivery or hysterectomy. Obstet Gynecol. 2006;108(1):27–31.

Humanization of Cesarean Section

Giorgio Capogna and Hans de Boer

13.1 Historical Perspectives

In the early 1980s, Professor Romano Forleo, the Head of the Department of Obstetrics at Fatebenefratelli Hospital in Rome, was one of the first in Europe to introduce in a Department of Obstetrics the so-called humanized childbirth (humanizing birth means considering women's values, beliefs, and feelings and respecting their dignity and autonomy during the birthing process). The idea was to introduce the "home in the hospital" rather than reproducing the home-like environment proposed by the birthing centers which sprung up in the USA in the 1970s, as alternatives to the heavily institutionalized maternity hospital [1].

A women-centered labor and delivery performed within a hospital department was thought to be more complete, adding the chance of a pain-free labor and delivery upon the woman's request. Therefore, in parallel, the anesthesia department was called on to contribute to this project, starting an epidural service and increasing the use of epidural anesthesia for cesarean section and creating one of the first full-time obstetric anesthesia departments in Italy, led by Prof. Giorgio Capogna. One of the major changes for all of us was the different way of considering the women as mothers rather than as patients, but also the involvement of the father and his presence in the labor and delivery room and in the cesarean section theater contributed to change and adjust our anesthetic procedures [2].

G. Capogna (✉)
Department of Anesthesiology, Città di Roma Hospital, Rome, Italy
e-mail: Dipartimento.anestesia@gruppogarofalo.com

H. de Boer, M.D., Ph.D.
Department of Anesthesiology and Pain Medicine, Martini General Hospital Groningen, Groningen, The Netherlands
e-mail: hd.de.boer@mzh.nl

© Springer International Publishing Switzerland 2017
G. Capogna (ed.), *Anesthesia for Cesarean Section*,
DOI 10.1007/978-3-319-42053-0_13

At that time, the UNICEF maternal best practice standards had not yet been published, but we already used to let the mother hug her baby immediately after birth after cesarean delivery, even if for only a short period of time and after the neonatologist's assessment, and the rooming-in was one of the most frequent maternal choices after delivery.

13.2   The Cesarean Section, A Normal Surgical Procedure?

Nowadays, cesarean section is one of the most frequent surgical procedures in many European countries and North America and it is perceived as a "normal surgical procedure," a routine practice that is not performed exclusively to save the life of the mother and of the baby, as it was originally designed for, or as a necessary or advisable procedure due to obstetrical reasons, but also for various nonmedical reasons, like the wish of the parents. The anesthesia approach is in favor of spinal anesthesia except for emergency cesarean section. One of the advantages is that both parents can experience the birth of their child. However, in many hospitals the cesarean section is still approached as a strict surgical procedure and therefore only the mother is allowed in the theater. Nowadays, in more and more hospitals the father is allowed to be present in the operating theater, but more can be done in order to satisfy both parents. Despite the general awareness of encouraging parent participation, rigid protocols define the appropriate behavior in the operating theater, and therefore the couple's participation is usually limited by the medical staff's needs as well as by the material and hygienic constraints of the surgical setting, according to the different hospitals' habits and procedures.

In addition, most frequently cesarean sections are performed as an emergency procedure or as an elective, programmed surgery due to pathological reasons, and therefore an immediate contact with the parents is often not possible or advisable, due to the neonatal or maternal conditions.

Even if the mother and the baby are doing well and are at term, an immediate maternal–neonatal contact might be denied for many not well-defined reasons. For example, although the mother is generally awake during the surgery, she usually does not see her baby coming out, because a drape separates her head from her abdomen. Unfortunately, in some institutions, the mother may be routinely under the effect of tranquilizers to help her face the atmosphere of the operating theater and the sensation of her body being operated on. In addition, it is not unusual for the baby to need assistance because he/she cannot breathe autonomously. Moreover, after the delivery, the baby is quickly shown to the mother and transferred to another room next to the theater together with the father. Subject to the health of mother and baby, the time of separation between the woman and her child after surgery can last one or more hours according to the hospital routines.

As a consequence, cesarean section does not allow the immediate skin-to-skin contact deemed beneficial in promoting bonding between mother and baby [3].

13.3   A More Human Approach

To increase the satisfactory birth experience, another approach is needed. In many years of research in cesarean section, the focus has been on improving the surgical technique and to reduce or to prevent complications. This has led to a reduced perioperative risk, but there was no focus on a very important point which is generally accepted in vaginal delivery, namely, the immediate skin-to-skin contact between the mother and her child. Also generally accepted is that due to this interaction several important factors are positively influenced like breastfeeding, bonding, glucose levels, and cardiovascular and respiratory stability [4–6].

Therefore, another approach in cesarean section is needed to improve not only the mother's satisfaction but also the maternal and neonatal outcome.

There are now a great number of studies [4–6] that demonstrate that mothers and babies should be together, skin to skin immediately after birth. The neonate's temperature, heart and breathing rates, and glycemia are more normal and stable. In addition, skin-to-skin contact immediately after birth allows the baby to be colonized by the same bacteria as the mother and this, plus breastfeeding, is believed to be very important factors in preventing allergic diseases. From the point of view of breastfeeding, babies who are kept skin to skin with the mother immediately after birth for at least 1 h are more likely to breastfeed without any help, which is seen in vaginal delivery. Prolonged skin-to-skin contact during the first few months after birth may also decrease total neonate crying, improve sleeping and decrease the incidence of maternal postpartum depression [7].

The first hour after birth after vaginal delivery, which is also to be expected in cesarean section, has been defined as the "sacred hour," a period of time during which skin-to-skin contact provides physiological stability and maternal attachment behaviors, favors optimal brain development, decreases the negative effects of separation, and increases breastfeeding rates and duration [8].

In 2008, the first steps were made to promote uninterrupted skin-to-skin contact immediately after birth after cesarean section by Professor Nicholas Fisk and coworkers at Queen Charlotte's Hospital in London, which signified a turning point in the humanization of the cesarean section [9]. Their approach described a number of measures mimicking as much as possible a vaginal delivery and called it "natural cesarean." These measures included among others the following: (a) parents can watch their baby immediately born since the surgical drape that separates the upper part of the mother's body from the birthing scene is dropped at the extraction time; (b) the baby is extracted slowly so that he/she is better able to start breathing unaided [10]; (c) the newborn is immediately handed to the mother for the skin-to-skin first contact, favoring maternal–infant bonding; (d) if requested, the father can perform a second cutting of the umbilical cord. The aim of this procedure is to encourage mother and father to be active participants in the birth of their child instead of undergoing the surgical event passively. This was a big step forward, as even little changes can make a big difference: for example, at Brigham and Women's Hospital in Boston, USA, the version of the "natural cesarean" or family-centered cesarean is called the "gentle cesarean," and mothers who choose this way of treatment can view the birth through a clear plastic drape, and immediate skin-to-skin contact follows.

The modification of the ordinary surgical technique to a more natural or better, woman-centered model is certainly a challenge and seems to indicate the current trend towards medical and social acceptance of cesarean section in many countries, where women as well as physicians regard surgery and more generally interventions during the birthing process as part of the necessary routine [11, 12].

The definition of "natural cesarean" may, however, be questionable since the definition of natural childbirth itself is very difficult, and there is no clear consensus about what "natural" or "normal" childbirth is but there is a general agreement about the fact that childbirth should be "woman centered," giving priority to her wishes and her needs, highlighting the importance of informed choice, continuity of care and the woman's involvement. For this reason, we feel it more appropriate to define all the attempts to perform a woman-centered cesarean section as a "humanized cesarean delivery" to emphasize that even if it is a surgical procedure it is still a "delivery" and not only a "section," and more like a birth than an operation.

13.4 The Challenge and Implementation of "Humanized Cesarean Delivery"

The clinical processes that support a mother- and baby-centered approach to cesarean section may vary between hospitals and countries and are a challenge to achieve. Although birth is a major life event for parents, a full parental involvement during cesarean section is still not common practice. Furthermore, we have to realize that apart from the cesarean section per se, the whole journey of the parents is a multidisciplinary team effort. Gynecologists, anesthesiologists, pediatricians, nurse anesthetists, obstetric nurses, and surgical nurses should be involved in the multidisciplinary approach of the humanized cesarean delivery [13, 14]. Each discipline contributes to the general protocol which describes in detail every step of the humanized cesarean delivery. The most important steps in the protocol are the parental participation, information for the parents (e.g., with video), a perfect neuraxial anesthesia (without any form of sedation), the 24-h staff availability for this procedure, and well-defined criteria of contraindications for this approach, in order to offer a humanized cesarean delivery also in the case of unplanned cesarean section due to nonprogressive labor without fetal distress. Usually this procedure is not recommended, or even contraindicated, with preterm births in emergency cesarean deliveries in cases where the baby is at risk of a low Apgar score.

There are some commonly used procedures and practices utilized among the hospitals to promote the humanization of cesarean delivery to transform a major surgical procedure such as a cesarean section into a mother–baby–family-centered experience. This includes the way it is performed. In addition to some procedures described in literature, some more specific aspects have to be highlighted, including (1) the placement of the ECG leads on the maternal back to favor skin-to-skin contact, (2) the temperature in the theater is kept optimal at 24 °C, (3) the gynecologists commence surgery with double sterile gloves and arm sleeves. The pediatrician is available in the neonatal resuscitation room and will treat the baby if neonatal distress occurs. Prior to the baby being born, the surgical drape is lowered for the parents to be able to observe the birth, which includes being born slowly, facing towards the parents and handed over to the mother's chest with the help of the obstetric nurse. If possible leave the baby's body in the uterus for a few moments in order to allow the contraction of the uterus around the body of the fetus [15]. This will favor the initiation of breathing and crying and the clearing of the fetal respiratory system of fluid. Delay cord clamping to permit auto transfusion and improve neonatal iron stores [16].

Before continuing the surgical procedure, the surgeon removes one pair of gloves and sleeves. The sterile barrier is restored by raising the surgical drape. The first neonatal assessment and monitoring on the chest of the mother can be performed by the neonatologist, the obstetric nurse, the midwife or the anesthesiologist, according to local clinical practice. If the baby shows no sign of distress, it stays on the mother's chest as long as possible [13, 14]. Encourage intraoperative breastfeeding. Routine care for the infant can be delayed until after the first feeding is completed and keep the mother and baby together. Rather than separating the mother and newborn for the trip to the recovery area, have the mother cradle the newborn on her chest during the transport process. Within an hour after birth the baby may be checked by the pediatrician in the recovery room. In this procedure there are a few very important questions to answer regarding the safety of the surgical site infections, more blood loss and maternal and fetal outcome. In the next section, the outcome of the humanized cesarean delivery will be described.

13.5 Neonatal and Maternal Outcome

The plan to promote early skin-to-skin contact and keep the newborn with the mother may need to be altered if the newborn needs more intensive support at the resuscitation table for symptoms of transient tachypnea, which will affect both the neonatal and the maternal outcome. Careful attention to ensuring that the baby is not left exposed to the cold operating room temperature is helpful to reduce the risk of hypothermia. Early skin-to-skin contact at cesarean section has been reported to improve maintenance of neonatal thermoregulation [17]. Forced air warmers may prevent thermal dispersion and are as effective as an incubator in preventing neonatal hypothermia while the newborn baby is on the mother's chest as she is undergoing surgery in the operating room, thus favoring very early skin-to-skin contact in a cold environment [18]. Nowadays, more data are published on the outcome of the humanized cesarean delivery [13–15]. Birth experiences of a more humanized cesarean delivery approach were rated higher when compared with the classical cesarean section. Moreover, with regard to humanized cesarean delivery neonatal outcome showed no differences in APGAR scores compared with the classical cesarean section performed; there were less admissions to the neonatal ward, and suspected neonatal infection was less frequent. The procedural surgical time may be a little increased but that is due to the lowering of the surgical drapes and to removing the gloves and arm sleeves. The maternal outcome was not affected by applying a humanized cesarean delivery. Maternal surgical site infections and blood loss are comparable between the humanized cesarean delivery and the classical cesarean section. However, the need for maternal blood transfusion is less in the humanized cesarean delivery compared to the conventional cesarean section. This may possibly be explained by the fact that the humanized cesarean delivery includes spontaneous delivery of the placenta which is associated with less maternal blood loss when compared to manual removal [19], and, in addition, neonates start to breastfeed earlier, most of the time already during surgery, and this may also increase uterine contractions [13–15].

Conclusion

As cesarean section rates are increasing worldwide, we have to realize that birth is a major life event for parents. It is our responsibility to increase the satisfactory birth experience for the parents and as such another approach is needed. The clinical processes that support a mother- and baby-centered approach to cesarean section may vary between hospitals and countries and is a challenge to achieve. The humanization of cesarean delivery to transform a major surgical procedure such as a cesarean section into a mother-baby-family-centered experience is a multidisciplinary challenge. Once the humanized cesarean delivery is well organized and more common practice the rating of the birth experience is increased. Moreover, the maternal and neonatal outcome is also improved and the satisfaction of the healthcare worker involved is increased.

References

1. Forleo R, Forleo P. Fondamenti di Storia della Ostetricia e Ginecologia. Verduci Editore. 2009;77–80.
2. Forleo R, Zanetti H. Il papà in attesa. Edizioni Paoline. 1987.
3. Odent M. New reasons and new ways to study birth physiology. Inter J Gynecol Obstet. 2001;75(Suppl 1):S39–45.
4. Moore E, Anderson G, Bergman N, Dowswell T. Early skin-to-skin contact for mothers and their healthy newborn infants. Cochrane Database Syst Rev. 2012:5. doi:10.1002/14651858. CD003519.pub3.
5. Stevens J, Schmied V, Burns E, Dahlen H. Immediate or early skin-to-skin contact after a caesarean section: a review of the literature. Mater Child Nutr. 2014;10:456–73.
6. Thukral A, Sankar MJ, Agarwal R, Gupta N, Deorari AK, Paul VK. Early skin-to-skin contact and breast-feeding behavior in term neonates: a randomized controlled trial. Neonatology. 2012;102:114–9.
7. Bigelow A, Power M, Maclellan Peters J, Marion A, McDonald C. Effect of mother/infant skin-to-skin contact on postpartum depressive symptoms and maternal physiological stress. J Obstet Gynec Neon Nursing. 2012;41:369–82.
8. Phillips R. The sacred hour: uninterrupted skin to skin contact immediately after birth. Newborn & Infant Nursing Research. 2013;13:67–72.
9. Smith J, Plaat F, Fisk NM. The natural caesarean: a woman-centred technique. Br J Obstet Gynaecol. 2008;115:1037–42.

10. Edwardes C. The new natural caesarean, The Times. 4 April 2009.
11. Green JM, Baston HA. Have women become more willing to accept obstetric interventions and does this relate to mode of birth? Data from a prospective study. Birth. 2007;34:6–13.
12. Habiba M, Kaminski M, Da Frè M, Marsal K, Bleker O, Librero J, Grandjean H, Gratia P, Guaschino S, Heyl W, Taylor D, Cuttini M. Caesarean section on request: a comparison of obstetricians' attitudes in eight European countries. BJOG. 2006;113:647–56.
13. Posthuma S, Korteweg FJ, van der Ploeg JM, et al. Risks and benefits of the skin-to-skin cesarean section - a retrospective cohort study. J Mater Fetal Neonatal Med. 2016;29:1–5.
14. Boer HD, Korteweg FJ, van der Ploeg JM, Wiersma Zweens M, Kremer P, van der Ham. Natural cesarean section: family centered multidisciplinary standard procedure for all term cesarean sections. Eur J Anaesth. 2015;32 (suppl 53): 121.
15. Armbrust R et al. The charite cesarean birth: a family oriented approach of cesarean section. J Matern Fetal Neonatal Med 2015;1–6
16. Andersson O, Helmström-Westas L, Andersson D, Domellof M. Effect of delayed versus early umbilical cord clamping on neonatal outcomes and iron status at 4 months of age: a randomised controlled trial. BMJ. 2011;343:d7157.
17. Gouchon S, Gregori D, Picotto A, Patrucco G, Nangeroni M, Di Giulio P. Skin-to-skin contact after cesarean delivery: an experimental study. Nurs Res. 2010;59:78–84.
18. Stirparo S, Farcomeni A, Laudani A, Capogna G. Maintaining neonatal normothermia during WHO necommended skin-to-skin contact in the setting of cesarean section under regional anesthesia. Open Journal of Anesthesiology. 2013;3:186–8.
19. Morales M, Ceysens G, Jastrow N, et al. Spontaneous delivery or manual removal of the placenta during caesarean section: a randomised controlled trial. BJOG. 2004;111:908–12.

Caesarean Section on Maternal Request and the Anaesthetist

14

Marwan Habiba

Caesarean section (or delivery) on maternal request (CSMR), patient choice caesarean or caesarean on demand all refer to elective caesarean section (ELCS) for singleton term pregnancy carried out at the request of the pregnant woman in the absence of medical maternal or fetal indications [1]. This may have parallels to 'prophylactic caesarean' which was proposed in 1985 as an alternative to what was termed 'passive anticipation of vaginal delivery' [2]. Renewed interest in the topic followed the report by Al-Mufti et al. that 31% of female obstetricians in London would choose a caesarean section for themselves in case of uncomplicated pregnancy [3]. The relevance of these expressed preferences is unclear as there is no evidence that they have translated into real actions at the relevant time. CSMR has been extensively discussed in medical literature and also in public discourse, where it is often referred to using somewhat derogatory phrases such as 'too posh to push' [4–8]. In the UK, recent guidelines to obstetricians issued by the National Institute of Clinical Excellence (NICE) state that: 'for women requesting a caesarean section (CS), if after discussion and offer of support (including perinatal mental health support for women with anxiety about childbirth), a vaginal birth is still not an acceptable option, offer a planned caesarean section'. The guidelines go on to advise that any obstetrician unwilling to perform a caesarean section under such circumstances should refer the woman to an obstetrician who will carry out the CSMR [9].

Consideration of ethical principles or of the place of respect for autonomy is not within the remit of NICE. Thus acceptance of CSMR in national guidance may or may not be indicative of a significant shift of attitude towards maternal choice. The conclusion reached by NICE was apparently based on the guidelines authors' interpretation of clinical evidence that is summarised as follows: ELCS may (1) reduce

M. Habiba
Obstetrics and Gynaecology, University Hospitals of Leicester and
Department of Health Sciences, University of Leicester, Leicester, UK
e-mail: mah6@leicester.ac.uk

© Springer International Publishing Switzerland 2017
G. Capogna (ed.), *Anesthesia for Cesarean Section*,
DOI 10.1007/978-3-319-42053-0_14

the risk of perineal and abdominal pain during birth and three days post-partum; (2) reduce injury to the vagina; (3) reduce early post-partum haemorrhage; and (4) reduce obstetric shock. But ELCS may (1) increase the risk of neonatal admission to intensive care; (2) result in longer hospital stay; (3) increase the risk of hysterectomy caused by post-partum haemorrhage; and (4) increase the risk of cardiac arrest. I will return to the discussion of the evidence base later in the chapter. It is interesting to note that NICE advises obstetricians who are not willing to perform a CSMR to refer the patient to another doctor. This demonstrates that NICE recognises the ethical dimension inherent in the guidelines but the view taken by NICE averts rather than resolves the dilemma. In effect, it leaves the ethical question unanswered whilst allowing CSMR to take place.

14.1   What Is the Incidence of CSMR?

Despite much effort to reverse the trend, caesarean section rates continue to rise. In the UK, the mean caesarean section rate in primiparous women was 22.1% and for multiparous women was 21.3% in 2013–2014 [10]. In the United States, there were more than 1.3 million caesarean deliveries (32.9% of all births) in 2009 [11]. As the proportion of caesarean section births continues to rise, debate continues on the status of CSMR. Estimates of CSMR vary widely. One quoted range puts that at 4–18% of all caesarean deliveries. CSMR was reported to account for 2.6% of all caesarean sections in Flanders [12] and 26.8% in Western Australia [13] and some have argued that the rate might be increasing. Both sides of the debate use selected estimates of prevalence to emphasise that this issue is either important from the public perspective or is a small-scale issue that should not be of public concern and should, therefore, be left to the individual woman concerned.

One study from the United States reported that there has been an increase of primary caesarean where there was 'no indicated risk' from 3.3% in 1991 to 5.5% in 2001. This study also suggested higher rates in older primiparous women, perhaps fitting with a stereotypical representation of this group of women [14]. But the study itself used national US birth certificate data that does not specifically document 'maternal request'. It is also reported that caesarean delivery without labour or some medical indication had increased in the United States from 1.9% of all deliveries in 2001 to 2.6% in 2003, but this estimate was based on statistical algorithms rather than actual reported cases [15].

Some of the difficulty in providing an estimate is related to problems inherent in the definition of CSMR. CSMR is a term that could be applicable to a range of scenarios where there has been a significant maternal preference or influence on the choices made. The American College of Obstetricians and Gynecologists (ACOG) proposed that CSMR be defined as a primary pre-labour caesarean delivery on maternal request in the absence of any maternal or fetal indications [11]. But even this remains open to interpretation. A common scenario where caesarean section delivery can be seen to fall within the ACOG definition is the group of woman who had a previous caesarean section. Allowing labour with the aim of achieving vaginal delivery in women with a previous CS (VBAC) has a recognised failure rate of between 20 and 40%. In case of failure, women will require emergency surgical delivery with added risk and disruption. Cumulatively, this may counter the potential benefits of VBAC. VBAC is also associated with a numerically small (about 1%) but serious risk of uterine rupture during labour. Whether a woman who indicates her preference for a repeat caesarean section rather than VBAC is classed within the category of CSMR will, to a large extent, be dependent on the attitude of the obstetrician. Indeed, the same may be applicable to most cases of ELCS because most indications of caesarean section are relative not absolute.

14.2 Medical Indication

Literature creates the impression that there is wide recognition of a sizable proportion of caesarean sections done purely on maternal request. It is debatable, however, whether these are a distinct subset or whether the categorisation only indicate a difference in emphasis. Caesarean sections done purely at the request of the obstetrician are probably very rare and, in Western societies, are likely to require court authorisation. The vast majority of caesarean sections are undertaken through agreement between obstetricians and patients. As might be expected, obstetricians are often the party who propose the intervention once the clinical scenario has reached the threshold of professional acceptance and thus comes to be recognised as 'medically indicated'. The list of medical indications has itself dramatically increased over time. It is perhaps helpful to refer to the early roots in order to appreciate the magnitude of this change. In 1849 Charles Meigs wrote that 'caesarean operation, in its spirit and intention, should be devoted absolutely to the conservation of the mother alone' and that 'no man has a right to subject a living, breathing, human creature to so great a hazard as that attending the caesarean section, from views relating to any other interests than those of his patient' [16]. By 1939 the indications for caesarean section had expanded to include a number of maternal conditions resulting in obstructed labour such as contracted pelvis, fibroids obstructing the birth canal, contraction ring, as well as severe preeclampsia or eclampsia where delivery is not imminent, and cases of severe maternal haemorrhage. Debate had then started around the acceptability of caesarean section in a limited number of fetal indications such as selected cases of cord prolapse or impacted shoulder where fetal decapitation might have been an alternative [17]. In 1980 Pritchard and MacDonald wrote: 'once delivery has been affected by caesarean section, delivery in subsequent pregnancy is usually performed the same way, although some obstetricians contest this policy' [18]. Thus acceptance of VBAC in obstetric practice is relatively recent. What is evident is that the appreciation of what is medically indicated has radically shifted. In many developed regions or countries between a fifth and a third of all babies are now being delivered by caesarean section. Arguably, wider acceptance of caesarean delivery reflects a strong emphasis on the safety of the baby and the appreciation of the huge increase in surgical safety. This is perhaps also affected by the risk of litigation. It is also the case that the increased acceptance of medical interventions is not limited to caesarean sections. This point here is that the determination of what is medically indicated is an evolving matter and that increased acceptability of caesarean section reflects a range of influences. The change in medical opinion could not have occurred in isolation and was accompanied by acceptance or perhaps was a response to a wider shift in public attitude away from fatalism and resignation and towards self-direction and control. This shift in attitude is not only expressed in the relation between society and medicine but in other aspects far beyond. This leads us to consider two aspects of the discussion about CSMR: those aspects that focus on facts as the important components of consent and those aspects that focus on value.

14.3 Against CSMR

Attempt to persuade the audience that CSMR is not justified focus on four arguments. One centres on the need to avoid the financial cost of an intervention that is seen as not essential as demonstrable by the lack of a medical indication. This is often linked to a perhaps exaggerated assessment of the magnitude of demand. Criticism for this argument stems from the real difficulties in distinguishing actual costs from provider charges. The question could also be asked whether an ethical question remains if the costs could be reduced—and some have argued that this is indeed achievable—or if the woman herself could self-finance any difference. Cost-based arguments could have different conclusions based on the source of funding be that public funding, insurance based or self-financed. This is not to deny the importance of the question of resource but to challenge whether there can exist separate ethical environments depending on the ability to pay. Arguments that focus on the question of resource need to develop a narrative that does not solely rely on whether an intervention is demanded by the patient or advised by the doctor as an arbiter of whether a procedure ought to be made available.

Those who argue in favour of natural birth because of it being natural advance the second argument. This is sometimes linked to fears raised against known, presumed or yet unknown risks linked to departure from nature. The argument typically starts by emphasising that pregnancy and childbirth are natural physiological processes that ought therefore to be viewed as such by the medical profession. In this context, vaginal birth is seen as the default option in that its occurrence cannot be stopped in the absence of intervention and it is thus argued that the burden of proof lies with advocates of intervention. The irrelevance of the argument that 'what is natural is good' must be apparent from the simple observation of the tragic outcomes of pregnancy and labour that still occur today in areas that have inadequate health care. In any case, such argument can hardly hold sway given the high prevalence of caesarean sections in modern obstetric practice. It would be hard to convince anaesthetists that pain in labour is good or desirable simply because of it being natural. In fact, this is not unlike arguments from the 1800s against pain relief in labour. Interventions to relief pain were, at the time, regarded by the Clergy as a sin against the will of God. Religious inference aside, pain in labour was regarded as a natural feature that ought to be suffered. It was assumed that such pain existed for a good, though undefined, reason and that it ought to be suffered by the well adjusted. Attitudes have changed and advocates of this viewpoint are more likely to be seen as marginal. Yet views against pain relief in labour continue to be expressed into modern times [19]. This is not to dispute that pain as a physiological process has an important function in relevant situations. For example, it alerts to danger and triggers avoidance of harm, but this is not a point that needs to be explored further in this chapter.

The third approach that is perhaps linked to arguments favouring the state of nature or that is perhaps linked to a particular perspective of feminism is that women ought to accept or celebrate their physiological bodily function including childbirth. This becomes inexplicably linked to a view that presents women who request CSMR as having a weak appreciation of self-worth or as associating their self-esteem or identity with vaginal anatomy. Bewley and Cockburn wrote: 'if a doctor performs a caesarean section purportedly to keep the vagina the same, not only may it fail to preserve a fragile relationship, it may reinforce problems of adaptation after birth' [20]. Arguably, there is a link rather than a contradiction between maintaining high self-esteem and seeking to preserve the body or to protect it from injury. Related to this are arguments that suggest that women who indicate a preference for caesarean section may be petrified of labour because of a type of phobia (tokophobia) or post-traumatic stress disorder [20]. This view is developed to advance that women requesting CSMR qualify to be brought to the attention of a psychiatrist with the aim to resolve their metal health, weakness or deficiency. Yet, there is no evidence of a high prevalence of psychiatric morbidity amongst this group.

The fourth approach to countering CSMR is by providing statistics and estimates of the various risks entailed in caesarean section compared to vaginal birth as a basis for rejecting CSMR. There are many examples of this in literature and is echoed in the approach adopted by NICE [9]. I will discuss some of these 'facts' below, but it is important to consider two general points. The first is that because CSMR is an infrequent occurrence in most institutions, assessing outcomes had relied on extrapolations from studies of caesarean section where there has been a clinical indication and the contribution of the underlying condition to the quoted risk profile is difficult to assess. The second and more important point is that whether CSMR is ethically justifiable is not a question that could be settled through an exposition of known or a search for unknown facts. The question of what is preferred is a valuation that does vary depending amongst other factors on peoples' perception, character, outlook and circumstances. Hume's assertion that moral conclusions cannot be derived from non-moral premises, or the 'no *ought* from an *is*' [21], rule is relevant here. But whilst arguments about the 'facts' relevant to caesarean section are not able to provide proof as commonly understood, they generate an 'impression' aimed at motivating action.

In 2002, Bewley and Cockburn wrote: 'new, unexpected long term risks of caesarean section continue to be reported such as ectopic pregnancy, haemorrhage and hysterectomy following uterine evacuation, latex allergy, cutaneous endometriosis, adenomyosis, increased hospital readmission and even an increase in gall bladder disease and appendicitis' [20]. The authors seem to justify their narrative by stating that: 'while the medical profession debates the risks and benefits for different modes of management, the press and the public hear that the debate is about rights and wrongs and so popular beliefs, myths and dogma are generated'. If anything, this type of argument demonstrates that medical profession is not itself immune from dogma and myths or from lack of critical analysis of fragments of information that is uncritically quoted in support of the adopted standpoint. It is also important to note that the medical profession is not the sole determinant or guardian for what is right or wrong.

14.4　FACTS and Their Relevance

The expression by about a third of female obstetricians in London and the United States that they would choose a caesarean section in an uncomplicated pregnancy is presented in support of CSMR [3, 22]. This acquired particular resonance because of it being the view attributed to doctors with close knowledge of the intervention and of its risks and benefits. There is some evidence that in ethical matters physicians' practices (i.e. 'what physicians do') reflect fairly closely what physicians 'say they would do' [23, 24]. But it is not clear if this applies when doctors come to make personal choices, which they have to negotiate with their own care provider. Also, there is no evidence of increased CSMR amongst obstetricians. A counter-argument is that obstetricians' views may be biased because of their higher exposure to complicated pregnancies. Obstetricians' expressed preference may in fact be indicative—not of personal choice—but of a more permissive attitude towards performing caesarean section generally or towards CSMR specifically as suggested by the study of the views of obstetricians in Europe [25]. Still, opinion remains divided, for while 69% of consultant obstetricians in England and Wales indicated that they would agree to perform an elective caesarean section on a woman with an uncomplicated pregnancy based on her request, and approximately 50% of obstetricians in Israel were willing to perform a CSMR in support for patient's autonomy, this continues to raise passionate protestation [26].

Bewley and Cockburn and the approach by NICE suggest that a key to resolving the dilemma resides in determining which is globally 'safer', a caesarean sections or a vaginal delivery, and that once the safety question is resolved, ethical stipulations will compel clinicians to offer the safer option to all [20, 21]. Curiously, one extrapolation of this is that if caesarean section were to be proven safer, obstetricians ought to offer it to all women. It is argued that the crux of the matter is that either: 'first of all, do no harm' or 'respect autonomy' must prevail [26]. But there is no mechanism for hierarchal ordering of competing obligations within the principlist approach to ethics and as previously argued, principlism does not help resolve the specific quandary posed by CSMR [27]. Hierarchal ordering can only be understood in relation to the prevailing determination, not from examining innate characteristics or from reference to morality. Interestingly, offering routine caesarean section has come to be the current accepted practice in relation to breech presentation [28] despite recognised techniques for vaginal breech birth and cogent arguments against the evidence on which caesarean section is offered [29–31]. It is interesting that various authors have reached divergent conclusions from their examination of the evidence base in relation to CSMR.

NICE presented a tabulated list of evidence in the form of various risks linked to each mode of delivery (Table 14.1). It is important to note that the guideline development group rated the quality of all the studies that were examined as either low or very low. Amongst this there was evidence in favour or against both modes of delivery, and the magnitude of benefit or harm was very small. Yet, the writers of the guideline had to reach a conclusion. Appreciating how the aggregated averages of likely benefit or harm may be applicable to any individual woman is not a matter that could be derived from studying policy or practice guidance. The surgical risk,

Table 14.1 List of factors identified in studies comparing low-risk CS and vaginal birth

Effects around the time of birth
Studies suggest may be reduced after a planned CS
Perineal and abdominal pain during birth
Perineal and abdominal pain three days post-partum
Injury to vagina
Early post-partum haemorrhage
Obstetric shock
Studies suggest may be reduced after planned vaginal birth
Length of hospital stay
Hysterectomy due to post-partum haemorrhage
Cardiac arrest
No difference found in studies
Perineal and abdominal pain four months post-partum
Injury to bladder/ureter
Injury to cervix
Iatrogenic surgical injury
Pulmonary embolism
Wound infection
Intraoperative trauma
Uterine rupture
Assisted ventilation or intubation
Acute renal failure
Maternal death
Deep vein thrombosis
Blood transfusion
Infection—wound and post-partum
Hysterectomy
Anaesthetic complications

NICE noted that the quality of evidence was low or very low in all these studies. Most outcomes were rare or very rare which is a main concern for CSMR, is also highly dependent on the skill of the obstetrician and the surgical team and on how they can operate to optimise safety.

There are only limited certainties linked to caesarean section (i.e. the presence of an abdominal and uterine scar, the need for an anaesthetic during delivery and for a recovery period that also varies widely). It has been advanced that as caesarean section carries more risk compared to vaginal delivery it constitutes a 'harm' which should not be performed in response to maternal request. Clearly, any suggestion that doctors are inducing harm must cause considerable moral disquiet. But equating doctors' concordance with patients' request for a caesarean section with inducing harm must necessarily be rooted in a narrow viewpoint of the sort of risk–benefit calculations both patients and doctors contemplate in decision-making. Patients who *request* caesarean section do not view this as a demand to be harmed but rather as a legitimate request for a widely practised mode of delivery and although it is true that some women may be misinformed, their preference for a caesarean section is not, in itself, indicative of that. Furthermore, it is argued that women are entitled to expect that their expressed preference be respected and considered irrespective of their ability or willingness to provide a reasoned argument. There ought to be a wider recognition that individuals with different backgrounds and experiences can arrive at divergent conclusions with regard to evaluative judgements. That this should occur is not *per se* symptomatic of a misconception or of a need for psychiatric or psychological support.

14.5 For CSMR

Given the limitations inherent in medical knowledge and also the concerns about litigation [25] it is not surprising that doctors have, to some measure, come to endorse patients' preferences and valuation. This is perhaps more commonly integrated within the taxonomy of 'medically indicated' interventions than is acknowledged. In fact, patient preference plays—as it ought to do—a distinctly decisive role in a large number of procedures. In gynaecological practice, this includes procedures performed for abortion, sterilisation, fertility treatment, hysterectomy for non-malignant indications or operations for prolapse: in short, in most elective surgery. I say to some measure because patients undergoing these procedures are still required to fit within a medically defined framework such as the requirement to try other forms of therapy or to reach a certain threshold of eligibility. So why should a *request* for caesarean section cause so much disquiet? The European multi-centre study (EUROBS) compared the attitudes of obstetricians from eight European countries, France, Germany, Italy, Luxembourg, the Netherlands, Spain, Sweden and the UK, to CSMR [25]. The clinical case description was of a 25-year-old woman who started labour at 39 completed weeks. The foetus was normal and in cephalic presentation. She insisted on a caesarean section despite being informed that a vaginal delivery was indicated, and of the higher morbidity and mortality associated with caesarean delivery. Compliance with this woman's request for caesarean section simply because this 'was her choice' was lowest amongst responders from Spain (15%), France (19%) and the Netherlands (22%), and was highest in the UK (79%) and Germany (75%). Respect for patient's autonomy was the most frequently reported justification for accepting CSMR. Fear of litigation and working in a university-affiliated hospital were associated with physicians' likelihood to agree to patient's request whilst female doctors who themselves had children were less likely to agree. Whilst this indicates a high level of acceptance of CSMR, it also indicated that opinion remains divided. The country differences may indicate differences in prevailing attitudes or cultures.

The perception of an intervention as being 'indicated' or 'not indicated' is necessarily agent relevant. At the core of CSMR is not that there is no maternal of fetal indication in absolute terms, but rather that (some) doctors do not share the same valuation of risk–benefit as viewed by the patient or that they do not regard the risk–benefit ratio favourable for the performance of caesarean section. As mentioned above, at the time when caesarean section was associated with high maternal mortality, Meigs articulated an opinion against caesarean section for any fetal indication. But the fact that the safety profile of caesarean section has changed is apparent to all, resulting in a shift of focus to quality of life considerations. Common reasons for women to request CSMR include the desire to avoid labour pain and stress, the wish to avoid uncertainty, fear of emergency interventions and the need to maintain a level of control, fear of forceps, concerns about fetal well being including the wish to avoid trauma or fetal distress in labour, as well as factors related to vaginal prolapse and urinary incontinence. Whilst literature may be able to provide a numerical estimate of these occurrences, it remains impossible to understand the value each individual woman places on them without directly seeking her view.

Amongst the considerations commonly debated are those relevant to vaginal function and continence. It is clear, including to ordinary people, that vaginal birth affects vaginal and perineal anatomy and that it results in 'physiological' perineal tears. Routine perineal incision or episiotomy has been abandoned in most obstetric practice, but the notion of a 'cut' or a 'tear' is recognised in lay language. Yet, fear of perineal trauma is cited as a good example of issues that 'scare and undermine' women's ability to successfully undergo a normal process [20]. Various extrapolations and interpretations of statistics are often produced in this area [32–34]. Rortveit et al. studied the prevalence of urinary incontinence in women younger than 65 years [35, 36]. They reported that the adjusted odds ratio for any incontinence associated with vaginal deliveries as compared with caesarean sections was 1.7 (95% confidence interval, 1.3–2.1), and the adjusted odds ratio for moderate or severe incontinence was 2.2 (95% confidence interval, 1.5–3.1). Only stress incontinence (adjusted odds ratio, 2.4; 95% confidence interval, 1.7–3.2) was associated with the mode of delivery. Still, they concluded by emphasising their viewpoint that: 'these findings should not be used to justify an increase in the use of caesarean sections'. It is interesting to note that those who oppose CSMR refer to patients' 'fear' rather than their wish to avoid 'risk' of a particular complication. This helps foster the impression of a contrast with a more detached or rational medical view that is expressed using the language of 'fact' and 'risk'.

Media interest in this topic remains high. On 12th April 2012, Reuters carried a news article reporting that: 'Women who have given birth vaginally are more likely to develop incontinence decades later than moms who delivered their babies via cesarean section, according to a new study from Sweden'. This was accompanied by a comment from a practicing urogynaecology specialist stating that: 'Anybody who has ever witnessed a vaginal delivery realizes the baby's head is quite large and the muscles that it passes through are not that large. And any time you stretch a muscle there's the potential for damage' [37]. The study subject to this press interest ([38]) reported that two decades after one birth, vaginal delivery was associated with a 67% increased risk of urinary incontinence, and that urinary incontinence for more than 10 years increased by 275% for vaginal delivery compared with caesarean section [38]. The authors calculated that based on their data, it is necessary to perform eight or nine caesarean sections to avoid one case of urinary incontinence. They also found no difference in the incidence of incontinence between those who had an elective or an emergency caesarean section. This suggested that incontinence arises following the passage of the fetal head through the birth canal. Other studies have also linked caesarean sections to a reduced risk of pelvic floor disorders [39]. Perhaps not surprisingly, the issue remains hotly debated. But whilst debates are likely to continue, it is important to consider that even if an exact risk figure, or the estimate of the number needed to treat or to harm were to be agreed, this cannot determine what ought to be done at the level of the individual. Space does not allow an extensive discussion about each of the factors that are considered in literature or the media, but it is important to point out how often weak or inconclusive scientific content provides the context for sensational media reporting.

14.6   Values: Listening to Patients

As discussed above, medical practice has shifted from the very restrictive early start to the stage where between one fifth and one third of all deliveries are conducted by caesarean section. The question must be asked as to why the insistence against accommodating maternal expressed wishes. A proposed answer may be that the professional view is a reflection of progress brought about through advancements in safety and that 'medical indication' is a reflection of where 'evidence' indicates a right balance which allows doctors to exercise their duty of beneficence and non-maleficence. This may seem plausible, except that assessments of benefit or harm are value judgements and, as such, are agency relevant. It has long been argued that doctors' training does not qualify them to become arbiters of best interest. Indeed, as Veatch points out, it is difficult to argue that a physician who is expert in only one component of well-being is able to determine what constitutes the good for another person or to propose a plan to which individual patients would offer mere consent [40, 41]. A patient's best interest is not an objective reality that could be elicited by a doctor based on the outcomes of clinical experiments performed on people with similar conditions, or based on the doctor's own evaluation of whether a particular outcome, complication or risk is preferable to another. Irrespective of the theory of good adopted, it appears that the only way of knowing what is good for a patient is to ask her individually. The idea that a clinician can determine what is a 'medically indicated' intervention or what is in the patient's 'best interest' must reside either in paternalism or reflect a misunderstanding of what a clinician can do [40]. The other critical factor in the debate concerns the place and valuation placed on autonomous choice and patient expressed preferences.

14.7 Autonomy and Paternalism

Paternalism is perhaps one of the more common criticisms levelled at the medical profession [42] and is one that is difficult to defend. The imposition of benefit is necessarily paternalistic, and this remains true irrespective of the nature or magnitude of benefit. It is argued that paternalism is wrong because it violates autonomy, it is a violation of one's perception of oneself, it is a hindrance to achieving self-determined objectives, or because it reflects lack of recognition of others as capable of independent choice. Berlin puts it as follows:

> 'Paternalism is despotic, not because it is more oppressive than naked, brutal, unenlightened tyranny, nor merely because it ignores the transcendental reason embodied in me, but because it is an insult to my conception of myself as a human being, determined to make my own life in accordance with my own (not necessarily rational or benevolent) purposes...' [43]

Autonomy is inextricably linked to the Western tradition of liberalism, and is given central status in Kantian moral philosophy and in Mill's utilitarian liberalism [25, 50]. The principle of *respect for autonomy* requires that the views of those who are capable of deliberation about their personal goals be sought and respected.

The ascent of autonomy in medical ethics is relatively recent. Schneewind traced this to the end of the eighteenth century when there was a shift from the conception of morality as obedience to a conception where individuals were seen as equally able to live together in a morality of self-governance [44]. The emerging view was that all individuals are, in principle, equally able to recognise for themselves what morality calls for and to act accordingly. This conception, which was not confined to the clinical interface, came to challenge the earlier view that most people are not able to see what morality requires or to understand the reason for moral dictates. The older conceptions that gave rise to the need for higher authorities from which ordinary (or most) people obtain guidance or instruction linked to threats of punishment or promises of reward have thus been superseded.

Beauchamp and Childress noted that although respect for the autonomous choices of a person runs as deep in today's common morality as any principle, there is little agreement about its nature, scope or strength [45]. They argued that autonomy should not be excessively individualistic, excessively focused on reason or unduly legalistic. They proposed that autonomy should allow for the social nature of individuals including their emotions, the impact of their choices on others, and that it should not be a mere front for the exercise of legal rights. Beauchamp and Childress also argued that at a minimum, *respect for autonomy* acknowledges the person's right to hold views, to make choices, and to take actions based on personal values and beliefs, and that it also involves or requires from others respectful actions that go beyond non-interference in others' personal affairs [45]. They argue that respect for autonomy entails acknowledging decision-making rights and enabling persons to act autonomously. The emphasis on autonomy within normative ethics generates a number of challenges to practising clinicians. A conflict may arise between the doctor's view of their role, their desire to respect autonomous choice and their other ethical duties such as beneficence and non-maleficence. It ought also to be recognised that autonomy is necessarily restricted by the practical confines within which it could be exercised. It may be possible to resolve the potential difficulty posed by non-availability of willing care providers, but cost differentials and other practical relevant factors are grounded in the real world. Questions of distributive justice can feature prominently in debates about provision in public or other insurance-based health care systems because individual demand is not usually seen as sufficient grounds for care provision, primarily because of the likely burden on others. Whether an intervention is seen as medically justified, a matter of choice or as a resource-based determination will have a bearing on provision in privately funded services. Doctors have traditionally endeavoured to maximise patient benefit as entailed within the Hippocratic tradition and have thus been hesitant to positioning themselves as arbiters in decisions that are primarily concerned with resource. This does not imply that resource implications do not factor into doctors' decision-making, arguably these ought to, but if cost or other practical considerations were the reason to limit or deny autonomous choice, this ought to be made explicit.

Current emphasis on autonomy may underpin those practices where patients are simply given information or a range of options and then left to choose. Arguably, this does not provide a convincing paradigm for the delivery of an obligation to benefit or to avoid harm and it would strain credibility to label a choice for caesarean section within such a construct as CSMR. Examples of this practice may have prompted criticism such as that by Hall and Schneider who argued that ethicists have moved towards what could be called mandatory autonomy or that patients should make their own decisions whether they want it or not or that the emphasis has shifted from what patients do want to what patents should want [46]. Empirical evidence is also advanced to support the idea that at least some patients do not want such 'unwanted' autonomy. But presenting examples where doctors are unwilling or unable to exercise their duties as a 'triumph of autonomy' can potentially mask the realisation that current practice readily accommodates patient choice only if that falls within the range of options predefined or delimited by the doctor. In today's practice, patients are seen to be free to accept or to refuse any of the options offered but barriers emerge against expressed preferences if these fall outside the orthodoxy.

It is though critically important that the medical encounter is not reduced to an interaction through which doctors simply provide learnt technical skill in response to determination by patients. Such would constitute a fundamental departure from the duties entailed within the Hippocratic Oath and subsequent medical codes of practice. There is a substantial risk that it would be detrimental to patients if their care were to be dictated by them, not because they are not the best arbiters of their needs, but because they usually lack the depth of knowledge or expertise that enables them to fully appreciate the implications of the various modalities of treatment. It is the need for such experience that drives patients to seek medical care. It would also be important to ensure that patients are not under undue influence or misconceptions when expressing their choices. Relevant to this are difficulties and challenges linked to providing non-directive counselling. It could be seen how preferences or biases held by clinicians or others can operate, covertly or overtly, to affect patients' choice or expressed requests. This is an area where safeguards are needed.

14.8 Consent

The traditional model of consent is for doctors to propose an intervention and for the patient to (mostly) agree and only rarely to decline. Consent within bioethical discourses is positioned as an ethical panacea that counteracts the danger of paternalistic and autocratic practices. Such valorisation is also evident in professional codes of practice and law, which regard obtaining consent as the means to the realisation of ethical ideals of respecting individual rights and autonomy. But women's accounts of consenting to surgery suggest that they rarely do anything when faced with consent forms other than obey professionals' requests for a signature. Indeed far from bolstering or safeguarding autonomy the consent process may reinforce rather than disrupt passivity [47]. The account of women of their experience of given consent in obstetrics indicates that they interpret the process as ritualistic. There is an overwhelming tendency to view consent as not primarily serving patients' needs [48]. Indeed the utility of consent as an antidote for medical paternalism or as an expression of patients' right to self-determination has been called into question. It is arguable that consent mostly fits within a dominant-subordinate relationship that is at odds with liberty or autonomy [48]. Unless this is recognised, consent risks becoming a restricting concept within which patients are expected to concord and acquiesce. It can thus be seen how a maternal request for a caesarean section came to represent a role reversal with the woman taking the initiative and seeking the concordance of the obstetrician.

Those who consistently refuse patients' choice as expressed through their own initiative as exemplified through CSMR probably base such opposition on a particular interpretation of the notion of 'best interest'. This interpretation is embedded in professional notion of clinical indication and is expressed though what is deemed acceptable by the profession. This may also provide doctors with a level of assurance or protection. The emphasis may be interpreted to be on what doctors—not patients—view as best and on what doctors are 'meant' to deliver (given consent). In this context it is illuminating to consider that the views of doctors and patients can diverge. Ordinary women are highly unlikely to be interested in those considerations or risk–benefit calculations advanced in medical literature that are most relevant at the population or policy level. How many caesarean sections are necessary to save one fetal life? How much maternal mortality, morbidity and future risk justifies saving the life of one baby? Whether the baby is of no or of infinite worth? And how does this compare to the mother's worth? Such questions can generate interesting debate but are unlikely to be helpful for a woman making her own life choices.

## 14.9	The Role of the Anaesthetist

Many of the most challenging problems in medical ethics arise within the clinical discipline of anaesthesia. These include life and death choices that face anaesthetists caring for the critically ill surgical patients and patients in intensive care. Particular difficulties arise when patients are unable to be party to decision-making or when there is need to take into consideration issues such as advance directives or the—perhaps conflicting—wishes of family and carers. Also, in modern medicine, anaesthetists are often at the centre of decision-making in a wide range of scenarios including the use of critical and dual effect drugs, resuscitation and determinations of death in relation to organ donation. There is a large body of literature that specifically addresses these issues. These are not within the scope of this chapter, but the distinction I need to draw here is between the role of the anaesthetist within such scenarios where they adopt the 'lead clinical role' at the interface with patients and family and their perhaps more common 'essential role' in the day-to-day practice of anaesthesia. Within routine clinical practice, anaesthetists rarely scrutinise the indication for operations to any great depth. They may enquire with the surgeon or the obstetrician who have the lead clinical role about the indication, but more often this is to clarify the degree of urgency or to confirm rather than challenge the indication. The underlying assumption is that the need for surgery is a matter for the exchange and agreement between the patient and the doctor with a lead role who is the expert in the relevant field. Within this scenario, some anaesthetists may view their ethical duty as being confined to the optimal discharge of their clinical skill and towards the safe administration of anaesthesia or pain relief. Surgeons typically reciprocate and leave matters related to anaesthesia to anaesthetists. Such division of responsibility or symbiosis may be due to a degree of trust acquired through close working relationships, but may also be a reflection of scripted social roles that emanate from the need or advantage of maintaining harmony and presentation.

Literature and guidance in medical ethics focus on the immediate interface or the relation between the doctor and the patient. Representations of decision-making and efforts directed at addressing uncertainties or dilemmas are often presented from the perspective of the lead role who—possibly in consultation with the patient, carer or others—agrees the action plan towards obtaining consent. There is relatively little consideration in literature of the role of other essential clinicians. There are perhaps few exceptions such as in relation to abortion which can invoke 'conscientious objection' arguments. This is a significant omission considering that ethical dimensions are entailed in all clinical decisions which means that concordance between lead role and other essential or supportive roles ought not to be taken for granted.

Guidance such as those from the UK General Medical Council [49] rarely, if ever, draw distinctions based on whether doctors have a lead or an essential role within any given scenario. Yet the manner by which each practitioner is able to exercise their duty and, arguably, the exact duties must be affected based on the doctor's particular relation to the patient. A distinction could be made between three roles: (1) the lead clinician role: is the person who agrees the management plan, (2) the essential clinician role: includes anaesthetists and others who have direct communication with the patient and a direct role in delivering the intervention; (3) the supporting clinician role: includes those who have less prominent roles whether or not they come into direct contact with the patient. The different perspectives that each party will have can and do create risk of conflict. Situations could be envisaged where an essential clinician harbors doubts or uncertainties about the utility of the planned intervention or about whether it satisfies ethical stipulates. CSMR could be one of those testing scenarios. The anaesthetists' role is essential for the fulfillment of CSMR, yet they are not commonly present at the point of decision-making. The distinction I draw here is between agreement to undertake CSMR and input into practical factors such as optimisation of preoperative work-up or decisions about the timing of interventions.

When agreeing to CSMR, the obstetrician may assume, perhaps based on prior knowledge, that the anaesthetist would also agree. Alternatively, the obstetrician may assume that an anaesthetist could be found who is willing to take part. The latter has parallels in the suggestion by NICE that an obstetrician who does not agree to CSMR should refer the patient to someone who will undertake the delivery [21]. But the question remains about how anaesthetists can discharge their ethical obligations within these scenarios. One important feature of ethical decisions is that they are—in a similar way to clinical decisions—individual and situation relevant. Thus it is conceivable that a doctor may be willing to become involved in delivery of care in one particular clinical scenario but not in another. This is, arguably, the reason why decisions about abortion are taken individually rather than via group directives. Clinical scenarios where there are generally accepted indications for the intervention can be less contentious as these provide doctors with a framework for judgement. An anaesthetist is unlikely to raise protestation about administering an anaesthetic when there is a clearly declared clinical indication, **for example, cases of** placenta previa, or where the decision rests with the clinical skill or expertise of the obstetrician as the specialist in the field, for example, fetal distress. Thus a prima facie acceptance of the need for the intervention provides a sound starting point for the anaesthetist to proceed to discharge his or her learnt skill. But the absence of medical indication removes this foundation and creates a higher level of uncertainty. Furthermore, obstetricians become lead clinicians in cases of CSMR solely because of their technical skill and their regard is somewhat weakened because the reason for intervention is outside their area of specialised knowledge.

Caesarean section on maternal request (CSMR) must therefore pose a distinct challenge to the symbiotic relationship. The risk–benefit assessment may be different from the anaesthetist's viewpoint. Whilst the obstetrician would normally have had the opportunity for a conversation with the patient leading to agreement to perform the operation, the question remains whether the anaesthetist can or ought to consider acceptance by the obstetrician as a sufficient safeguard. If not considered sufficient, this calls for a separate conversation which patients may view as overbearing, repetitive or unnecessary.

14.10 How Best to Proceed?

There are familiar arguments, which invoke the notion of conscientious objection in relation to refusal to provide anaesthesia for termination of pregnancy. But the clinical scenarios are sufficiently different that drawing analogies or extrapolations will be problematic. It is thus arguable that decisions about CSMR are best made with reference to doctors' duties as articulated in codes of ethics including reference to the duty of beneficence and non-maleficence. Conscientious objection is recognised as grounded in freedom of thought, conscience, disability and/or religion. It is, therefore, unlikely that a convincing articulation could be made against CSMR with reference to conscientious objection. After all, the issues under consideration primarily concern evaluations of risk and benefit or of hierarchical ordering of competing values or demands.

Landau and Yentis explored the question of CSMR and concluded that they would be agreeable to care for a lawyer in her mid-40s who requested CSMR following the success of her fourth attempt at IVF [50]. Arguably, some obstetricians would view caesarean section in this particular scenario as clinically appropriate and perhaps would themselves advocate caesarean section if not requested by the woman. Thus examining the dilemma at the core of CSMR requires consideration of cases where there are no confounding factors. Here, the decision becomes more challenging and requires a more in-depth exploration of patient's motivation and rationale. It is arguable that ethical decision-making could not be delegated. This calls for a workable solution that would enable anaesthetists to satisfy themselves of the merit of the procedure to which they input. But any adopted solution should spare the patient the need for repeat conversations, insurmountable obstacles or challenges.

In 2006, the US NIH (National Institute of Health) produced a consensus statement on CSMR (Table 14.2) [15]. Like most consensus statements this was more successful in describing what is widely established than in resolving what was not generally agreed prior to the publication.[1] The consensus statement is open to considerable challenge because if, as it is by definition, CSMR is not supported based on the current state of knowledge, future discovery or research as called for by the NIH is unlikely

---

[1] Consensus: 'The process of abandoning all beliefs, principles, values, and policies in search of something in which no one believes, but to which no one objects; the process of avoiding the very issues that have to be solved, merely because you cannot get agreement on the way ahead. What great cause would have been fought and won under the banner: 'I stand for consensus?' (Margaret Thatcher, Speech at Monash University October 1981)

Table 14.2 Summary points of the NIH consensus statement on CSMR

Statement 1: There is insufficient evidence to evaluate fully the benefits and risks of caesarean delivery on maternal request as compared to planned vaginal delivery, and more research is needed
Statement 2: Until quality evidence becomes available, any decision to perform a caesarean delivery on maternal request should be carefully individualised and consistent with ethical principles
Statement 3: Given that the risks of placenta previa and accreta rise with each caesarean delivery, caesarean delivery on maternal request is not recommended for women desiring several children
Statement 4: Caesarean delivery on maternal request should not be performed prior to 39 weeks of gestation or without verification of lung maturity because of the significant danger of neonatal respiratory complications
Statement 5: Maternal request for cesarean delivery should not be motivated by unavailability of effective pain management. Efforts must be made to assure availability of pain management services for all women
Statement 6: NIH or another appropriate Federal agency should establish and maintain a Web site to provide up-to-date information on the benefits and risks of all modes of delivery

to eliminate all subsets to which this definition is applicable. Neither can further research bridge the core conflict between doctors' and patients' valuation of risk–benefit. Contrary to the assertion in the consensus statement, the question is not whether CSMR should be consistent with ethical principles, but rather how could that be determined. Optimising the provision of pain relief (Statement 5) and emphasis on explaining the risks for women (Statement 3 and 6) who desire larger families are issues of resource or of information provision. Addressing these would not address the underlying ethical issues, nor would it provide a way forward for the individual woman who, despite such effort, maintains her preference for caesarean section. A reading of the NIH consensus statement indicates that CSMR whilst not fully integrated within the list of accepted medical indications is not totally rejected. Finally, it remains a possibility that the increasing acceptance of CSMR can translate into it being recognised amongst the list of medical indications for caesarean section. Should this happen the need will arise for safeguards to ensure that a woman's request is not a response to remediable adverse circumstance or third-party interests.

Conclusion

The traditional patient–doctor relationship commences when autonomous patients approach doctors seeking advice or a solution to given problems: a *request*. Yet, current medical practice places consent at the centre of the exchange. Although what one wants and what one agrees to often concur, the underlying concepts are different and this generates the tension at the core of professional response to CSMR. There is evidence of a shift in attitude towards CSMR and this is not totally based on respect for patient's autonomy. There is a need to balance acceptance of autonomous choice with other professional duties such as beneficence and non-maleficence. It is important to develop mechanisms that enable anaesthetists to exercise their ethical duties in a situation where they have an essential rather than a lead role in clinical care. CSMR, because of the absence of medical indication, is outside the sphere of obstetricians' specialist knowledge and, as such, provides an interesting and arguably unique clinical scenario to assess how clinicians who have an essential role ought to exercise their duties.

References

1. Viswanathan M., Visco AG HK, Wechter ME, Gartlehner G, Wu JM, Palmieri R, Funk MJ, Lux LJ, Swinson T, Lohr KN. Cesarean delivery on maternal request. Evidence Report/Technology Assessment No. 133 (Prepared by the RTI International-University of North Carolina Evidence-Based Practice Center under Contract No. 290-02-0016). AHRQ Publication No. 06-E009. Rockville, MD: Agency for Healthcare Research and Quality. March 2006.
2. Feldman GB, Freiman JA. Prophylactic cesarean section at term? N Engl J Med. 1985;312:1264–7.
3. Al-Mufti R, McCarthy A, Fisk NM. Survey of obstetricians' personal preference and discretionary practice. Eur J Obstet Gynecol Reprod Biol. 1997;73:1–4.
4. Brink S. Too posh to push? Cesarean sections have spiked dramatically. Progress or convenience? US News World Rep. 2002;133:42–3.
5. Hopkins S, Chivers L, Bassett C, Lehane M. Too posh to push. Nurs Stand. 2004;18:22–3.
6. Leeb K, Baibergenova A, Wen E, Webster G, Zelmer J. Are there socio-economic differences in caesarean section rates in Canada? Healthc Policy. 2005;1:48–54.
7. Tully KP, Ball HL. Misrecognition of need: women's experiences of and explanations for undergoing cesarean delivery. Soc Sci Med. 2013;85:103–11.
8. Weaver J, Magill-Cuerden J. "Too posh to push": the rise and rise of a catchphrase. Birth. 2013;40:264–71.
9. National Institute for Health and Clinical Excellence. Caesarean Section, Clinical guideline CG132.Manchester, UK, NICE, 2011. https://www.nice.org.uk/guidance/cg132.
10. Royal College of Obstetricians and Gynaecologists and London School of Hygiene and Tropical Medicine. Patterns of Maternity Care in English NHS Hospitals 2011/12. London, RCOG, 2013.
11. American College of Obstetricians and Gynecologists. ACOG committee opinion no. 559: Cesarean delivery on maternal request. Obstet Gynecol 2013; 121(4): 904-7.
12. Jacquemyn Y, Ahankour F, Martens G. Flemish obstetricians' personal preference regarding mode of delivery and attitude towards caesarean section on demand. Eur J Obstet Gynecol Reprod Biol. 2003;111:164–6.
13. Quinlivan JA, Petersen RW, Nichols CN. Patient preference the leading indication for elective caesarean section in public patients—results of a 2-year prospective audit in a teaching hospital. Aust N Z J Obstet Gynaecol. 1999;39:207–14.
14. Declercq E, Menacker F, MacDorman M. Rise in "no indicated risk" primary caesareans in the United States, 1991-2001: cross sectional analysis. BMJ. 2005;330:71–2.
15. NIH State-of-the-Science Conference Statement on Cesarean Delivery on Maternal Request. NIH Consens Sci Statements. 2006. Mar 27-29; 23(1) 1–29.
16. Meigs CD. Obstetrics: the science and the art. Philadelphia: Lea and Blanchard; 1849.
17. Munro Kerr JM, Johnstone RW, Young J, Hendry J, McIntyre D, Baird D, Fahmy, E.C. Combined textbook of obstetrics and gynaecology for students and medical practitioners. Third edition. Edinburgh, E&S Livingstone,1939; p 705-708.
18. Pritchard JA, and MacDonald PC. Williams Obstetrics. 16th edition. New York: Appleton-Century-Crofts; 1980, page 866-868.

19. Campbell D. It's good for women to suffer the pain of a natural birth, says medical chief. In: The Guardian. Vol. 2016. London: The Observer; 12 July 2009. https://www.theguardian.com/lifeandstyle/2009/jul/12/pregnancy-pain-natural-birth-yoga

20. Bewley S, Cockburn J. The unfacts of 'request' caesarean section. BJOG. 2002;109:597–605.

21. Hume, D. A Treatise of Human Nature: Being and Attempt to introduce the experimental method of reasoning into moral subjects. Volume 3: Of morals. Part 1: Of virtue and vice in general. London: Thomas Longman, 1739; p 233-246.

22. Gabbe SG, Holzman GB. Obstetricians' choice of delivery. Lancet. 2001;357:722.

23. Sprung CL, Cohen SL, Sjokvist P, Baras M, Bulow HH, Hovilehto S, et al. End-of-life practices in European intensive care units: the Ethicus study. JAMA. 2003;290:790–7.

24. Vincent JL. Forgoing life support in western European intensive care units: the results of an ethical questionnaire. Crit Care Med. 1999;27:1626–33.

25. Habiba M, Kaminski M, Da Fre M, Marsal K, Bleker O, Librero J, et al. Caesarean section on request: a comparison of obstetricians' attitudes in eight European countries. BJOG. 2006;113:647–56.

26. Bewley S, Cockburn J. The unethics of 'request' caesarean section. BJOG. 2002;109:593–6.

27. Nilstun T, Habiba M, Lingman G, Saracci R, Da Fre M, Cuttini M. Cesarean delivery on maternal request: can the ethical problem be solved by the principlist approach? BMC Med Ethics. 2008;9:11.

28. Hannah ME, Hannah WJ, Hewson SA, Hodnett ED, Saigal S, Willan AR. Planned caesarean section versus planned vaginal birth for breech presentation at term: a randomised multicentre trial. Term Breech Trial Collaborative Group. Lancet. 2000;356:1375–83.

29. Alarab M, Regan C, O'Connell MP, Keane DP, O'Herlihy C, Foley ME. Singleton vaginal breech delivery at term: still a safe option. Obstet Gynecol. 2004;103:407–12.

30. Kotaska A. Inappropriate use of randomised trials to evaluate complex phenomena: case study of vaginal breech delivery. BMJ. 2004;329:1039–42.

31. Glezerman M. Five years to the term breech trial: the rise and fall of a randomized controlled trial. Am J Obstet Gynecol. 2006;194:20–5.

32. Volloyhaug I, Morkved S, Salvesen O, Salvesen K. Pelvic organ prolapse and incontinence 15-23 years after first delivery: a cross-sectional study. BJOG. 2015;122:964–71.

33. Leijonhufvud A, Lundholm C, Cnattingius S, Granath F, Andolf E, Altman D. Risks of stress urinary incontinence and pelvic organ prolapse surgery in relation to mode of childbirth. Am J Obstet Gynecol 2011;204:70 e1-7.

34. Dolan LM, Hilton P. Obstetric risk factors and pelvic floor dysfunction 20 years after first delivery. Int Urogynecol J. 2010;21:535–44.

35. Rortveit G, Daltveit AK, Hannestad YS, Hunskaar S. Vaginal delivery parameters and urinary incontinence: the Norwegian EPINCONT study. Am J Obstet Gynecol. 2003;189:1268–74.

36. Rortveit G, Daltveit AK, Hannestad YS, Hunskaar S. Urinary incontinence after vaginal delivery or cesarean section. N Engl J Med. 2003;348:900–7.

37. Grens K. C-section tied to lower incontinence risk. Reuters: Reuters, 12 April 2012. http://www.reuters.com/article/us-c-sections-incontinence-risk-idUSBRE83B1C420120412

38. Gyhagen M, Bullarbo M, Nielsen TF, Milsom I. The prevalence of urinary incontinence 20 years after childbirth: a national cohort study in singleton primiparae after vaginal or caesarean delivery. BJOG. 2012;120:144–51.

39. Lukacz ES, Lawrence JM, Contreras R, Nager CW, Luber KM. Parity, mode of delivery, and pelvic floor disorders. Obstet Gynecol. 2006;107:1253–60.

40. Veatch RM. The concept of 'Medical Indications'. In: The patient-physician relation: the patient as partner, Part 2. Bloomington: Indiana University Press. 1991; p. 54–62.

41. Veatch, RM. Abandoning Informed Consent. Hastings Center Report, 1995;25(1): 5–12.

42. Redfern, M. The Royal Liverpool Children's Inquiry. London, The Stationery Office, 2001.

43. Berlin I. Four essays on liberty. Oxford: Oxford University Press; 1969.

44. Schneewind JB. The invention of autonomy. Cambridge: Cambridge university Press; 2008.

45. Beauchamp TL, Childress JF. Principles of medical ethics. 5th ed. Oxford: Oxford University Press; 2001.
46. Hall MA, Schneider CE. How should physicians involve patients in medical decisions? JAMA. 2000;283:2390–1. author reply 1-2
47. Dixon-Woods M, Williams SJ, Jackson CJ, Akkad A, Kenyon S, Habiba M. Why do women consent to surgery, even when they do not want to? An interactionist and Bourdieusian analysis. Soc Sci Med. 2006;62:2742–53.
48. Habiba MA. Examining consent within the patient-doctor relationship. J Med Ethics. 2000;26:183–7.
49. General Medical Council. Good Medical Practice. London, GMC, 2013.
50. Landau R, Yentis S. Maternal-fetal conflicts: cesarean delivery on maternal request. In: Van Norman GA, Jackson S, Rosenbaum SH, Palmer SK, editors. Clinical ethics in anesthesiology: a case-based textbook. Cambridge: Cambridge University Press; 2011. p. 49–54.

Maternal Expectations and Satisfaction with Caesarean Section

15

Amanda Hutcherson and Susan Ayers

15.1 Introduction

Human reproduction is a critical and life-changing process which depends on complex biological, psychological, social, and environmental factors. Pregnancy and birth are surrounded by many cultural beliefs and rituals which influence women's expectations and experiences [1, 2]. Maternal mortality and morbidity are low in high-income countries and reducing in low-income countries. Surgical intervention in the form of caesarean section has certainly increased the safety of birth with the World Health Organisation estimating caesareans are necessary in 10–15% of births to reduce mortality and morbidity for women and their babies [3]. However, the overall rate of caesarean has risen well above this in high-income countries: the USA and the UK seeing rises to 25–32% over a 20-year period to 2015. Rapidly developing countries such as Brazil and China have seen even greater increases with no significant improvement in perinatal outcomes. There are many possible reasons for the consistent increase in caesareans, including an increase in risk factors such as maternal obesity, maternal anxiety over the risks of vaginal birth [4, 5], convenience for medical staff or women of scheduled births [6, 7], and the popular phenomenon cited in the media of women being 'too posh to push' for which there is very little evidence [8]. None of these factors

A. Hutcherson
Centre for Maternal and Child Health Research, City University London,
London EC1R 0HB, UK

S. Ayers (✉)
Centre for Maternal and Child Health Research, City University London,
London EC1R 0HB, UK

School of Psychology, University of Sussex, Brighton, East Sussex, UK
e-mail: Susan.Ayers.1@city.ac.uk

© Springer International Publishing Switzerland 2017
G. Capogna (ed.), *Anesthesia for Cesarean Section*,
DOI 10.1007/978-3-319-42053-0_15

consider the risk of the anaesthetic and surgical procedure. Although the numbers of maternal deaths from anaesthetic complications are small and falling [9, 10], surgical procedures of any type carry a risk, which can be exacerbated by pre-existing comorbidities and also by pregnancy itself [11]. With these factors in mind, this chapter looks at what women expect in relation to birth and caesarean section, how they experience birth by caesarean section, and how caesareans can be managed to improve the experience for women.

15.2 Expectations of Birth and Caesarean Section

Birth is a significant life event for women and their partners, and women have detailed expectations of events of pregnancy, labour, and birth. Expectations are important because they influence a woman's choices about where to give birth, how to give birth, and use of pain relief. The widespread provision of antenatal classes during pregnancy is partly driven by the assumption of a causal relationship between a woman's expectations and her experience of birth. The first proponent of antenatal classes, Read [13], believed that expectations of pain caused fear and that this fear resulted in increased tension and therefore pain during labour. Read argued that if women are educated so they change their expectations and learn relaxation techniques to combat tension, then pain will be reduced. Although research does not provide unequivocal support for the attendance at antenatal classes leading to a reduction of pain in labour [13], the incorporation of antenatal classes is now an accepted part of antenatal care.

Women's expectations of birth are complex and dynamic. Research shows most women have well-formed expectations of many aspects of childbirth, the baby, their own role as a parent, and their partner's role as a parent. Women hold both positive and negative expectations of different aspects of birth, such as emotions, control, pain, and obstetric events, as well as detailed expectations regarding assistance with baby care, household tasks, emotional support, financial help, and their relationship with the baby [14]. These expectations are continually refined and developed with new information and experience [15].

The expectations a woman has will influence her birth experience and satisfaction with birth [16]. Positive expectations of birth are associated with greater control in birth, greater satisfaction, and emotional well-being [16–18]. Conversely, negative expectations are associated with finding birth less fulfilling, being less satisfied with birth, and reporting less emotional well-being after birth [17, 18]. There is also evidence that if a woman's expectations are not met they are more likely to report negative experiences and poor satisfaction. For example, a study of 1700 women in Norway found that women who wanted an elective caesarean but had a vaginal delivery had significantly more post-traumatic stress symptoms following birth, compared to women who wanted and had a vaginal delivery. Interestingly, women who wanted a caesarean and had one, or who wanted a vaginal delivery but had a caesarean, did not have greater symptoms of traumatic stress [19]. The authors suggest these results may be due to women who are frightened of childbirth requesting elective caesareans and being more likely to have negative experiences and symptoms of traumatic stress if they are denied a caesarean. It is therefore important to listen to maternal requests for caesarean and identify if there are psychological reasons underlying these.

The way in which the baby is delivered is one of the most significant factors in the healthy completion of pregnancy [20] and important in terms of women's choices and expectations. It is important to emphasise that most women expect their baby to be born vaginally [1, 21]. The majority of women also expect labour and birth to be painful. For example, a study in Jordan found that the majority of primiparous women expected childbirth to be a frightening, long, and painful process. However, most of these women still expected to have a normal vaginal birth [22]. A review of the literature on women's expectations and experiences of pain found many women underestimate the pain they will experience and hope to cope without pharmaceutical pain relief [23]. Women differ in their choices and expectations of pain relief with some preferring pharmaceutical methods and others preferring non-pharmaceutical methods. However, evidence suggests the majority of women who say in pregnancy that they want to try to cope without pain relief end up having some form of analgesia [24]. The review of expectations and experience of pain therefore concluded that 'women may have ideal hopes of what they would like to happen with respect to pain relief, control and engagement in decision-making, but experience is often very different from expectations' [23].

An important influence on women's expectations and experiences is anxiety and fear of childbirth. Fear of childbirth occurs in between 7 and 26% of pregnant women [25, 26], with a smaller proportion developing extreme fear or tokophobia [27]. The BIDENS study of 7200 women in six European countries found significant differences between countries with prevalence of severe fear of childbirth ranging from 1.9 to 14.2% [28]. Symptoms include high levels of anxiety about pregnancy and birth, fear of harm or death during birth, poor sleep, and somatic complaints. As with most psychological problems, the cause of fear of childbirth is multifactorial. It has been associated with factors such as nulliparity [29], increased gestation [29], poor mental health [26, 30], a history of abuse [31], younger age [26], lower education [26], and low self-efficacy [32]. Although fear of childbirth is more common in nulliparous women, women who have a negative or traumatic experience of birth are almost five times more likely to report fear of childbirth in a subsequent pregnancy [33]. The importance of traumatic birth experiences and fear of childbirth is apparent from the impact it has on women's preferences for intervention during birth. There is good evidence from large epidemiological studies that women with fear of childbirth are more likely to want interventions such as epidural analgesia and caesarean sections [27, 29].

15.3 Experience of Birth and Caesarean Section

How women experience caesareans and the impact of caesarean on their satisfaction and mental health is not straightforward. Al Nuaim [34] observes from clinical experience in Saudi Arabia that women who deliver by caesarean are often less satisfied with their experience, and with themselves. Al Nuaim argues they might experience feelings of resentment towards the physician, profound disappointment at the treatment expectation, and loss of the happy moment of natural birth which may lead to post-partum depression. Caesarean delivery also carries considerable disadvantages in terms of pain and trauma of an abdominal operation and complications associated with it. This is an interesting comparison to the conclusions drawn by Hobson [35] in which when exploring the psychology of successful caesarean birth, she proposes that well-supported women with a successful outcome rationalise this after the event to assimilate the caesarean birth as a personal, positive event that was right for her in these circumstances.

Whether a woman's birth matches her expectations might also be important. Retrospective studies that ask women whether their birth was as expected consistently find that poorer psychological outcomes are associated with birth being worse than expected. Findings from prospective studies where expectations are measured in pregnancy so a more 'objective' measure of the difference between expectations and experience can be calculated are more rigorous. Findings from these studies are mixed but increasingly provide support for the importance of the match between a woman's expectations and experience. For example, a prospective study of over 700 women in Israel found lowest satisfaction in women whose deliveries were different to how they planned. Poor satisfaction was reported by women who planned a natural birth but experienced emergency caesareans or unplanned epidural use, and/or women who felt they had low control over what staff were doing or over the birthing environment [36].

An emergency caesarean is likely to be frightening for most women and their partners. There is now substantial evidence that women who have assisted deliveries or emergency caesareans are at greater risk of experiencing birth as traumatic and suffering from post-traumatic stress symptoms after birth [37], as well as developing severe fear of future childbirth. This is supported by Jolly et al.'s [38] work on the sequelae of caesarean section and its effect on future pregnancies, birth, and neonatal outcomes for the women concerned. Fear of further pregnancy stands out in this study with 13% more women who had a primiparous caesarean section not having a second child after 5 years when compared to those who had a normal vaginal birth. Similarly, as we have seen, severe fear of childbirth is associated with preference for an elective caesarean. The literature on evidence for medical and psychosocial reasons for requesting an elective caesarean currently makes opposing recommendations. On the one hand, a Cochrane review concluded there is no robust medical evidence to support the recommendation of caesarean for non-medical reasons [39]. On the other hand, a review of women's reasons for requesting elective caesareans found most women do so because of a previous traumatic birth experience [40]. The latter review also found that most women chose caesarean surgery in the belief that it would enhance safety for themselves and their infant [40] indicating a need to listen to women and discuss their preferred option, along with information on risk and safety for this and other options.

However, it is clear that not all women who have emergency caesareans develop post-traumatic stress symptoms or fear of birth. Research also shows that women who have elective caesareans do not have the same low satisfaction [41] or traumatic stress response [19] as women who have emergency caesareans. This led Spaich et al. [42] to conclude that the actual mode of delivery may not have a direct influence on women's satisfaction with childbirth but is mediated by maternal involvement in decision-making, support during labour from a person of trust, and effective analgesia, all of which play a major role in providing a positive birth experience for women. Hobson [35] and Hobson et al. [43] add to this list the importance of providing information to women. The way we care for women before, during, and after caesarean is therefore critical.

15.4 Improving Satisfaction with Caesarean Birth

Patient satisfaction has become an important factor for all areas of health care in industrialised societies [44, 45]. Problems conceptualising and measuring satisfaction have been widely discussed and need to be borne in mind when interpreting the evidence [46]. However, despite these problems there is substantial evidence that a satisfied patient will be significantly more likely to engage with healthcare services, be amenable to treatments and recommendations and achieve more successful health outcomes. In the UK, the Department of Health (DH) has emphasised the importance of choice in maternity services. Reports on *Maternity Matters, Choice, Access and Continuity of Care in a Safe Service* [47] and *Making It Better for Mothers and Babies* [48] both emphasise that all women should be able to choose their place of birth in terms of home birth, midwifery-led birth units, or obstetric units. A recent extensive review of maternity services in England which consulted with women and stakeholders over a year concluded that consistent support for women, coupled with an individually tailored maternity service, is important and likely to increase safety and positive birth outcomes as well as satisfaction with care [49].

As we have seen, it is important not to conflate caesareans with poor satisfaction or negative psychological outcomes. Although poor psychological outcomes are more likely following a caesarean, the evidence shows this is not necessarily a causal relationship. Emergency caesareans can be stressful due to the context in which they are needed, but a woman's experience can still be positive if staff provide support, information, and involve women in decision-making. This is illustrated by the case study in Box 1 of a mother who had two babies by caesarean, one of which was a traumatic experience and the other a very positive experience. This case study also illustrates the potential long-term impact a traumatic experience can have on the mother and the baby. Guidelines from the Birth Trauma Association on how to reduce the likelihood a woman will find birth traumatic are shown in Box 2.

Box 1. Case Study a Woman's Experience of Two Caesarean Births
Caesarean 1

Louise[a] had two children by caesarean section. The first baby was born after a long labour (36 h latent phase and 20 h in established labour). The baby was in an occipito posterior (OP) position with an asynclitic head. Although she had an epidural, it wasn't effective and was not re-sited because the anaesthetists had time constraints. After 2.5 h of pushing, she went to theatre for assisted delivery. In theatre it took 90 min to site the spinal block. Louise says 'this was the most traumatic experience of my life. I had planned for a homebirth and nothing could have prepared me for the outcome. I felt completely out of control and scared. The worst part was the fact that the spinal took 1.5 hours to be sited. I was fully dilated with an ineffective epidural and pushing with each contraction, and there were 6 people holding me in left lateral and telling me to be completely still for the whole time because they were trying to get the spinal sited. My glasses were dirty through all the tears I was crying and I couldn't see. I was petrified, tired and I just wanted it to be over. No one communicated with me while this was going on, apart from telling me to stay completely still, which was awful. I remember one person who took my glasses off and cleaned them for me so I could see, this meant a lot to me'.

Eventually, the spinal anaesthesia was sited with Louise in a seated position. A vaginal forceps delivery was unsuccessful so Louise had a caesarean with Barton's forceps to the fetal head, followed by a post-partum haemorrhage of 1.6 L. After the birth, Louise and the baby were both traumatised. Breastfeeding did not go well. Louise did not bond with her baby and said 'The whole experience was extremely traumatic for me and it took me nearly 2 years of counselling and help to bond with my son'.

Caesarean 2

For the birth of her next child, Louise planned a vaginal birth at home. However, her membranes ruptured before labour and after 72 h she had to go to hospital to be induced. In hospital, the forewaters were artificially ruptured, and there was thin meconium staining. Louise had contractions for 6 h, but there was no progress in terms of dilation. She was given the option of having Syntocinon or a caesarean. She opted for a caesarean and agreed a plan for a 'gentle caesarean'[b] with the consultant beforehand so everyone was aware. Louise was in a seated position for the insertion of the spinal anaesthetic, and it was sited in 4 min. The lights were low in theatre (with only the theatre overhead lights on), music was playing, and the theatre team were friendly and chatty. Before the baby was born, the screen was lowered so Louise could see her baby being born, and he was passed straight to her. Cord clamping was delayed for 2+ min, and the baby remained skin to skin until the surgery was completed. Louise did not have exceptional blood loss (EBL 500 mL) and breastfeeding went really well. She was discharged after 24 h. Louise says 'this was such a healing birth for me. Even though it didn't go to plan, I felt completely in control and listened to. I was still in labour and contracting as they did the spinal—but they listened to what I wanted and made sure it happened. Everyone took care to talk me through what was happening, and take care of me. Seeing my baby being born and having him passed straight to me felt like I had birthed him naturally. It was the most amazing feeling in the world and I immediately bonded with him. He was calm as a result and we both had a brilliant, healing experience because of it. The care from the team made such a difference, and the gentle nature of the c section made me feel empowered and stronger than I ever had. Even though I had c sections with both my babies, they were worlds apart in terms of the impact on me and my babies'.

[a]Pseudonyms have been used to protect the identity of people involved

[b]Also referred to in the literature as 'natural caesarean' [50] or 'skin-to-skin caesarean' [52]

Box 2. Preventing Births Being Traumatic for Women (Birth Trauma Association)
http://www.birthtraumaassociation.org.uk/policy.htm

1. Women must be fully informed of their options, of details of obstetric procedures, and their associated physical and psychological risks.
2. The woman must be central to the decision-making process.
3. Women need to be presented with their choices in plain words and be allowed to make their own decisions.
4. Women need to be given as much time as possible to talk through their decision with appropriately qualified staff.[a]
5. The woman and her partner should be treated sensitively. Their decisions should be supported appropriately.
   Care should be individualized; this includes pain relief provision and complete information about the well-being of their baby because fear and lack of trust are commonly associated with the birth becoming traumatic.

[a]In emergency situation when it is not possible to give women time to talk through decisions about their birth they should be given time after birth to talk through why the decisions were made and the consequences

In the rest of this section, we look at how to improve satisfaction with caesarean through providing information, including women in decision-making, and providing support and compassionate care.

15.4.1 Providing Information

Providing clear information is associated with parents having more positive experiences and greater satisfaction in a wide range of settings and high-risk groups. The Birth Trauma Association guidelines (Box 2) have information as their first priority, stating that women should be fully informed of their options, details of obstetric procedures, and their associated physical and psychological risks. Similarly the UK National Institute for Health and Care Excellence [51] recommends that the risks and benefits of caesarean section and vaginal birth are discussed with women, including risks of placental problems with multiple episodes of caesarean surgery. The American Congress of Obstetricians and Gynecologists also provides information on their website about Safe Prevention of the Primary Cesarean Delivery [53].

15.4.2 Decision-Making

It is clear that the circumstances surrounding a caesarean will affect the decision-making process and how easy it is to involve women and their partners in these decisions. Caesarean section decisions may also vary between primiparous and multiparous women, the latter possibly involving a decision about vaginal birth after caesarean section (VBAC) [54, 55]. Decision-making for VBAC has been studied in some detail over the past 10–15 years. A Cochrane review of interventions for supporting women's decisions about mode of birth after caesarean found a variety approaches to help women's decision-making about whether to have a VBAC. These include Web-based decision-making tools and one-to-one coaching for maternity care providers. Women who used decision-making tools had greater knowledge and less decisional conflict about their choice of birth. However, no differences were found in the uptake of VBAC following interventions [56].

When the decision about type of birth has been made and if a woman wants an elective caesarean, the type of anaesthesia will need to be decided upon, ideally in a partnership between the woman and the anaesthetist [35]. This is not a new concept to anaesthetists working in general surgery, with several pieces of research investigating how to increase recipient satisfaction with anaesthesia and also how to measure it. Flierler et al. [58] consider this in some detail, thinking about the use of recognised satisfaction tools and also measuring the anaesthetist experience of the shared decision-making process in planned orthopaedic surgery. As with obstetric surgery, the decisions to be made here were largely those of general versus regional anaesthesia and post-operative pain relief. Whilst questioning factors that may impact on the research process such as expert leading and professional view, they arrived at the conclusion that the majority of the 197 patients surveyed were happy with their involvement in the decision-making process.

15.4.3 Support and Compassionate Care

The care a woman receives during birth can impact on her physically and psychologically for the rest of her life [57]. This is illustrated by the case study in Box 1 and throughout the world with the cultural expectation that birth will be a supported process in some form or another.

There is substantial evidence from many countries that women who have continuous support during pregnancy and throughout labour are more satisfied with the healthcare service and have increased confidence in their own ability to give birth and to parent a child [59–61]. For example, a Cochrane review of evidence from 22 randomised controlled trials of continuous support for women during labour involving 15,280 women found that women who receive continuous support are less likely to have intrapartum analgesia or report dissatisfaction with birth [62]. Varied types of continuous support were considered for this review, including hospital staff (such as nurses or midwives), women who were not hospital employees and had no personal relationship with the labouring woman (doulas or women who were provided with a modest amount of guidance), or companions of the woman's choice from her social network (her husband, partner, mother, or friend). The main criteria were that a continuous presence was maintained and aspects such as emotional support, comfort measures, information, and advocacy were provided.

Support from the parenting partner is also likely to play a major role in satisfaction with care. The UK Royal College of Midwives draws on the evidence base to recognise that a well-prepared father has a positive effect on his partner promoting a satisfying birth experience and reduced the need for pain relief [63]. It is highly likely that this would apply to other parenting and birthing partners in their provision of support. Pregnancy and birth are the first major opportunities to engage partners in appropriate care and upbringing of children [64]. This early and continuing involvement of the parenting partner in the child's life has a massive impact on developmental outcomes, as well as providing informed support for the birthing woman.

Women highly value support as illustrated in Box 1. This is illustrated effectively by Spiby et al who obtained the views of a range of stakeholders on the provision of support for women during labour this from a range of stakeholders including volunteer doulas who provided support to women. Some of the most important factors were those of being listened to and having their fears allayed by someone who was non-judgemental. Many of the women who were included in the study highlighted that support during birth had given them a feeling of wellbeing and a building of their self-esteem as well as increasing satisfaction with their birth process. Conversely, women who are not supported during birth were more likely to report post-traumatic stress symptoms [37]. Chapman [65] considers the role of the obstetric anaesthetist for women who have had previous traumatic births and whether use of self-hypnosis and relaxation during pregnancy might help women cope. However, at present there is very little evidence on effective interventions for women with severe fear of birth.

Considering the importance of support during birth in a woman's experience, it is fair to say that the attitude and actions of healthcare staff are critical. As caesareans take place in operating theatres with the anaesthetist and operating department technician as the woman's main carers, they can be key in terms of supporting women and consequently women's experiences. A friendly anaesthetist and technician will make a huge difference both to the mother and her partner. The role of the anaesthetic team is to support physiological homeostasis, ensuring patient comfort and safety throughout the process. They are therefore well placed to notice women's emotional and psychological state and provide the support women need.

15.5 Summary and Conclusions

This chapter shows how women have detailed expectations about pregnancy and birth that shape both their decisions about birth and their subsequent experiences of birth. Most women do not expect to have a caesarean although they do expect birth to be painful. However, in industrialised countries rates of caesareans are increasing and are higher than the WHO recommendations for reducing maternal and infant mortality and morbidity.

For most women, caesarean is unexpected and women who have caesareans are more likely to have a negative birth experience, poor satisfaction, and symptoms of post-traumatic stress. However, this is mediated by the way in which women are cared for during and after the caesarean. Supportive, compassionate care with good communication is critical [66]. For women planning a caesarean section, this is closely followed by involvement in decision-making, with clear information about what to expect and the pros and cons of specific anaesthetic techniques. In common with other hospital episodes and surgical procedures, women demonstrate higher levels of satisfaction with their caesarean section when they are provided with sufficient information to enable their involvement in a decision-making process. They benefit from having the ability to guide decisions about their birth, timing of that birth, and type of analgesia or anaesthesia that is used. Effective anaesthesia and postnatal pain relief delivered with caring support can help women have a positive birth experience even when caesarean might not have been what she planned or expected. Their satisfaction in the process and the likelihood of positive birth outcomes for mother and baby are further enhanced when they are supported in a kind and caring manner by healthcare professionals, their chosen birth partners being supported to help them. Healthcare provision is a provider business, depending on user satisfaction, positive publicity, and public confidence all of which are successfully supported by patient involvement and responsive carers.

Ultimately, it is important to try to conduct all caesareans in a way that minimises negative experiences for women. Anaesthetists are well placed to provide information and compassionate care during caesareans. Other promising initiatives which have the potential to promote more positive experiences include 'gentle caesareans' (also referred to as 'natural caesareans' [50] or 'skin-to-skin caesareans' [52]). This is a relatively new approach to caesareans, and there is currently limited evidence on the impact on women's experiences. However, research suggests there are no adverse effects on maternal or infant outcomes, and it might be beneficial in terms of reducing rates of infant infection and admission to NICU [52]. Other initiatives include providing neonatal life support close to the mother [67, 68] and kangaroo/couplet care for preterm babies. Compassionate, friendly support is a major factor in patient satisfaction, particularly when coping with the difficult and frightening process of surgical birth. This support needs to be provided by the staff and, where possible, those who have significant meaning for the woman to have maximum effect.

References

1. Iravani M, Zarean E, Janghorbani M, Bahrami M. Women's needs and expectations during normal labor and delivery. J Educ Health Promot. 2015;4(6). Published online. http://www.ncbi.nlm.nih.gov/pmc/articles/PMC4355842/. Accessed 20 Feb 2016.
2. Jordan B. Birth in four cultures, a crosscultural investigation of childbirth in Yucatan, Holland, Sweden and the United States. Long Grove, IL: Waveland Press; 1993.
3. World Health Organisation. Caesarean sections should be performed only when necessary, News release. 2015. http://www.who.int/mediacentre/news/releases/2015/caesarean-sections/en/. Accessed 19 Feb 2016.
4. Faisal I. Matinnia N. Hejar AR.Why do primigravidae request caesarean section in a normal pregnancy? A qualitative study in Iran. Midwifery: February 2014, 30, 2, 227–233.
5. Spiby, H.; Green, J.M.; Darwin, Z,; Willmot, H.; Knox, D.; McLeish, J. Multisite implementation of trained volunteer doula support for disadvantaged childbearing women: a mixed-methods evaluation. Source Health Services and Delivery Research: 2015, 3, 8,.
6. O'Driscoll K, Meagher D, Robson M. Active Management of Labour. Elsevier Mosby. 2003.
7. Palmer WL, Bottle A, Aylin P. Association between day of delivery and obstetric outcomes: observational study. Br Med J. 2015;351(8035):20.
8. Weaver J, Magill-Cuerden J. "Too posh to push": the rise and rise of a catchphrase. Birth. 2013;40(4):264–71.
9. Knight, M., Kenyon, S., Brocklehurst, P., Neilson, J., Shakespeare, J., & Kurinczuk, J.J. (Eds.) (2014). MBRRACE-UK. Saving Lives, Improving Mothers' Care—Lessons learned to inform future maternity care from the UK and Ireland Confidential Enquiries into Maternal Deaths and Morbidity 2009–12. Oxford: National Perinatal Epidemiology Unit, University of Oxford.
10. Rollins M, Lucero J. Overview of anesthetic considerations for Cesarean delivery. 2012. http://bmb.oxfordjournals.org/.
11. Arbous MS, Grobbee DE, van Kleef JW, de Lange JJ, Spoormans HH, Touw P, Werner FM, Meursing AEE. Mortality associated with anaesthesia: a qualitative analysis to identify risk factors. American Society of Anesthesiologists. 2016. https://www.asahq.org/. Accessed 16 Mar 2015.
12. Read GD, Childbirth without Fear: The Principles and Practice of Natural Childbirth. London: Pinter & Martin; 1933.
13. Gagnon AJ, Sandall J. Individual or group antenatal education for childbirth or parenthood, or both. Cochrane Database Syst Rev. 2007; doi:10.1002/14651858.CD002869.pub2.
14. Levitt M, Coffman S, Guacci-Franco N, Loveless S. Social support and relationship change after childbirth: an expectancy model. Health Care Women Int. 1993;14:503–12.
15. Gupton A, Beaton J, Sloan J, Bramadat I. The development of a scale to measure childbirth expectations. Can J Nurs Res. 1991;23(2):35–47.
16. Ayers S, Pickering AD. Women's expectations and experience of birth. Psychol Health. 2005;(1):79–92.
17. Green J, Coupland V, Kitzinger J. Expectations, experiences, and psychological outcomes of childbirth: a prospective study of 825 women. Birth. 1990;17(1):35–47.

18. Green JM, Coupland VA, Kitzinger JV. Great expectations: a prospective study of women's expectations and experiences of childbirth. Cheshire: Books for Midwives; 1998.
19. Garthus-Niegel S, von Soest T, Knoph C, Simonsen TB, Torgersen L, Eberhard-Gran M. The influence of women's preferences and actual mode of delivery on post-traumatic stress symptoms following childbirth: a population-based, longitudinal study. BMC Pregnancy Childbirth. 2014;14:191. doi:10.1186/1471-2393-14-191.
20. Akarsu RH, Muckuk S. Turkish women's opinions about caesarean delivery. Pak J Med Sci. 2014;30(6):1308–13.
21. Brodrick A. Exploring women's pre-birth expectations of labour and the role of the midwife. Evidence Based Midwifery. 2008. https://www.rcm.org.uk/learning-and-career/learning-and-research/ebm-articles/exploring-women%E2%80%99s-pre-birth-expectations-of. Accessed 20 Feb 2016.
22. Oweis A, Abushaikha L. Jordanian pregnant women's expectations of their first childbirth experience. Int J Nurs Pract. 2004;10(6):264–71.
23. Lally JE, Murtagh MJ, Macphail S, Thomson R. More in hope than expectation: a systematic review of women's expectations and experience of pain relief in labour. BMC Med. 2008;6:7. doi:10.1186/1741-7015-6-7.
24. Soliday E, Sayyam J, Tremblay K. Pathways to violated expectations of epidural uptake. J Reprod Infant Psychol. 2013;31(4):413–25. doi:10.1080/02646838.2013.830175.
25. Fenwick J, Gamble J, Nathan E, Bayes S, Hauck Y. Pre- and postpartum levels of childbirth fear and the relationship to birth outcomes in a cohort of Australian women. J Clin Nurs. 2009;18:667–77. doi:10.1111/j.1365-2702.2008.02568.x.
26. Laursen M, Johansen C, Hedegaard M. Fear of childbirth and risk for birth complications in nulliparous women in the Danish National Birth Cohort. BJOG. 2009;116:1350–5. doi:10.1111/j.1471-0528.2009.02250.x.
27. Nieminen K, Stephansson O, Ryding EL. Women's fear of childbirth and preference for cesarean section—a cross-sectional study at various stages of pregnancy in Sweden. Acta Obstet Gynecol Scand. 2009;88:807–13. doi:10.1080/00016340902998436.
28. Van Parys A, Ryding EL, Schei B, Lukasse M, Temmerman, M. Fear of childbirth and mode of delivery in six European countries: the BIDENS study. In: 22nd European Congress of Obstetrics and Gynaecology (EBCOG), Book of Abstracts (S14.4); 2012.
29. Rouhe H, Salmela-Aro K, Halmesmaki E, Saisto T. Fear of childbirth according to parity, gestational age, and obstetric history. BJOG. 2009;116:67–73. doi:10.1111/j.1471-0528.2008.02002.x.
30. Storksen HT, Eberhard-Gran M, Garthus-Niegel S, Eskild A. Fear of childbirth; the relation to anxiety and depression. Acta Obstet Gynecol Scand. 2012;91:237–42. doi:10.1111/j.1600-0412.2011.01323.x.
31. Lukasse M, Vangen S, Oian P, Schei B. Fear of childbirth, women's preference for cesarean section and childhood abuse: a longitudinal study. Acta Obstet Gynecol Scand. 2011;90:33–40. doi:10.1111/j.1600-0412.2010.01024.x.
32. Salomonsson B, Gullberg MT, Alehagen S, Wijma K. Self-efficacy beliefs and fear of childbirth in nulliparous women. J Psychosom Obstet Gynaecol. 2013;34:116–21. doi:10.3109/0167482X.2013.824418.
33. Storksen HT, Garthus-Niegel S, Vangen S, Eberhard-Gran M. The impact of previous birth experiences on maternal fear of childbirth. Acta Obstet Gynecol Scand. 2013;92:318–24. doi:10.1111/aogs.12072.
34. Al Nuaim LA. Views of women towards cesarean section. Saudi Med J. 2004;25(6):707–10.
35. Hobson JA. Satisfaction with caesarean section: a literature review and an exploration of the relationship between preoperative anxiety and postoperative satisfaction and recovery in elective caesarean section. 2002. Doctoral thesis, University of Sheffield.
36. Benyamini Y, Gozlan M, Preis H. Fulfilment of birth expectations and the subjective birth experience. In: 18th Conference of the International Society for Psychosomatic Obstetrics & Gynecology; May 2016, Malaga, Spain; 2016.
37. Ayers S, Bond R, Bertullies S, Wijma K. The aetiology of post-traumatic stress following childbirth: a meta-analysis and theoretical framework. Psychol Med. 2016;46(6):1121–34.

38. Jolly J, Walker J, Bhabra K. Subsequent obstetric performance related to primary mode of delivery. Br J Obstet Gynaecol. 1999;106(3):227–32.
39. Lavender T, Hofmeyr HG, Neilson JP, Kingdon C, Gyte MLG. Caesarean section for non-medical reasons at term. Cochrane Database Syst Rev. 2012;3:CD004660.
40. Gamble JA, Creedy DK. Women's request for caesarean section: a critique of the literature. Birth. 2000;27(4):256–26.
41. Handelzalts JE. The association of worries, mode of birth and reasons for possible intervention with subjective birth experience. In: 18th Conference of the International Society for Psychosomatic Obstetrics & Gynecology; May 2016, Malaga, Spain; 2016.
42. Spaich S, Welzel G, Berlit S, Temerinac D, Tuschy B, Sutterlin M, Kehl S. Mode of delivery and its influence on women's satisfaction with childbirth. Eur J Obstet Gynecol Reprod Biol. 2013;170:401–6.
43. Hobson JA, Slade P, Wrench IJ, Power L. Preoperative anxiety and postoperative satisfaction in women undergoing elective caesarean section. Int J Obstet Anesth. 2006;15:18–23.
44. Aitken AH, et al. Patient safety, satisfaction, and quality of hospital care: cross sectional surveys of nurses and patients in 12 countries in Europe and the United States. BMJ. 2012;344:e1717.
45. Bleich SN, Özaltin E, Murray CJL. How does satisfaction with the health-care system relate to patient experience? Bulletin of the World Health Organization. 2009. http://www.who.int/bulletin/volumes/87/4/07-050401/en/ Accessed 20 Feb 2017.
46. Bell DM, Halliburton JR, Preston JC. An evaluation of anesthesia patient satisfaction instruments. AANA J. 2004;72(3):211–7.
47. Department of Health. Maternity matters, choice, access and continuity of care in a safe service. Department of Health. 2007. www.dh.gov.uk/pulications.
48. Department of Health. Making It Better for Mother and Baby. Department of Health. 2008. www.dh.gov.uk/pulications.
49. NHS England. The National Maternity Review. 2016. https://www.england.nhs.uk/wp-content/uploads/2016/02/national-maternity-review-report.pdf. Accessed 24 Feb 2016.
50. Smith J, Plaat F, Fisk NM. The natural caesarean: a woman-centred technique. BJOG. 2008;115(8):1037–42.
51. NICE, (2013) National Institute for Health and Care Excellence. Caesarean Section Quality standard [QS32]
52. Posthuma S, Korteweg FJ, Marinus van der Ploeg J, de Boer HD, Buiter HD, van der Ham DP. Risks and benefits of the skin-to-skin cesarean section—a retrospective cohort study. J Matern Fetal Neonatal Med. 2016;30(2):159–63. doi:10.3109/14767058.2016.1163683.
53. American Congress of Obstetricians & Gynecologists. Safe Prevention of the Primary Cesarean Delivery. American Congress of Obstetricians and Gynecologists. 2014. http://www.acog.org/Resources-And-Publications/Obstetric-Care-Consensus-Series/Safe-Prevention-of-the-Primary-Cesarean-Delivery.
54. American Congress of Obstetricians & Gynecologists. Vaginal Birth After Previous Cesarean Delivery. American Congress of Obstetricians and Gynecologists. 2015. http://www.acog.org/Resources-And-Publications/Practice-Bulletins/Committee-on-Practice-Bulletins-Obstetrics/Vaginal-Birth-After-Previous-Cesarean-Delivery. Accessed 9 Mar 2016.
55. Royal College of Obstetricians and Gynaecologists. Birth after previous caesarean birth. 2015. Green-top Guideline No. 45.
56. Horey D, Kealy M, Davey MA. Interventions for supporting pregnant women's decision-making about mode of birth after a caesarean. Cochrane Database Syst Rev. 2013;(7): CD010041.
57. NICE, National Institute for Health and Care Excellence. Intrapartum Care for Healthy Women and Babies: 2014.
58. Flierler WJ, Nubling M, Kasper J, Heidegger T. Implementation of shared decision making in anaesthesia and its influence on patient satisfaction. Anaesthesia. 2013;68:713–22.
59. Koumouitzesdouvia J, Carr CA. Women's perceptions of their doula support. J Perinat Educ. 2006;15(4):34–40.

60. Lungren I. Swedish women's experiences of doula support during childbirth. Midwifery. 2011;26(2):173–80.
61. McGrath SK, Kennell JH. A randomized controlled trial of continuous labor support for middle-class couples: effect on cesarean delivery rates. Birth. 2008;35(2):92–7.
62. Hodnett ED, Gates S, Hofmeyr JG, Sakala C. Continuous support for women during childbirth. Cochrane Database Syst Rev. 2013;7:CD003766.
63. Royal College of Midwives. Reaching out: involving fathers in maternity care. 2010. https://www.rcm.org.uk/sites/default/.../Father's%20Guides%20A4_3_0.p. Accessed Mar 2016.
64. Department of Health. National service framework for children, young people and maternity services. London: Department of Health & Department for Education, Skills and Families, HMSO; 2004.
65. Chapman KSA. Post-traumatic stress disorder and the obstetric anaesthetist. Int J Obstet Anesth. 2015;24:207–9.
66. NHS England. Compassion in Practice: the 6C's for Compassionate care. 2012. https://www.england.nhs.uk/wp-content/uploads/2012/12/6c-a5-leaflet.pdf. Accessed 2 June 2016.
67. Sawyer A, Ayers S, Bertullies S, Thomas M, Weeks AD, Yoxall CW, Duley L. Providing immediate neonatal care and resuscitation at birth beside the woman: parents' views, a qualitative study. BMJ Open. 2015;5(9):e008495. doi:10.1136/bmjopen-2015-008495.
68. Yoxall CW, Ayers S, Sawyer A, Bertullies S, Thomas M, Weeks AD, Duley L. Bedside neonatal care at birth: clinicians views, a qualitative study. BMJ Open. 2015;5:e008494. doi:10.1136/bmjopen-2015-008494.
69. National Institute for Health and Care Excellence. Caesarean section NICE guidelines CG132. 2011.
70. National Patient Safety Agency. Placenta Praevia after Caesarean Section Care Bundle. 2010. http://www.nrls.npsa.nhs.uk/resources/?EntryId45=66359. Accessed 21 Feb 2016.

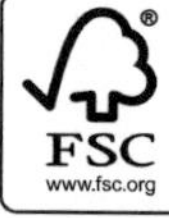

FSC
www.fsc.org
MIX
Papier aus verantwortungsvollen Quellen
Paper from responsible sources
FSC® C105338